Thriving
with Your
Autoimmune
Disorder

A Woman's
Mind-Body Guide

SIMONE RAVICZ, Ph.D., M.B.A.

New Harbinger Publications, Inc.

Distributed in the U.S.A. by Publishers Group West; in Canada by Raincoast Books; in Great Britain by Airlift Book Company, Ltd.; in South Africa by Real Books, Ltd.; in Australia by Boobook; and in New Zealand by Tandem Press.

Copyright © 2000 by Simone Ravicz, Ph.D., M.B.A.
               New Harbinger Publications, Inc.
               5674 Shattuck Avenue
               Oakland, CA 94609

Cover design by SHELBY DESIGNS & ILLUSTRATES
Text design by Tracy Marie Powell

Library of Congress Catalog Card Number: 99-75284
ISBN 1-57224-189-6 Paperback

New Harbinger Publications' Web site address: www.newharbinger.com

02   01   00

10   9   8   7   6   5   4   3   2   1

First printing

Contents

Preface

Thriving with Your Autoimmune Disorder, by Dr. Simone Ravicz, is an excellent, well-written, comprehensive survey of a complex yet common phenomenon. It is the best book targeted to the educated layperson that I have read on this topic. I cannot cite a more sophisticated and comprehensive work by a nonphysician.

I specialize in treating patients with chronic fatigue syndrome (CFS), also known as chronic fatigue immune dysfunction syndrome (CFIDS); fibromyalgia syndrome (FMS); and related disorders, which I term "neurosomatic." Dr. Ravicz discusses diverse research, clinical experience, and opinion about such illnesses, fortunately omitting a vast body of useless research that has hindered advancement and would be of no use to the reader. I congratulate her on her review of the literature and her synthesis. *Thriving with Your Autoimmune Disorder* will be an informative guide for patients and their families.

Many books on the subject belong in the junkpile. This one should be in your bookcase.

—Jay A. Goldstein, M.D.

Acknowledgments

There are many to whom I owe a great deal for their assistance and sharing.

I would like to thank my family, first and foremost, for their continued support and patience while I was immersed in a project so emotionally and intellectually challenging.

My admiration and thanks go to the women who were courageous and generous enough to share their stories with me and with all those who will read and learn much from their tales and their strength.

Thanks also to the many organizations that provided me with much valuable information. In particular, I would like to thank Virginia Ladd and the American Autoimmune Related Diseases Association, Inc., for their invaluable assistance, generosity, and responsiveness to my queries. I feel confident that with such a dedicated, caring organization, the many mysteries of autoimmune diseases and related conditions will be solved in the not too distant future.

Introduction

If you're among the many women who have been diagnosed with an autoimmune disease or related condition (ARC), or if you know somebody who has, you might try to educate yourself as so many of us do these days; namely, by walking into a bookstore and searching through title after title on the subject. On the other hand, you could sit in the luxury of your home combing through the online bookstores that are proliferating daily. Of course, there are those of us who prefer the good old library, where we can look through the stacks and catalogs. Whether you try any or all of these approaches, you could become quite frustrated locating a book on ARCs. If you did locate some, you might become equally frustrated with their extremely technical presentations and high prices. This reflects the fact that, until recently, this topic was primarily under the purview of scientists and researchers. Even for these individuals, it has only been within recent decades that an improved understanding of the autoimmune system, ARCs, and their prevalence has developed. While science has gained important knowledge about these conditions, considerable mystery remains as to the underlying dynamics of the disorders. In addition, there has been little attention paid to one major fact: These disorders affect women in far greater numbers than men. When considered in light of other trends in our society and medicine in particular, this gap isn't surprising. Such trends and reasons are explained in this chapter and throughout the book.

Why I Wrote This Book and How It Can Help You Optimize Your Journey

I cannot tell you how many times I asked myself the former of these two questions. I can tell you that it was a great many times. Other people asked me this question too . . . and the more they saw the time, effort, energy, and spirit I was pouring into it, let alone the inevitable periods of frustration and exhaustion, the more they asked. With respect to many of these people, I'm not wholly certain what they were really asking. Why are you spending so much of your precious free time working so incredibly hard on this subject (i.e., so serious and so, from their point of view, unexciting)? Or, why not write a simple pop psych book that will sell?

Perhaps I'm not in touch with all of the reasons why I chose to dedicate so much of my time to this subject. However, I am completely aware of some. For one, I have a personal tie with the topic as I have several of the conditions described here. I've gone through (and continue to go through) many of the same very difficult experiences that both you and the women who generously offered to share their stories herein with us have had to contend. So, first off, I hope to help you feel you're not all alone in feeling picked on by the system, particularly doctors, insurance companies, and the like. Secondly, I'm hoping that by getting the word out about such harassment, we women can band together in effective ways, and thereby effect a change in the system. I've never agreed with the notion of treating people with less consideration because of their sex, race, health, social status, socioeconomic status, or any of the other labels our society loves to cut and paste. With regard to ARCs, as in general, the effects of such differential treatment are incredibly harmful. While some medical professionals are experts in these conditions and wonderfully supportive of women dealing with these challenges, the majority continue to indulge in disbelief, stereotyping, and minimizing the seriousness of mind-body debilitation, fatigue, and pain. Women with ARCs often hear statements such as, "Say, I have someone great you should go talk to . . . ," from doctors who think, "Oh no . . . another neurotic, probably depressed woman! She looks okay. Can't these women see I have really sick people who need my time and attention?" Such attitudes contribute to our painful, debilitating conditions and worsen our mind-body health.

A third reason for my setting out on this challenging path involves my desire to disperse the knowledge I've gained from the many women I've worked with, whether as individual clients or members of workshops and seminars. I've also learned much from and felt great empathy for the many women I've chatted with for hours as we've duly waited to be called in by our doctors. With the women with whom I work in particular, I've noted the undeniable efficacy of applying the notions of holistic healing and mind-body intervention in beating the odds against these tricky illnesses, which don't play by the rules and lure our bodies into working against us. The more female clients I was referred with these physical conditions, and the more I researched and learned as a result, the more disgusted I became with the shocking dearth of information about these complex conditions. Particularly lacking is the type of information that women need to improve the quality of their mind-body health. My goal is to provide sufficient data and suggestions to help in this quest so women like you and I can learn, make changes, improve our mind-body health, derive new meanings for our lives, and thus thrive rather than just survive.

There are two more reasons I believe you'll derive benefits from this book. One is that when people learn and understand more about their particular conditions, they derive a sense of control and involvement—both of which improve recovery and healing. Secondly, from my varied roles in working with women with ARCs, whether as therapist, lecturer, e-mail correspondent, interviewer, and comrade, I've seen one noticeable trait that can't be ignored. These women are among the most ardent pursuers of knowledge regarding their conditions I have ever seen. Perhaps we're motivated by frustration brought on by the denial from the medical system as to the reality and pain of our conditions, as well as the insulting comments we've received, ranging from "It's all in your head" (known by the inner circles of patients as IAIYH) and "You look too good to be sick" to "Insurance doesn't cover that." I believe this book will help in our dedicated quest for knowledge and tools that can reduce our cycle of pain, illness, guilt, depression and the resulting further dampening of our immune systems.

I've included stories from women like us, hoping the information helps create a sense of sharing that will mitigate the aloneness and hopelessness many of us feel. Also, I asked each thriving woman for techniques and tools that helped her mind-body healing and her ability to cope with her new life. Each woman also shared what she had learned from her illness and how she had changed and grown. Talking about their experiences helped these women more clearly see their progress in the face of adversity, their strength, and their continued hope. The point is that no matter how ill you are, there are things you can do to assume control over improving your mind-body health. Too many women have experienced intense distress and pain from their illnesses and then have had to endure negative forecasts or demeaning comments from doctors or loved ones. Feelings of hopelessness and worthlessness are easily comprehensible in this light. I recall finally receiving my diagnosis after having made the typical exhaustive rounds of doctors. The doctor who gave me the news was right on with the diagnosis but completely off with the delivery: "You have fibromyalgia and chronic fatigue syndrome. They're chronic—you'll have 'em for the rest of your life . . . pain and fatigue. There's really nothing you can do about it." This is worse than poor practice, given that there is much evidence that negative, disheartening messages like these can worsen mind-body health.

I received encouragement to write this book from others based on my experience with women and health psychology, as well as the knowledge and understanding I gained in writing my previous book, *High on Stress: A Woman's Guide to Optimizing Stress in Her Life*. It's my hope that this knowledge and understanding, as well as some shared experiences, will help you develop a sense of trust and willingness to work with me, particularly in the sections entitled What You Can Do. These are composed of alternative and conventional, allopathic techniques and recommendations to reduce symptoms and pain, to heal, and to go beyond enduring to actually thriving in the face of real obstacles and difficulties.

Please try to use a notebook or journal during your healing process. Actually writing down thoughts, feelings, memories, images, dreams, plans, assumptions, realizations, progress, letters to people in your life (whether or not they're sent), lists of goals and priorities, schedules, and charts showing your pain in conjunction with stress, diet, exercise, and medications, are among the most effective tools you can use as you journey along your self- and health-optimization course (SHOC).

At this point, I would like to explain two other reasons I took on such a technically and emotionally challenging topic. I suggest you write them down in the very beginning of your personal notebook.

- I want this book to empower you by helping you understand what is going on within your mind-body system. The greater your understanding, the more informed your decision making. You'll also feel a greater sense of control (over your symptoms, responses to your ARC, and the whole medical system–self interaction), and won't be so overwhelmed by fears of the unknown. Each of these three elements (greater understanding, a sense of control, less distress regarding the unknown) directly reduce negative stress (distress).

- The less distress you experience, the less immune-system suppression you'll experience, and the more energy you'll have available for positive purposes such as extinguishing your negative, irrational thinking and replacing it with positive, rational thinking; designing and leading a balanced, harmonious lifestyle; getting in touch with the priority goals for your life and ensuring you follow those that are *consistent with your values, enhance your sense of self, and allow you to grow in the direction you choose rather than in the ways you believe you "should"*; educating yourself about your ARC and the most effective conventional and alternative techniques (the combined whole yields results greater than the sum of its parts); participating in activities involving social support and human interaction; finding or rewriting the purpose and meaning of your illness and your life in ways that are relevant and motivating to you; including essential, appropriate prostress activities for you whether these are skydiving, mountain climbing, learning a new language or hobby, writing, or getting involved in a volunteer program.

One of the positive consequences of taking personal responsibility and assuming control of your life is reduced distress and suppression of your immune system. The healthful suggestions above complete the picture as they involve and generate positive emotions and power and can enhance your immune system functioning, enjoyment, and life growth. Amidst the tears of the women I interviewed came the ring of beautiful, healing laughter. May this book also help you on your journey toward healing.

PART I

Women and Autoimmune Disorders

CHAPTER 1

Women & Autoimmune Disorders and Related Conditions

In our sleep, pain, which we cannot forget, falls drop by drop upon the heart, until, in our own despair, against our will, comes wisdom, through the awful grace of God.

—Aeschylus, *Agamemnon*

A recent explosion of interest in women's health has shaken the medical, social, and political communities. For far too long, the majority of dollars and resources have gone toward studying diseases more likely to strike men. In addition, the subjects participating in research studies exploring the causes and potential cures of illnesses have been predominantly male. Why look at the health of women? Besides all of those "hormonal things," aren't the majority of our health issues the same as those of men? In fact, given that we typically live seven to eight years longer than men, doesn't this mean we're healthier overall?

Is This a Women's Issue?

While it's true that women live longer, we also have higher rates of painful, debilitating chronic illnesses. Given this difference in longevity, many of us out-live our husbands or partners and must deal with extremely difficult circumstances, including the financial, social, and emotional costs associated with poor health. Women tend to see doctors more frequently throughout their lives and purchase more prescription medications; this together with their higher incidence of chronic illness, can rapidly deplete any financial savings, pensions, or limited funding in the form of Medicaid, Medicare, or private insurance. However, illnesses and conditions discussed in this book aren't limited to women of greater years. ARCs often hit us in our twenties, thirties, and forties—years during which we typically need all of our energy for working, giving birth, raising children, building relationships, loving, growing, and just living day to day.

Whether you live alone or with a family, whether you have few or many financial resources, whether you're a woman of greater years or a younger woman, living with an ARC can be a nightmare. It can be . . . but with the right kind of hard work, knowledge, and faith, it doesn't have to be. I've often heard women with chronic illnesses say things like, "If I'd known that my life was going to be like this, I would have checked out long ago" or "I just don't know if it's worth it anymore. It's such a struggle . . . if this is life, is it really worth sticking around?" You may have voiced these very comments and queries.

On a positive note, each passing day seems to bring new medications that can help partially relieve symptoms and pain of some of the ARCs. However, it's just as necessary that there be governmental, insurance, societal, and labor changes so we receive the financial, educational, social, and medical support and thus the simple yet powerful acknowledgment of our real pain and distress, which can to help transform the "living nightmare" experience into a positive, tolerable healing one. In essence, this is downright necessary because the longer the human lifespan becomes, the more common chronic illnesses will become. This fact is probably partly responsible for some of the rapid explosion of interest in women's health.

Research Inequities

Another reason for the increased focus on women's health is that we have begun to respond and communicate that the continued downplaying of our importance, clearly evident in the bias in financial allotment and number of studies favoring men's health issues, just isn't okay anymore. Certainly there were some earlier efforts to communicate the inequity of these circumstances but, for various reasons, these movements were not vocal or organized enough to change the status quo. One change strengthening and lending credibility to the current trend is that many more female psychologists, medical doctors, psychiatrists, and others are spreading the word about such inequities in attention and resources allocated to women's conditions and health. The fact that they can do so using empirically validated studies and impressive figures has enhanced the validity of our claims. Changes within the fields of medicine, psychology, and biology, together with growing numbers of women working within them, have expanded the chances for us to generate mutual support, stand up for ourselves, and highlight such biases in an increasingly effective way. There are also growing numbers of male professionals joining arms with us to communicate the dearth of studies and funding for women and health.

Although it's not quite equal to the burgeoning wave of interest in women's health, the subject of ARCs has recently begun to gather popularity and interest. This may be related to the wave of attention to women's health, as approximately 80 percent of those with ARCs are women, and many more than the self-admitted underestimate of 8.5 million Americans are affected by autoimmune diseases (Jacobson, Gange, Rose, and Graham 1997). Many more are affected by autoimmune-related conditions (Whitacre, Reingold, O'Looney, and the Task Force on Gender, Multiple Sclerosis and Autoimmunity 1999). According to Virginia Ladd, president of the American Autoimmune Related Diseases Association, Inc., approximately fifty million Americans experience both autoimmune diseases and autoimmune conditions that do exhibit autoantibodies and autoimmune dynamics but remain the subject of some debate. Out of eighty ARCs, there are about twenty-eight that all agree are so-called autoimmune diseases. (Note that the fifty million figure does not include the many women who have chronic fatigue immune dysfunction syndrome or fibromyalgia syndrome.)

Are ARCs Related to AIDS?

There appear to be a few other reasons underlying the somewhat sudden widespread interest in these disorders. For one, the worldwide impact of AIDS, an illness centrally involving the immune system, has made research in this area a worldwide priority and a public interest. Some people who pick up this book may search through it looking for some discussion or exploration of AIDS. It's important that you understand from the beginning that while there are certain similar dynamics involved, ARCs are not immediately related to AIDS. Interestingly, a recent article by Gail Kansky (1999) suggested that chronic fatigue immune dysfunction syndrome (CFIDS), an ARC presented in this book, may someday be found to be a cousin of HIV. This is based on the possibility that the two share the presence of human herpes virus 6. It has also been noted that this strain seems to be involved in multiple sclerosis (MS), an ARC also discussed in this book. Perhaps CFIDS and AIDS share similar dynamics in terms of immune system dysfunction underlying onset or maintenance. However, at this writing nothing definitive can be stated.

We can finally say that AIDS is obtaining significant amounts of research monies; unfortunately, we cannot say the same regarding ARCs. While financial support is increasing gradually, particularly with respect to a few of the conditions, this area remains seriously underfunded. Because of this, anything we can do to increase attention to and awareness of ARCs and the plight of women is essential.

How about the Mind-Body Connection?

The upswing of interest in mind-body dynamics, often spurred on more by the public than by most medical professionals, has led to the dissemination of information produced by the field of science called psychoneuroimmunology. This field's advancement has also been aided by the development of complex measurement and monitoring technology that allows skeptics to see there do indeed exist complex interactional pathways among seemingly independent systems within the body. Basically, this field focuses on the interaction between the mind, the immune system, and the endocrine system. These scientific and technological advances have offered researchers an increased understanding of the incredibly complex, intricately balanced world of the immune system. One of the biggest challenges remaining is for those with a predominantly Western, conventional medicine orientation to modify their usual beliefs and perceptions so they can comprehend and accept multicausal, multidirectional influences and the impact of each unique person's mind-body state on illness and health.

Almost daily, it seems, new linkages among our immune, neuronal, and hormonal systems are being discovered. Let's take one simple example. IL-1, a chemical messenger involved in the immune process, has the ability to trigger a fever, calling into play the central nervous system. This may not sound significant to you, but for centuries and even throughout the last several decades, researchers and physicians would not believe any interaction was possible between the immune system and the central nervous system. I'll be discussing the discoveries in the field of psychoneuroimmunology throughout this book, as they're powerful in illustrating mind-body unity. They will also prove essential in your efforts to heal and thrive.

Just What Are ARCs?

At this point, it's important to understand what ARCs are and how your immune system works. As you read about the immune system, consider that its functioning includes the brain, lymph nodes, thymus, spleen, and bone marrow. There is no single location of the immune system; it's truly spread throughout the entire mind-body system. To complicate things further, and as you've probably figured out, many factors impact the immune system—genes, toxins, hormones, nutritional deficiencies, moods, stress, infectious agents, or any combination thereof—and these are only the ones of which we're currently aware. My favorite description of the immune system that truly conveys its mind-body nature is from Norman Cousins' *Head First*: "The immune system is a mirror to life, responding to its joy and anguish, its exuberance and boredom, its laughter and tears, its excitement and depression, its problems and prospects." (1989, 35–36).

Calculating estimates of individuals with autoimmune disorders is extremely difficult due to variations among geographic locales, ethnic groups, changing diagnostic criteria, the influence of viral or bacterial factors, and the like. In the U.S. and most European countries, it is assumed that about 5 percent of the population (one out of twenty people) will have an autoimmune disease during their lives (Isenberg and Morrow 1995). In addition, it has been estimated that the cost of ARCs is as much as eighty-six billion dollars per year! They are also the fourth leading cause of disability in women.

Despite these staggering numbers, these disorders don't receive the research or attention they require and, in fact, particular types are still not yet completely accepted by the medical field as true illnesses. One of the reasons for this is that these conditions manifest throughout different medical areas, such as endocrinology, neurology, cardiology, gastroenterology, rheumatology, and dermatology, and researchers working within these areas tend to focus on singular diseases falling solely within their boundaries. Another reason underlying the lack of acceptance of this category of disease is that its representatives are baffling, complex illnesses stemming from a still poorly understood breakdown in the immune system's functioning, with the end result being either a rapid or gradual self-destruction. Finally, because ARCs typically target women, they have not received as much scientific research and support as they likely would have had their primary targets been men.

How Things Go Wrong

There are two types of illnesses in which the autoimmune system goes awry:

- Autoimmunity occurs when the immune system erroneously labels organs, systems, or substances of its own body as invaders and thus sets out to destroy itself.

- Immunodeficiency occurs when the immune system actually fails to label an intruder as dangerous and thus does not kick into action to eliminate it.

This book focuses on disorders of the first type, in which the immune system betrays the very body it occupies.

Nonimmunologic Defenses

The immune system, which is extremely complex, plays a central role in our ability to resist disease. In general, its responsibility is to defend its home turf (the body) against foreign invaders intent on destroying or taking over this homeland.

The body has several ways to protect against and destroy outside invaders without having to bother the immune system. For example, a virus or bacteria may gain access to your body through your mouth or nose as you breathe. However, the invader is far from being home free. It has to contend with mucous (which interferes with its efforts to attach to cells), with entrapment by cilia in your lungs, and with ejection by your coughing or sneezing reflexes. If the pathogen gets into your gastrointestinal (GI) tract, there are a number of acids there that can kill bacteria. In addition, the greatest concentration of white blood cells in your body is in your GI tract. If these preliminary defenses fail, the invader can make it into your immune system by traveling along the blood stream to reach the spleen, entering the GI or respiratory tract and lodging in their lymphoid organs, or getting into lymphatic vessels and nodes.

The First Line of Immune System Defense

Margaret Kemeny, an expert in the field of psychoneuroimmunology, uses the term "the first line of immune system defense" to indicate the immune system's first activity should the former nonimmunologic defenses fail. What happens during this stage? Inflammation, a central process of the immune system, can draw immune cells into the area of damage so that they can carry out their destructive role. There are several phases of inflammation, including fever, tissues holding fluids, immune cells entering tissues, increased blood flow and vascular permeability, destruction of invader (antigen), and ultimate repair of damaged tissues.

Inflammation is one of the most important activities involved in immunity; however, it can go awry, as in the case of ARCs, and cause significant problems. Much of the pain and breakdown of the body in some of the autoimmune disorders stems from excessive inflammation. Our white blood cells, which include lymphocytes, macrophages, and neutrophils, are central to the immune response. During this first line of defense, the macrophages detect the invading antigen. These foreign invaders may include bacteria, viruses, parasites, and fungi.

Let's look at an example of this process. Imagine that a virus enters the body and, because it does not have the materials to reproduce itself, it looks for a host cell to invade, take over, and turn into a factory to reproduce itself. As this occurs, the new offspring viruses leave the pirated cell in search of their own host cells to attack, take over, and turn into more virus-propagating factories. However, these intruders don't have full reign. The macrophages in our bodies generally detect and attack the intruders, put some of the destroyed intruder on their surface for display so other immune system cells can determine just who the invader is, and digest them to break down the proteins. These cells then present them to other cells, such as T and B cells, to obtain additional backup self-defense. Also, the macrophages release important substances called cytokines at this time. (For instance, the cytokine called interleukin 1 [IL-1] stimulates the activity of other cells, such as helper T cells with a marker of CD4. These markers will be discussed further below.) There are also natural killer (NK) cells involved in this stage. These kill virally infected cells and generate interferon, which increases the ability to kill and inhibit the reproduction of viruses. A final formation during this nonspecific stage is that of complement (discussed below). All of these measures may not be enough to protect the body from a particular invader and thus the second line of defense, involving specificity, may be required.

Specific Second Line of Immune System Defense

Why the word "specific" here? This process differs from the nonspecific first-line defense in that there must be a match between the immune cell receptor and the invader or antigen. Both the T cells and the B cells involved in this phase have particular structures on their surfaces that allow them to interact only with specific antigens. When the match is made, the immune response is triggered. Let's look first at the various T cells that have different functions during this phase. The macrophages present the digested invaders or antigens to various T cells. At times, they will present to T helper cells, which causes an antibody response. Sometimes, the macrophages will present the digested antigens to cyto-toxic/suppressor T cells, which causes a cytotoxic response. Helper T cells (CD4) that release substances such as interleukin 2 (IL-2) improve the workings of cyto-toxic cells and assists B cells to multiply. Cytotoxic cells are similar to natural killer cells in that they can destroy our cells that have been infiltrated by, for example, viral cells. However, unlike the nonspecific natural killer cells, the cyto-toxic cells can only destroy the viruses within cells to which they're specifically matched. Your genetic pattern dictates the types of structures that will develop on the outside of your T cells throughout your life. Because our T cells can respond to millions of different antigens, we can conclude that millions of T cell receptors have had to be formed.

The helper cells can also increase the rapidity with which B cells mature and are ready to produce their particular antibodies (to be elaborated upon below). On the other hand, helper T cells may also suppress these activities if their jobs are complete. One of the most important functions of T cells (as well as of macro-phages) is their release of cytokines, which are protein molecules that act as mes-sengers or communicators. Cytokines are central in activating many other immunological cells. Macrophages produce interleukin 1 (IL-1), a cytokine that triggers helper T cells to differentiate and produce IL-2 and cause the prolifera-tion of B cells. Another cytokine is gamma interferon, generated by helper T cells. This cytokine also stimulates cytotoxic T cells, macrophages, and natural killer (NK) cells. (I have artificially separated B cells into a different discussion just for ease of description.) Just like T cells, the B cells are essential throughout this spe-cific immune phase. B cells compose about 25 percent of the lymphocytes. After the B cells are apprised of the enemy presence, they rush to carry out their duties. The job of B cells is to produce proteins called antibodies, which bind to the invader or antigen.

What is truly amazing is that, in order to produce the appropriate antibody that can "match" and thus attack the antigen, our immune systems have evolved hundreds of millions of antibodies which can be selected through activating par-ticular B cells, which can produce antibodies matching the particular pathogen. The particular B cells that can generate the antibody to match the perceived anti-gen develop into plasma cells, which produce the requisite antibody. Antibodies differ from some of the other immune system cells, such as killer cells, because they operate by simply coating and thus neutralizing the infected cell. As the antibody shares the engulfed pathogen's receptors, the killer T cells or natural kil-ler cells attach and kill both the cell and virus inside. When the antibodies specifi-cally selected to combat the antigen are through and the invader has been destroyed, the macrophages sweep through the area to gather up and dispose of the antigen-antibody pair (also called the complex).

A Model for Autoimmune Disease

As you can see, the immune system's functioning is incredibly complex and relies on each cell and process functioning accurately within the interdependent system if it is to be effective. While the immune system functions incredibly well in defending our bodies against innumerable threats, it cannot always be successful. There are numerous "entry points" at which if something goes awry with the immune system, the door is opened to the potential development of an autoimmune syndrome or disease. The following discussion clarifies these entry points.

B cell activity is one of the entry points that can disrupt the immune system. If your B cells don't produce sufficient antibodies, your risk for developing an autoimmune disorder increases. If your B cells generate too much of an antibody, the extra may attach to a part of your own tissues or organs, thereby forming destructive "self-antigens" or autoantibodies. They can attack DNA (linked with lupus), thyroid tissue, acetylcholine receptors (linked with myasthenia gravis), and white blood cells (Isenberg and Morrow 1995). Recent evidence has shown that many of these types exist within the blood of perfectly healthy individuals.

Most B cells are covered with molecular structures, "markers," but some people with Sjogren's syndrome, type I diabetes, and rheumatoid arthritis have B cells covered with the marker CD5. B cells with this marker have a tendency to make autoantibodies that attach to one's own DNA, which can cause the production of rheumatoid factors seen in ARCs.

Invading infectious organisms may resemble body cells or tissues, causing the immune response to attack its very own cells and tissues. Another place things can go awry and lead to the development of an ARC occurs when there is a problem in the complement system. The complement system stimulates neutrophils and macrophages to clean up or dispose of the destroyed invading antigens by depositing them in the spleen. The complement system is central to the initiation and maintenance of the inflammation response, and since the genetic process determining types of HLA molecules (class I and II) is associated with the elements of the complement system and its functioning, one's genetic predisposition may again underlie the dysfunctions.

How may things go wrong? If the neutrophils and macrophages in charge of "cleaning up" after a battle with a virus or other antigen or the complement system are inadequate, then autoimmunity and inflammation can result. Two ARCs associated with problems in this phase are systemic lupus erythematosus and myositis.

Other white blood cells, the T cells, also play a central role in the immune system response. Three types of T cells we will examine include the T helper cells, T killer cells, and T suppressor cells. T helper cells are involved in apprising the B cells of the presence of an invader (antigen) through producing small proteins called cytokines. Cytokines up the response of B cells so that they produce increased amounts of antibodies. Too much T helper cell activity seen in some ARCs and related to genetic inheritance can cause excessive production of self-antigens.

An interesting discovery that mirrors this dynamic but has surprised many researchers is that cytokine levels in fibromyalgia syndrome and chronic fatigue immune dysfunction syndrome seem higher than normal. Wouldn't more active immune systems mean greater health of those with FMS and CFIDS? The answer is no. What we need to realize is that just as balance is so important in every aspect of health and well-being, so, too, is it vital in the functioning of the immune system. Overactive immune systems cause as many autoimmune related problems as deficient immune systems. In fact, CFIDS may well be associated with excessive immune activation. This has been explored with relation to cytokines released during inflammation. Studies done on rodents have shown that these cytokines can pass into the brain and cause "sickness behavior," such as sleep problems, fever, memory problems, and exhaustion, greatly resembling chronic fatigue syndrome in people.

Other types of T cells, such as the suppressor or killer (cytotoxic) cells, work in different ways to conduct the business of the immune system. Suppressor T cells can suppress the production of antibodies by the B cells when they are no longer necessary, as when a virus has been eliminated from the body. There are times, however, when the suppressor T cell is unable to stop the continued production of antibodies even after the defeat of the intruder. When suppressor T cells function properly, they tell B cells to stop antibody production. On the other hand, suppressor T cells can also directly terminate the cells maintaining the immune response. In addition, killer T cells can directly damage intruding cells or other tissues. The T helper cells, which tell the B cells to increase their antibody production, can also cause the T killer cells to rapidly reproduce and multiply dramatically. The killer T cells then rush to the sites of attack and help by killing off many infected host cells.

The T suppressor cells seem to be the mechanism by which the immune system can distinguish foreign invaders from "self" tissues, cells, and organs. In possibly all of the ARCs, it has been found that there are either too few T suppressor cells or that their functioning is impaired. Therefore, the mechanism to suppress the continued generation of antibodies or continued activity of killer cells is unable to function properly and excessive antibodies continue to be produced. Large numbers of them can cause many problems in the body. However, problems with T suppressor cells have also been found to exist in healthy relatives of people who have systemic lupus erythematosus (Isenberg and Morrow 1995). As with T helper and B cells, a genetic twist may affect the T suppressor cells, but an activating trigger is also necessary if an autoimmune disease is to develop.

While the suppressor T cells communicate to the B cells and killer T cells that the battle is over and they can return to normal levels of activity, the scavenging macrophages (functioning as phagocytes) come to clean up the destroyed matter after the battle. Some T and B cells remain in the area to act as "memory" cells to ensure that the same virus, bacteria, or other antigen cannot mount a second invasion. If the invaders do manage to get inside, the body's cells are already primed to respond immediately and effectively. So, when infectious disease is the issue, the immune system "learns" after exposure and the infectious disease has little chance of successfully reoccurring. For example, people who have illnesses such as chicken pox, mumps, or measles while young are no longer susceptible to these diseases in later life.

Based upon this principle, immunizations are given to trick the immune system into thinking the body is being attacked by a foreign invader. The body generates the "right" antibodies (in a mysterious process still not understood) to attack the small amount of invader injected, the typical immune system responses are activated, and a memory is established. Through this method, immunity is introduced artificially and future invaders of this type will be immediately recognized and destroyed, usually prohibiting this particular disease from ever again taking hold.

What Can I Do?

As I mentioned in the introduction, I want you to feel empowered by this book and the techniques you'll learn. I want you to play an active, central role in your own physical and mental healing. What others (and even many of us with ARCs) may see as *less* of a life can actually be *more*. Certainly, your life will be different from before, but as you'll see in reading the case stories, it doesn't have to be less.

You will develop a set of tools to use in your self- and health-optimization course (SHOC). I include the term "self" because if you truly incorporate these strategies into your life, you'll improve more than your physical health. You will truly optimize your whole self with the new knowledge of your strength and abilities, the new meaning you find in your life, and the growth you obtain by working on and from your illness—this is what I call healing. I use the word "course" to symbolize the journey you are undertaking. Sometimes the course will be smooth, but often it will appear rough or blocked, as if a great brick wall spanned unmoving across your path. It's your choice whether you retreat or instead challenge yourself to find different ways around, above, and under blockages you encounter. I'm not saying everything you experience with your illness is under your control. It simply isn't, and I don't want to do the damage some have done by suggesting that if you just try hard enough, you can overcome everything and your symptoms will disappear. This message has caused many of us to blame ourselves harshly and call ourselves weak if we don't vanquish all symptoms, increase our energy, or regain our former physical state. As you'll learn from this book, you have an immense ability to create positive effects on yourself and your health if you choose to focus on your mind-body state in healing ways. If this book helps you simultaneously understand that you can control certain things and benefit from striving in these areas, and accept that many things aren't under your control and you can free yourself by letting go, I will have accomplished much and you more.

What Healing Means to You

The variety in definitions of the word "healing" is amazing yet understandable, as it is an intensely personal experience. For some, healing simply means getting rid of symptoms of an illness or injury and getting back to "normal." To people with ARC, the very idea of being pain and symptom free is a wondrous notion and a marvelous, worthy goal. But given the nature of ARCs and our ignorance as to causes and cures, this may not be completely attainable. Given the potency of words in guiding us and forming our expectations and actions, what happens when we change the words we use to describe healing? Is our reality thus changed? Will we obtain different goals or at least make progress in different directions? I've learned the answer is yes.

Some of the incredibly strong, resilient women I interviewed described healing as "getting in touch with my body and my self"; "growing and changing"; "learning important lessons about life and love"; and "understanding the real meaning of life and being able to express gratitude for what I do have."

As you read, ask yourself some questions: "How will I know if I'm making progress in healing? What is it that I want? What does 'healing' mean to me? What lessons have I learned? What will I do with this knowledge?" Understanding these issues is central to accepting your challenges and choosing to thrive and grow rather than focusing on the times past, things now lost, or what you "can't" do anymore. Jot down in your SHOC notebook answers to the questions above. You and your SHOC are a work in progress, so look back at your answers often and feel free to add to or change them as you advance.

The Role of Spirituality

Lynn Andrews (1989) discusses the importance of including the sacred and the spiritual in our concepts of healing. She talks about enlightenment as a component to healing, one most of us claim to seek but of which we're most afraid. I see this over and over in my work with clients. They say they can't take their lives or their personalities anymore, they want to change, they'll do anything. But problems arise when it's time for change and they're terrified to venture forward, to walk unseeing into the darkness, not knowing what awaits them. When people have spirituality, it's easier to move forward. They know the darkness no more than others, but they have faith they will pass toward the light, not necessarily unscathed, but for a purpose and a meaning. Andrews supports the use of shamanism for healing and describes it as an effective, pragmatic approach to heal the psychology of the person and move into the spiritual realm. Her description of shamanism, the ancient way of healing, may help put us in touch with the female aspect we all share. She sees our world as nonharmonious and unbalanced, as she believes a patriarchal world is linear rather than cyclical. Feminine consciousness is what we need to heal ourselves and the world, and the aim of healing is to bring balance back to the earth. Of course, to do this we must heal ourselves first. Let us take on this challenge.

What Causes ARCs?

Most experts concur that the reason for women's greater vulnerability to ARCs isn't clear-cut. Among the most popular theories is that a genetic predisposition is involved. It's also thought that triggers are necessary to produce an ARC in someone who is genetically predisposed. There is much debate when it comes to which triggers are the "right" ones, but perhaps this is the wrong question. From reviewing the literature and studies, I see the accurate question as, "What are the triggers in this particular case?" Some of these triggers include hormonal factors, genetic elements, societal influences, negative stress, personality variables, viruses and bacteria, allergies, cigarette smoking, medications, toxins, and even sun exposure. Whenever a gap exists between men and women with respect to characteristics like these, the first thing that comes to mind is hormones. In this case, they do seem to play a strong role. You'll read about hormones and other triggers of ARCs in general below, while triggers linked with specific ARCs appear in later chapters. Some triggers are more clearly linked with ARCs than others, but you'll learn what you can do about various triggers and how to turn them around for your own benefit.

Most of you reading this book are probably familiar with ARCs, whether you yourself have one or know someone who does. Common examples of ARCs are multiple sclerosis (MS), systemic lupus erythematosus (SLE), rheumatoid arthritis (RA), and Graves' disease (GD). The table below shows the extreme gender differences. Two ARCs garnering increased attention with the highest prevalence in women are FMS and CFIDS (9:1, female to male). Their initial causes, whether viral or bacterial, or involving sleep disorders, toxin exposure, information-processing problems, or immune system malfunctioning, are not yet clear. However, as of July 1998, the AARDA rated these disorders, often appearing in conjunction with autoimmune diseases and disorders, as second and third most important in their list of issues to tackle. The role of the immune system is not clear here, but studies indicate that disruptions in immune system functioning are integral to the conditions. While distress and other psychological factors are involved with these disorders, they are clearly not psychosomatic ailments appearing in hysterical women. While initially we were told such fatigue and pain were "in our heads," growing consensus exists that these are true biologically-based disorders. Depression often associated with FMS and CFIDS is now rightfully deemed to be the *outcome* of these painful, debilitating disorders, and possibly part of the disease process itself (i.e., through deficiencies of neurotransmitters and chemicals).

Autoimmune-Related Diseases/Conditions (ARCs)	Ratio of Women/Men
Multiple sclerosis (MS)	2:1
Rheumatoid arthritis (RA)	4:1
Systemic lupus erythematosus (SLE)	9:1
Ankylosing spondylitis	1:3
Graves' disease (GD, hyperthyroiditis)	7:1
Hashimoto's hypothyroiditis (HT)	5:1
Sjogren's syndrome (SS)	9:1

Fibromyalgia syndrome (FMS)   9:1

Chronic fatigue immune dysfunction syndrome (CFIDS)   9:1

Now let's look at some of the elements underlying ARCs.

Genes: Important But Not Enough

According to the AARDA, the development of autoimmune-related conditions can be based on genetic inheritances passed on through families. The AARDA maintains that the ability to develop an ARC is determined by a dominant genetic trait that seems quite widespread, existing in approximately 20 percent of the population. For most of the ARCs, a single gene causing the illness either does not exist or has not yet been found. Instead there appear to be multiple genes that can be involved in creating the predisposition often underlying the development of an ARC. As you learned in the section about the immune system's functioning, there are many places at which a genetic inheritance can cause parts of the immune system to malfunction. Somehow there is a breakdown in the controls of the immune system, which leads it to begin attacking the body's tissues or elements as though they were foreign invaders. In terms of efforts to explain the greater prevalence of ARCs in women, it has been suggested that certain genes that are particularly important in controlling the immune system occur on the X chromosome. Given that the X chromosome exists only in women, this might explain why we have more frequent disturbances and disorders of our immune system functioning.

Other Factors Count

While there are many puzzling elements about ARCs, one is particularly interesting: In families with the genetic predisposition, we don't necessarily see the development of the same ARC, but instead often see the appearance of different autoimmune disorders. Even among those who believe that genetics is the primary explanation for the development of such disorders, most concur that additional factors need to be present before such a disorder appears. Some of these include the factors that others hold forth as explanations for ARCs. So, for example, a researcher who supports the genetic model as primary might also believe that triggers, such as viruses, bacteria, hormonal changes, physical and emotional stress and trauma, chemical exposure, and possibly food allergies, are necessary to actually jump-start the development of an ARC. The trigger is in some way a negative stressor to the person's physical and emotional health, which, when combined with the genetic vulnerability, is the right mix to cause the manifestation of a particular ARC.

What Role Do Genes Play?

A great deal of progress has been made recently in specifying how genes may have a role in the development of ARCs. The use of animal studies, although the subject of great debate, has been invaluable in assisting with this progress. In animals, researchers found a specific location on a particular chromosome that controls many immunological functions. This region is called the major histocompatibility complex (MHC). Shortly thereafter, a similar location was found in humans. In people, this region has been called the HLA region, and it is located on the sixth chromosome of every cell. Within the HLA region there exist a number of subregions that appear differentially within different people. According to the AARDA, HLA is the major group of genes that distinguishes one person from another. It exemplifies the single genetic trait of greatest import in appraising vulnerability to autoimmune conditions.

It may help you to think of these HLA types as blood types directly determined by one's genetic inheritance. Researchers have been able to clearly associate certain of these HLA types with certain ARCs—a tremendous accomplishment. For example, among those with ankylosing spondylitis, a marker called HLA-B27 was found to exist in 80 percent of patients, as compared to 10 percent of people without the disorder. As more research is done, the evidence supporting the genetic role in predisposing individuals to ARCs becomes stronger. While we cannot yet say to a person that because she has a particular HLA type she's going to develop an autoimmune-related condition, we can say that she has a greater chance of doing so. However, as you read about in the discussion of hormones and other factors, genes, while important, do not explain the whole story.

How Do Trigger Factors Work?

Different factors can be sufficient to trigger an ARC if a person has the particular genetic backing required. One woman with a genetic predisposition toward autoimmune disease might develop one type after a severe emotional loss, such as the loss of her partner or children. Another woman also genetically predisposed might develop a completely different disorder. Or, she might develop such a condition after exposure to a virus or toxin. The similarities of a number of the autoimmune conditions are too notable to ignore. Just as there are similarities among ARCs in the mechanisms of their onset, there are also commonalties in certain symptoms.

Many of you have probably heard of chronic fatigue immune dysfunction syndrome and one of its central complaints of extreme fatigue and weakness. (I emphasize "one" as we've gotten so much bad press that this condition is just about fatigue that we could overcome if we tried hard enough.) CFIDS shares this symptom of great fatigue with lupus, fibromyalgia, and Sjogren's syndrome, among other ARCs. It has been suggested that the same mechanism underlies this symptom in the various ARCs. In 1989, Dr. Robert Schwartz explained that the inflammation typical of ARCs causes certain white blood cells, the lymphocytes, to emit specific signals. A lymphokine or peptide called interleukin-1 (IL-1) causes particular brain cells to emit another peptide that causes sleep. When your immune system is functioning accurately, this response is a good one, in that it helps you to get the sleep you need in order to heal when you're ill. However, in ARCs, the immune system is often overactive, and the inflammatory response occurs all over the body. The last thing you need in this case is further tiredness and loss of energy.

What's the Family Connection?

There is a great amount of evidence indicating that ARCs run in families, which manifests as a tendency toward ARCs. For example, this means that different family members don't necessarily all develop SLE. This is one reason for the confusion during the diagnostic process. The patient with symptoms may know her aunt has scleroderma and her mother has Graves' disease, but may have no idea about the common thread of autoimmunity. Thus, when she presents her family history of illness to her doctor, she may not mention these ARCs, even though the knowledge would significantly help her doctor in diagnosing her autoimmune condition.

Research is underway into the genetic links of various conditions. Multiple sclerosis has been studied in a specific geographic region, and results indicated clear genetic propensities passed through family members. When a family member has the disease, the chances of other members developing it are as follows: sister or brother—4 percent chance; parents—3 percent chance; offspring—2.5 percent chance. Well, you may say, these numbers don't sound all that high. However, when we compare these numbers to the general risk in that geographical area, we see that unrelated individuals have only a .1 percent risk.

In addition to familial factors, lupus is tied to ethnicity, and is manifest far more frequently in Caucasians than in Asians, Africans, and other groups with little Caucasian genetic contribution. If you have lupus, your siblings or parents have a 10 percent chance of also having it, but your children have only a 5 percent chance, assuming your partner doesn't also have it. Studying identical twins has been enlightening as well. When one member of an identical twin set has lupus, the chance the other will develop it is a bit less than 30 percent. Among twins without the same genetic material—fraternal twins—the chances of one developing the disease after the other has it are much lower, at 5 to 15 percent.

When studying genes and ARCs, we can't restrict ourselves to examining full-blown cases. Other factors to look at are types and numbers of autoantibodies in the blood. Healthy relatives of people with lupus themselves manifest some of the same autoimmune system characteristics of their relatives with lupus. For instance, about 20 to 30 percent of healthy relatives also have autoantibodies (antibodies to their own DNA) characteristic of people with lupus (Isenberg and Morrow 1995). This again shows that genes are important but don't explain the whole story. If so, all of those with characteristic genetic components would have ARCs, which isn't the case. The AARDA concludes that genes account for 50 percent of the chance of developing an ARC.

Brain Structures and Functioning

In addition to the role of genetics, there's good evidence indicating problems with brain functioning and neurotransmitter levels in the brain. Modern technology, such as PET and SPECT scans, allows researchers to detect differences between the brains of those with and without ARCs. These dynamics may also be viewed with respect to the issue of gender. Preliminary evidence suggests that the

brains of healthy men may generate significantly more serotonin as that generated by healthy females' brains. The neurotransmitter, serotonin, has a central
role in many aspects affected by or involved in ARCs, such as sleep, mood, and
levels of substance P (the pain neurotransmitter). Other researchers theorize that
some ARCs stem from information-processing problems in the brain. This is a
fairly recent area of research and offers promising results in our understanding of
and ability to treat ARCs.

Viruses, Bacteria, and Parasites

The immune system serves as the body's defense against harmful external
invaders like bacteria, viruses, and parasites. However, the immune system can
malfunction in its efforts to protect the body. Sometimes this happens when the
external invader tricks the immune system and ends up using its mechanisms for
its own benefit. Sometimes the infection caused by an external agent leads to the
development of a short-lived autoimmune reaction or to the onset of various
symptoms characteristic of ARCs. A good example of the latter is the reaction of
the body to infection by the human immunodeficiency virus (HIV), which causes
AIDS. When somebody is battling AIDS, many autoimmune symptoms arise,
such as diabetes, Sjogren's syndrome, arthritis, and even thyroiditis. (You will be
reading about these symptoms as they are manifested in full-blown ARCs in later
chapters.) The body's immune system is usually no match for HIV. Part of its failure results from the triggering of the typical autoimmune reaction, causing the
immune system to turn against its own body.

In the earlier description of a model for autoimmune disease, you read about
another way in which autoimmunity can arise. In this case, the invading agent,
such as a virus, bacteria, or parasite, has characteristics similar enough to those
within one's body's cells or tissues that the autoimmune system is confused and
attacks this part of its own body as part of the attack against the invader. The
exact nature of the relationship underlying these observations isn't yet clear,
though there are some ARCs for which strong evidence suggests a bacterial, viral
or parasitic infection as the trigger. In fact, there are cases in which ARCs are
greatly increased in a geographic region after a widespread battle with a virus.

A good explanation of how bacteria interacts with the autoimmune system
is given by Ronald Hoffman (1993). He discusses how unhealthy bacteria and the
resulting toxic waste in the digestive tract and colon can precipitate the onset of
ankylosing spondylitis, a painful disorder believed by some to be an ARC. The
actual onset is dependent upon the individual having a genetic predisposition for
such a disorder. Hoffman proposes several methods by which harmful bacteria
can proliferate and overwhelm our healthy bacteria. It can begin with the bottle-
feeding rather than breast-feeding of an infant, which doesn't allow the baby
access to the mother's colostrum, a substance containing immune factors and antibodies. As the baby's immune system isn't fully developed at birth, an essential
function of colostrum is that it goes directly to the digestive tract (with its own
immune system components) and assists in the development of the baby's
immune system. Without benefit of colostrom, bacterial overgrowth may occur.

In addition, while chlorinating and fluoridating tap water serves a purpose, treated water may kill helpful bacteria in the digestive tract.

Antibiotics, which we usually look to as health boosters, can be disastrous for the immune system (as well as for babies' developing attentional abilities). They don't distinguish between good and bad bacteria, and end up destroying good bacteria whose function is to protect the stomach and other organs. The result: The doors are opened to harmful yeast and bacteria and the onset of candida and fungal illnesses. Hoffman adds that besides ingesting our own antibiotics, many of us ingest the milk and meat of livestock treated with the same. Women are often exposed to an additional risk factor if they are taking hormone-related medications such as birth-control pills. Such hormones can actually increase the levels of damaging fungi and yeast. Other risk factors include consuming alcohol and medications such as aspirin, acetaminophen, and ibuprofen. Does it sound like there is no way out? As you'll read later, there *are* things you can do to reduce your exposure to risk factors and decrease the development and continued presence of such harmful bacteria, fungi, and parasites.

A Cancer Connection

Another important area being researched is the link between ARCs and cancer. There are several ways in which the cancer process seems related to the autoimmune system process. For example, lymphomas are malignant tumors comprised of B cells that have not yet developed into their usual role of secreting antibodies. Thus, lymphomas can be thought of as solid tumors of the immune system, and patients with lymphomas cannot react against some types of foreign invaders. Obviously then, the immune system is malfunctioning in some way. In fact, lymphomas are one of the potential long-term harmful outcomes experienced by those who have been battling ARCs, including Sjogren's syndrome, rheumatoid arthritis, and lupus. Echoing this relationship is the fact that some people with lymphoma develop autoimmune symptoms like arthritis and certain antibodies (Isenberg and Morrow 1995). For an in-depth exploration, refer to David Isenberg and John Morrow's 1995 book, *Friendly Fire: Explaining Autoimmune Disease*. I highly recommend this book as one of the few that attains a balance between being informative and understandable for the layperson.

Hormones

Because ARCs present with a ratio so overwhelmingly female, it's natural to consider the role of hormones. Or so one would think. However, as mentioned earlier, when I commenced writing this book in 1998, the scarcity of information for women—or about the gender discrepancy—was shocking. It wasn't until my book's first draft was completed that an awakening had begun within this sorely ignored area.

There are a few professionals in the medical field who aren't at all surprised by this needless delay. For example, Dr. Elizabeth Lee Vliet (1995) asserts that doctors of all types have never paid attention to women in terms of research or treatment. As an M.D. in a time during which she sees women turning away from traditional Western doctors and treatments, she holds a tenuous position. However, she bridges this gap by valuing alternative medicines as well. Her focus is on the role of hormones in causing various disorders. She sees that women have gotten short shrift because men, largely directing the medical system, don't understand hormonal changes and so have avoided, ignored, or minimized the potency of such factors in illness and health.

Vliet explains that after years of seeing women develop conditions like chronic fatigue syndrome and fibromyalgia, often in their forties just after the onset of menopause or after tubal ligations or hysterectomies, she could no longer ignore the role of lowered estrogen levels in explaining these conditions. This is particularly so given that her clients with these disorders had less than normal levels of estrogen, which can lead to low levels of testosterone and DHEA. Low estrogen seems to work in a few different ways to trigger the onset of ARCs. First, it interferes with sleep. We know from various studies that just interfering with delta level, or deep restorative, sleep among healthy individuals prompts body aches, trigger point pain, and other symptoms characteristic of FMS. Besides disturbing sleep, low estrogen reduces levels of neurotransmitters such as serotonin, which is linked with mood and pain regulation. Vliet's approach includes increasing amounts of estrogen in the body and she maintains that sleep, thinking, fatigue, and pain all improve within six to nine months. She warns that increasing testosterone or DHEA levels (which women might do by taking over-the-counter preparations) before rectifying estrogen levels can worsen pain. She prefers using Ovcon 35 and believes that many birth control pills have too much progesterone and too little estrogen. If this isn't suitable for the woman, she uses Estrace or the Climara patch. You would do well to familiarize yourself with the information in her book and then talk to your doctor about her findings.

Let's take a quick look at hormones in general. Hormones, which are emitted by glands, travel through the bloodstream to particular locations in the body. Hormones are essential because they control the activities that perpetuate cells and tissues. As mentioned earlier, ARCs may be genetically linked. Winifred Conkling (1996) notes that when the effects of female hormones, notably estrogen, are thrown into the mix, the result is the significantly greater likelihood of ARCs in women. Hormones, genes, and the interaction between the two may be powerful influences in the development of such illnesses. So, women might come out ahead in terms of longevity, but we don't necessarily do so with respect to overall health. We have more costly chronic illnesses, and greater rates of consulting doctors, undergoing operations, using medications, and staying in hospitals.

On the one hand, female hormones such as estrogen can have beneficial consequences by reducing the reactivity of our cardiovascular systems to stress, thereby lowering the rates of heart disease until menopause. But in a strange, ironic twist, most studies of the role of estrogen in heart disease have been conducted on men! This isn't to say that heart disease poses no risk for women. Approximately 233,000 women die from coronary heart disease annually; it is still the leading killer of women in the U.S. It has been estimated that *up to two-thirds of medical doctors do not diagnose heart disease in women accurately*. This is because most of the research on heart disease has been done on men, and doctors are educated on the male model of heart disease. Women show different patterns of symptoms from heart disease and heart attacks. Essential tests and treatments routinely ordered for male patients are often not even considered in the case of female patients!

Let's look at the other side of female hormones and their role in women's health. The same female hormones that protect us from some problems backfire in terms of other illnesses. Estrogen has been linked with breast and uterine cancer and also seems to be associated with the onset of ARCs. One solid theory is that estrogen triggers the immune system to respond excessively. Indeed, there are indications that a woman's immune system is different from a man's. Women have a greater ability to fight off infections, and when their immune system is triggered, its reactions are more powerful. However, in these "strengths" may lie the kernels of "weakness" leading to ARCs.

As discussed earlier, there has been a very recent upswing in interest in gender issues and autoimmune-related conditions. An article by Whitacre et al (1999) attests that it's time to convene a panel of experts to send out the word that research about the gender gap of ARCs is critical. While this is progress, I must wonder why it has taken until now for the medical community to give the go-ahead for research that's been desperately needed for years. At any rate, what these experts suggest is that women's systems have greater amounts of substances that induce inflammation. A disruption in the inflammatory processes is one of the central dynamics of many ARCs. Because of the gender gap in the prevalence of these disorders, sex hormones have been extensively explored. While both men and women have both male and female sex hormones, women have more estrogen and progesterone, while men have more androgens. These sex hormones may have differential impacts on the immune system. For example, testosterone has anti-inflammatory characteristics. Immune responses in women are stronger and lead to greater antibody production, and we also have more prolactin and growth hormone, which increase autoimmunity.

Not much is known about the detailed interaction between sex hormones and autoimmune disorders, but several studies have produced telling findings. It is well known that pregnancy and birth, times during which hormones fluctuate greatly, can be associated with the development of several ARCs. Women with lupus often go through a worsening in their condition during pregnancy. On the other hand, women with rheumatoid arthritis and multiple sclerosis may experience a reprieve during their pregnancy; however, there is frequently a flare following delivery of the baby. Basically, after a woman gives birth, the level of estrogen in her body decreases, but the level of progesterone decreases to a much greater degree. Using lupus as an example, it has been found that many men and women with lupus have elevated levels of estrogen. In addition, the men also have lower than normal levels of testosterone (primarily a male sex hormone). It appears that male sex hormones offer protection against ARCs, as castrating male mice leads to autoimmune thyroiditis identical in incidence and severity to that developed by female mice. However, when testosterone was given to these castrated males and to female mice, clinical improvement was observed. As improvement was related to the dosage of testosterone, there may well be something to the hypothesis that *the levels or proportions* of sex hormones determine propensities toward ARCs (Isenberg and Morrow 1995).

Thymic hormones have also been studied to determine their relationship to autoimmune conditions. These hormones are important because they're involved in differentiating T cells into suppressor cells or helper cells. Through this mechanism, they exert a great deal of influence over the functioning of the immune system. The thymus is incredibly important in the early stages of development of the immune system. If it is removed in a young animal, the animal will show a decline in immune functioning and will eventually die from infection. While there is a great deal of evidence from animal studies that removal of the thymus is linked to the development of autoimmune disorders, far less evidence is available for humans. One point that implicates low levels of thymus hormones in partially contributing to the development of at least one autoimmune disease is that Lupus sometimes develops in people upon removal of their thymus. There also seems to be a link between the sex hormones discussed above and thymic hormones. For example, estrogen sometimes decreases thymic hormone in the body. This may help explain why women are more prone to developing ARCs.

Thus, further research into the role of hormones in triggering ARCs is essential. At least there is evidence that while hormones aren't the only causes of ARCs, they may be a trigger and certainly affect the type and severity of disease that develops. You'll read more about theories on hormones and their relation to dysfunction of the immune system in chapter 2.

Triggers in the World Around You

What do society and one's environment have to do with ARCs? A great deal. They can be the source of triggers and stressors, which, when combined with a genetic inheritance, may precipitate an ARC. Environmentally, there are endless lists of toxic chemicals, germs, viruses, bacteria, and the like that can trigger an ARC in somebody predisposed to developing one. For example, Dr. Furio Pacini (1998) notes that young adults who were children during the 1986 nuclear accident at Chernobyl may be at heightened risk for developing the autoimmune disease hypothyroidism. He asserts that children with greatest nuclear exposure have the highest levels of antibodies to the thyroid gland. Pacini speculates this may lead to the development of thyroid disease in the future. Obviously, long-term studies will be needed to explore this area. You will find that in each chapter focusing on a specific disorder, the issue of whether environmental events, toxins, chemicals, medications, and the like can serve as triggers for the development of that particular autoimmune condition will be discussed in greater depth.

In terms of external forces, our society is certainly a source of negative stress, as well as stereotypes and prejudices that are particularly detrimental to us as women. In addition, triggers such as drugs (illegal or prescription), nutritional deficiencies, and unhealthy lifestyle choices can contribute greatly to the likelihood of our becoming ill. In terms of negative stress, the incredible rapidity of the pace of our lives, the hurry sickness assailing most of us, the never-ending, ever-increasing cycle of change in technology, information, and even in our roles and responsibilities, can be too overwhelming for our physical bodies and mental processes to tolerate. In addition, the stressors that trigger the arousal of our bodies (i.e., the fight-or-flight response) these days are quite different from those to which our bodies adapted in earlier times. No longer do we see a predator approaching us as the threat, triggering the rapid arousal of the stress process in our bodies. The threats to us nowadays are much more subtle and insidious. Nor do we have the opportunity to react, thereby dispersing the arousal of the fight-or-flight response and regaining bodily balance, as human beings evolved to do.

The messages often passed on to women raised in our society can also have direct, negative effects upon our bodies and minds. Many of us are taught to avoid conflict and respond with passivity—a pattern of behavior that leads to suppression of true feelings and continued, unhealthy arousal of our bodies. Another message we may receive is that we are to forget about our needs and desires and work only to satisfy and support those of other people. In this case, a rift develops between a woman's self and her true wants and goals. The continuous denial of her needs and self leads to chronic distress, anxiety, and low self-esteem.

Further conflicts are internalized as women today also receive messages that we can (and "should") have it all: loving marriages, respectful children, high-powered careers, beauty, health, and on and on. Indeed, there are a large number of now disheartened women who have followed this call and ended up with suffocating job responsibilities and pressures while finally realizing they never wanted to be career women in the first place. The opposite pattern has also emerged. Women who enjoyed working followed directions and stopped, married, and had kids because this is what women "do." What happened? The external voices had internalized and their volume overwhelmed the woman's personal internal voice. Subdued by societal and familial messages, it turned into a mere whisper.

All of these so-called mental phenomena are entrenched in our body's functioning. When we expend our energy in nonbeneficial areas, we clear the path for the onset of physical weakness and illness. Other negative stressors involving the conflicting demands that can arise from the many roles we occupy these days, together with our internal conflicts about success and our traditional ways of interacting, caretaking, and being (which are societal and familial in origin), all add to the troubled mix. Make no mistake about the incredible toll these dynamics can take on our mind-body well-being. On a positive note, there are techniques and tools you can use to decrease the impact of such negative stress. If you so choose, you can use the information presented in this book to reconnect with your true desires and regain control over your thoughts, emotions, and behaviors in ways that benefit your mind-body system and give you the strength to protect yourself to some degree from disease or, when necessary, to accept its presence yet continue to grow intellectually and emotionally.

In terms of toxins and pollutants in our environment, most of us are all too aware of their ever-increasing presence and harmful results. Lifestyle choices such as burning the candle at both ends, smoking cigarettes, drinking excessive alcohol or caffeinated drinks, not exercising, using prescription or illegal drugs excessively, and eating unhealthy diets of fast foods, fatty substances, and refined sugars can all disrupt our mind-body balance sufficiently to allow the entry and takeover by ARCs in those of us who are genetically predisposed. When this does occur, we are left to fight a difficult battle with insurance companies, disbelieving physicians, critical onlookers, and our own self-doubts and old expectations. As you'll learn in later sections of this book, the healthiest thing you can do is accept the fact that there are some situations and people that you can't control and who won't believe the truth of your illness. You must do your best to protect your interests in these situations. What you can control, however, is your thoughts, emotions, and behaviors about these situations and people. You don't have a choice in developing your illness, but you do have a choice in how you decide to respond. It is in this choice that the winners, those who can actually grow, learn, and develop from a challenging experience such as chronic illness, take their stand.

Personality Characteristics

Also important for women is the suggestion that certain personality characteristics are linked with the onset of diseases such as autoimmune disorders and cancer. This area of study is complex and very controversial. However, there is evidence that certain personality and behavioral characteristics are associated with illness, its rate of progression, and with the process of recuperating and healing. As mentioned, one of the autoimmune disorders seen more frequently in women than in men is rheumatoid arthritis. Bernie Siegel (1986) suggests that chronic RA is seen in people manifesting a lifelong pattern of self-denial. Siegel maintains that, as with cancer, rheumatoid arthritis also develops from a life of self-minimization; those with RA were described as having consciously restricted their own achievements during their lives. This pattern is one that many women end up adopting because we have been socialized to put our needs and wants after those of others. Siegel also suggests that individuals at high risk of developing cancer tend to be very hard on themselves and blame themselves while forgiving others.

As you can imagine, the theory that personality plays a role in causing disease is highly charged and much debated. Probably the most frequently studied association between personality and illness is that between individuals called Type As and heart disease. Type As have been described as aggressive, short-tempered, fast-moving, loud, stressed-out, extremely competitive workaholics who continuously attempt to do more and more in less and less time. You've probably heard about the studies that indicate a relationship between Type A *behavior* and heart disease. However, when these studies were examined more closely and such relationships were not always found some researchers took a different approach. They teased apart different characteristics of Type As, such as hostility, aggression, time pressure, competition, and so on and attempted to determine which of these particular components were actually related to heart disease. It was found that it's actually the hostility and aggression of these individuals that seems to be associated with illness. In a study I conducted of Type As (1996), the results indicated that feeling good about oneself and the resulting relationship with stress was a significant factor in distinguishing between "healthy" and "unhealthy" Type As. Unfortunately, most of the research has tried to further the understanding of this linkage in men, while very little attention has been paid to high rates of heart disease in women.

Efforts have also been made to find a relationship between personality and cancer. According to Bernie Siegel in *Love, Medicine & Miracles* (1986), past research and his own experiences have suggested that people who end up developing cancer experienced a deficiency in unconditional love as children and thus never developed a good sense of self or self-esteem. For the purposes of this book, let's take the case of a female child. If this child didn't receive necessary acceptance and validation as she grew up, she would instead depend heavily on external reinforcement and strive to behave in such a way as to ensure sufficient attention or affection, in order to make herself feel worthy and good. As a young woman, she would find work or a lover or group of friends to give her a temporary sense of self-worth. Underlying such externally driven self-esteem, however, are the hidden feelings of insecurity and inferiority. By continuing to focus on others and satisfying their needs while suppressing her own, this woman is able to feel she is functioning adequately in the world. At some point, however, something happens to break up her delicately constructed world. It's likely to be a stressor such as losing a job, losing a husband or lover, or no longer finding fulfillment in her life. There she is, left alone, overwhelmed by her previously carefully hidden feelings of inferiority, low self-worth, fear, and dependency.

Siegel suggests that cancer is the disease of "nice" people, those who continually strive to satisfy others so that they themselves feel accepted and valuable. After a loss such as those mentioned, frequently within approximately two years, Siegel maintains that this person is highly likely to become ill. Siegel also summarizes research studies indicating that people who developed cancer rated high on hopelessness, had experienced a recent emotional loss, and were restricted in expressing their own emotions, particularly those related to their own needs. Siegel describes one questionnaire covering such issues that achieves 88 percent accuracy in identifying those who turn out to have a biopsy-confirmed cancer.

Those of you with rheumatoid arthritis and other ARCs may have extremely differing reactions reading this. Some of you may be furious and state that your personality has absolutely nothing to do with the fact that you developed an illness. Others of you may feel you've gained a glimpse of personality characteristics you've tried to ignore or hide. As always, each person is so individual and unique that there is rarely, if ever, a single description or model that can explain the whys and hows of a person's emotional and physical health. Researchers and scientists have argued for centuries over whether the individual or the disease was primary. The answer that is probably most accurate overall is "it depends." Now, I know that isn't a very fulfilling answer, but suffice it to say that there is significant evidence substantiating the role of personality and stress in illness. Even if you don't believe that your personality had anything to do with the onset of your ailments—and it very well may not—I hope you believe that you can benefit physically and emotionally by modifying certain characteristics and beliefs. You'll learn more about this in the subsequent section on stress and in the portion of this book that provides techniques and tools for coping with and even growing from your illness.

Diet

We all know how central diet can be to determining our relative good or poor health. Your body needs specific types and amounts of nutrients so that all of its systems, including the autoimmune system, can function effectively. As with hormone research, most of the research on diet and autoimmunity has been done on animals. One food that none of us would probably suspect as being potentially harmful is alfalfa, but animal studies have shown that diets high in alfalfa have been associated with blood changes reminiscent of those in humans with lupus. The conclusion was that alfalfa sprouts have high amounts of a particular amino acid that may be the culprit. In addition, Virginia Ladd, president of AARDA, informed me that a study in which men were given a great amount of alfalfa in an effort to reduce cholesterol resulted in some autoimmune disease symptoms in some of the men.

Another suspect in our diets is one that we already know can be physically harmful in a number of ways: fat. The culprit we must really strive to minimize is animal fats. Isenberg and Morrow (1995) discuss a telling study, again involving mice, in which diets high in fat have produced disturbances in lymphocyte (a type of white blood cell) functioning and elevated levels of autoantibodies (antibodies targeting one's own body). On the other hand, when animals with tendencies toward developing lupus are fed low-fat diets, reductions in both kidney inflammation and autoantibody levels are seen. In addition, these animals tend to live longer. Fat may somehow affect the synthesis of such chemical messengers as prostaglandins and leucotrienes, thereby affecting autoimmunity.

The type of fat you consume is also an important variable. For example, you may have heard about the value of having some fish oils in your diet. In addition to food sources, you can find a variety of forms of fish oil in any health food store, pharmacy, or supermarket. Giving mice a low-fat diet that includes fish oils can protect female mice against developing inflammation of the kidneys. Some research has been conducted on humans as well, providing diets low in fat but including some omega-3 fatty acids. These fatty acids have an anti-inflammatory effect and may well have protective effects on rheumatoid arthritis and irritable bowel syndrome. The amounts used were 10 to 20 grams/day, and they were derived from cold-water fish. On the other hand, omega-6 fatty acid, often found in vegetable oils, may increase unwanted inflammation, thereby worsening certain autoimmune disorders. This area seems a fruitful one for exploration and definitely warrants further research. You're probably aware that caffeine and refined sugar disrupt sleep, but you might not know they also trigger the stress, or fight-or-flight, response in our bodies. Both of these effects are unhealthy, increase the levels of negative stress experienced, and can lead to disruptions in the functioning of our immune systems. Keep this in mind when planning your meals.

Vitamins and Minerals

None of us can escape the bombardment of news, advertising, and statements by friends or family, all advising about the amazing benefits of various vitamins. However, some people who go by the premise that if some is good, more is better, have actually overdosed on vitamins, including the B vitamins and vitamin D. While there are only certain vitamins on which people can overdose, it's always best to check with your health care professional about the types and amounts of vitamins you should be taking. Some types of vitamins when taken in combination can cancel beneficial effects of one or both. You also need to be aware of how certain types and amounts of vitamins might interact with other medications you're taking.

Vitamin D

Several vitamins, including vitamin D, which has myriad interactions with the immune system seem to offer promising effects on autoimmunity. As you may know, this vitamin's central role is to maintain an appropriate level of calcium in the bloodstream. Both deficiencies and excesses of calcium can lead to a variety of negative physical consequences. Vitamin D and a hormone called parathormone, produced by the parathyroid glands, manage the input and output of appropriate amounts of calcium. In addition, disturbance in the generation of vitamin D may be associated with the development of autoimmunity, because vitamin D prevents excessive production of both T cells and B cell–generated antibodies. When B cells generate too much of an antibody, the extra antibodies may attach to a part of one's own tissues or organs, thereby forming destructive "self-antigens." Possible targets of the body include DNA (which could eventually lead to lupus), thyroid tissue, acetylcholine receptors (in individuals with myasthenia gravis), and white blood cells (Isenberg and Morrow 1995). If the production of antibodies by B cells can be diminished, it's less likely that there will be excess antibodies to bind to and destroy body tissues.

Vitamin D also gives a boost to the body's white blood cells, primarily the macrophages, thereby making them more potent killers of invading bacteria. Vitamin D may have a greater role in certain conditions than in others. For example, people with rheumatoid arthritis tend to have normal vitamin D levels. On the other hand, patients with type I diabetes (insulin-dependent) and Grave's disease have much lower levels of vitamin D3, a type of vitamin D.

Antioxidants

Vitamins A, C, and E also provide protection against autoimmune disorders. Studies on the effects of these vitamins have most frequently involved the use of animals, but the results are quite promising. These three vitamins are antioxidants, and they are important in deactivating free radicals, which are single electrons that damage our cells and can change the DNA inside them. Where do these damaging free radicals come from? They can come from chemicals, pesticides, cigarette smoke, pollution, radiation, and even the natural processes of the immune system's functioning.

Vitamin E has been studied in humans, and it's been found that increasing the amount of vitamin E in the diet can benefit those with conditions like scleroderma, polymyositis, and lupus. A critical thing for you to know about vitamins A, C, and E is that they must be consumed in a balanced way. For example, smokers who take vitamin A may be creating a dangerous imbalance, because cigarette smoke depletes vitamins C and E. Such an imbalance can increase cancer risk.

Other Substances

Certain medications or drugs may be related to the onset of ARCs. In exploring such possibilities, we've gathered further evidence about the complexity and multiple etiologies involved in the onset of these conditions. In particular, simply ingesting a particular medication doesn't necessarily lead to autoimmune symptoms or disorders. Just as in all cases, other factors such as genetic influences, hormone levels, environmental influences, and the like are involved in the mix.

Alcohol

I am not saying that you must abstain from alcohol; however, there is sufficient evidence indicating negative consequences that you owe it to yourself to really take a look at this drug. Certainly, it has been shown that alcohol increases the risk of certain cancers. It's important to acknowledge the fact that as mentioned earlier, more than a few researchers believe there is some kind of link between cancer and ARCs. In animals, alcohol has been shown to decrease the responses of B cells. In addition, alcohol is associated with a decrease in the percentages of autoimmune T cells and natural killer cells (Kemeny 1998).

Illegal Drugs

So-called recreational drugs, such as cocaine and marijuana, may also increase the chances of developing ARCs. For example, it has been shown that cocaine interferes with B cells' and T cells' immune responses in mice. Marijuana, also studied in animals, decreases natural killer cell activity and the production of interferon, as well as lowering resistance to cancer proliferation.

Tobacco

A mention of tobacco here is certainly relevant. You will read in subsequent chapters how tobacco can play a role in certain immune system dysfunctions. Here's a statistic that really drives home what we do to ourselves and our loved ones when we smoke: Tobacco is the estimated cause of up to 30 percent of cancer deaths, and one study indicated that smokers live a whopping eighteen years less than comparison nonsmokers (Kemeny 1998). It's likely that smoking negatively impacts the immune system because we know that smoke has a number of negative effects on various systems within the body. The relationship between smoking and the development of autoimmune symptoms is a complex one and research is lacking. One of the few tentative conclusions is that smoking reduces the number of Langerhans' cells that exist in the respiratory system. The suspected decrease in these cells due to smoking is thought to increase the risk of viral infection, as well as to reduce the ability of these cells to respond sufficiently to negative changes in the system.

Prescription Drugs

Let's take a brief look at just a few of the drug-induced ARCs. It is easy to understand how one type of medication, namely the immune suppressors, can increase the chances of developing ARCs. These are typically given to people who have received an organ transplant, in order to put the immune system on hold so that it doesn't perceive the new organ as a foreign invader. The existence of drug-induced myasthenia gravis was initially discovered when a number of individuals with rheumatoid arthritis developed myasthenia gravis, an association that is quite rare. It was eventually discovered that these individuals had been given D-penicillamine to assist with their arthritis. Fortunately, this outcome is quite infrequent, and the vast majority of people who take this medication do not develop myasthenia gravis or related symptoms. Another positive aspect is that even when this condition does arise, it seems to completely disappear when the individual is taken off of D-penicillamine. Other medications that can trigger myasthenia gravis include: quinidine, propanolol, trimethadone, dephenylhydantoin, and lithium. Again, such linkages are very infrequent.

D-penicillamine is also the culprit in potentiating the development of some other medication-induced ARCs, including scleroderma; myositis; and drug-induced lupus. Drug-induced lupus is one of the most well-studied of these types of conditions. This type of lupus differs from the true autoimmune disorder (SLE) as it affects men and women equally, doesn't lead to kidney disease, and disappears when the offending medication is terminated. Substantial progress has been made in terms of understanding some of the underlying dynamics of developing lupuslike symptoms from certain medicines. For example, just as genetics are involved in determining the possible development of the true autoimmune disorder of lupus, so too are they involved in the possibility of developing medication-induced lupus.

Several characteristics have been isolated as being associated with increasing the risk of developing such a medication-induced disorder (Isenberg and Morrow 1995). For example, individuals with a genetically determined propensity for the slow metabolism of certain substances have a greater likelihood of developing drug-induced lupus. In addition, as discussed earlier, each human being has a unique pattern of human leucocyte antigens (HLA). Evidence suggests that a person's type of HLA is related to the risk of developing drug-induced lupus. Unlike the case with drug-induced myasthenia gravis, the length of time an individual has been taking the triggering medication does matter. People may need to have taken the triggering medication for up to one or two years before certain symptoms, such as joint pains or skin rashes, first appear. This delayed onset is one of the reasons that health care professionals may not be sufficiently concerned as to whether such a situation is developing. Thus, it's essential you be aware of such potential relationships so that you can discuss these possibilities with your doctor. Of course, once this is determined or even considered a possibility, your doctor must take appropriate steps such as weaning you off of the detrimental medication.

Chemical Exposure

Isenberg and Morrow (1995) describe other external chemicals and elements associated with the development of ARCs. While there is a clear relationship between the silicate exposure of gold miners and the onset of scleroderma, the debate rages on with respect to a potential similar relationship between the silicon in breast implants and symptoms reported by some women that typify lupus and scleroderma. As you'd expect with the monetary amounts involved, there are many who support and just as many who oppose the suggestion of such a relationship. In addition, chemicals used as solvents in aromatic products; in vitamin, organic, and pharmaceutical synthesis; and for other purposes, such as in polyvinyl chloride, benzene, and xylene, have all been associated with skin changes like those occurring in scleroderma. Even our hair coloring treatments are suspect.

CHAPTER 2

Stress and the Immune System

It's better to know the patient that has the disease than the disease that has the patient.

—William Osler, *Lancet*

In our hectic times, we experience traffic jams and post office lines as threats. In line with our extreme interpretations, our bodies jump into full gear to prepare for a life-threatening stressor. However, these days we don't usually fight or flee even though our bodies rev up to do so. Instead, we end up sitting still, confined within our motorized metal cocoons, or standing still in slow-moving lines with no outlet for the extra energy produced by changes in our body chemicals. As a result, we have no opportunity to regain balance and harmony within our bodies.

Negative Stress

Over time, our bodies are aroused so many times by mild or inconsequential threats, with no opportunity to release this bodily tension, that our systems permanently remain at an elevated level of arousal. This is incredibly taxing to both our physical and emotional resources, and our systems can begin to break down.

For example, the onset of Crohn's disease is linked to stressors like divorce and bereavement. Also, children who develop type I diabetes have often experienced a parent's death or divorce. Dr. R. L. Swank, an ARC expert, sees distress as second only to unhealthy, fatty diets in causing multiple sclerosis, an ARC linked with nutritional deficiencies (1990). The development and onset of rheumatoid arthritis has also been shown to be related to the experience of distress. Distress directly interferes with the optimal functioning of our immune systems, and thus often primes us to develop illness, such as an ARC, if we are genetically predisposed.

Modern technology helps us understand the negative impact of distress on our health. For example, we've learned that one central physical event occurring during the stress response is the release of stress hormones called glucocorticoids. While these are adaptive in "real" negative stress situations (i.e., life-threatening), most of us face few if any such stressors anymore. Instead, we experience daily hassles piling up one after the other. With each hassle comes the stress response's arousal, usually incomplete discharge of tension, in addition to residual elevated levels of glucocorticoids. New research suggests elevated levels of these hormones can kill certain brain cells, including those associated with memory and recall. Also, as mentioned, immune functioning is suppressed. In addition, bodily functions, such as digestion, repair, and growth, slow down or stop during the stress response. I can't help but think of fibromyalgia, in which three common symptoms are memory loss/disturbance, muscle tissue repair deficiencies, and gastrointestinal distress. As you read the FMS chapter, you'll see that changes in brain structure and functioning, stress, and neurotransmitter and hormonal changes have all been suggested as causing FMS. Other ARCs involve symptoms such as these as well.

Self-Knowledge Is Key

Various biological functions and events differentiate men and women and can be potent sources of distress for some women. These include menstruation, pregnancy, postnatal depression, and other difficult psychological and physical consequences of childbirth, premenstrual symptomatology, and menopause. I say "some of us" in the previous sentence to acknowledge that not all of us go through the same physical experiences, and even when we do, we can experience them in completely different ways. Throughout this book, I ask you to recall there are major differences among women and how we experience and perceive situations and stress. It's essential that you begin to understand your patterns of interpreting and responding to potentially stressful situations. Do you tend to react excessively to mere hassles? If so, you're probably telling yourself something bad is going to happen. Start reassessing situations more realistically, or your resulting hurry-and-worry sickness can do real damage to your body. You'll be learning tools to help you accomplish these aims in later sections of the book.

It's also essential to know the dual nature of stress. Negative stress (distress) occurs when you're faced with a situation and have the following reactions: you have little or no control; you don't have resources or abilities to meet the demands; and you see the situation as a threat and want to avoid it or at least minimize its impact. Positive stress or "prostress" (the name I coined for positive stress in my book, *High on Stress: A Woman's Guide to Optimizing Stress in Her Life* [1998]) arises when you're facing a situation and feel like this: you have some control; you have abilities or resources to meet the demands of the situation; and you feel challenged and want to be actively involved as you perceive the chance for growth or other positive results. As you read, strive to find the dynamics and elements that resonate with your experience, to understand your particular "distressors," to learn how they negatively affect your mind-body, and to learn how to cope with them to reduce the experience and drawbacks of distress. Later you'll learn more about the flip side of stress, prostress, and its hows and whys.

Hormone Happenings

What does all this have to do with ARCs? Although personality variables and coping skills don't cause illness by themselves, they interact with potentially stressful situations to increase or decrease your chances of becoming ill. Because some attitudes and behaviors increase distress, they can affect likelihood of illness. One theory explaining this link is that negative stress causes disruptions along the hypothalamic-pituitary-adrenal axis (HPA). This axis is central to the workings of the immune system and brain, and disruptions here could explain ARC characteristics like increased pain and fatigue. Your hypothalamus regulates temperature, hunger, thirst, weight, and, importantly, the fight-or-flight stress response. When you experience distress, your hypothalamus' neurons release corticotropin releasing hormone (CRH), most of which travels directly to pituitary cells. The pituitary gland responds by releasing ACTH hormone into the bloodstream. ACTH affects parts of the adrenal gland, causing the release of a third hormone, cortisol. People with high distress manifest high levels of cortisol. Normally, high levels of cortisol feed back to the hypothalamus and pituitary glands, signaling them to stop generating CRH and ACTH. However, distress interferes with this feedback loop and may cause all three hormones to continue being released, with inevitable mind-body damage.

Individuals with HPA problems and a tendency toward *low* cortisol levels may be vulnerable to ARCs. Doesn't this contradict what was just described about stress and high cortisol? Acutally, no. If you continue experiencing distress over time, your cortisol levels eventually decline. Cortisol is an anti-inflammatory, and it's thought that insufficient cortisol may underlie the inflammatory response seen in ARCs. It has also been suggested that chronically depressed people have lower than normal levels of cortisol, while those suffering from brief, time-limited depression manifest more normal levels.

Another way distress harms the immune system is by interfering with the production of cytokines. Cortisol, released during the distress response, particularly during situations in which one feels helpless and out of control, inhibits the release of cytokines like interleukin 2 and interferes with the ability of macrophages to produce interleukin 1 or tumor necrosis factor (Kemeny 1998). While we now know that many people with ARCs have lower than normal amounts of cytokines, this doesn't necessarily clarify our understanding. It may not be a simple fact of quantity of cytokines determining health. We can't directly link low cytokine levels with ARCs, as FMS and CFIDS seem to manifest in those with high cytokine levels. Fortunately, actual clinical treatments have been developed for ARCs, and it's now possible to increase amounts of antibodies to specific targets, like those going after CD4 molecules, and the cytokine TNF alpha being used to treat RA and Crohn's disease.

External Triggers

If you have an ARC, you're probably very aware of the fact that while the pain and other illness-related symptoms increase negative stress, they're not the only triggers. Many external situations we have to deal with as patients and human beings—such as interacting with cold, disbelieving medical staff; attempting to gain assistance from resisting insurance agencies and managed care companies; trying to obtain emotional support from family members with beliefs similar to the doctors' or who resent the inevitable changes in the family unit's functioning; facing financial losses, and experiencing discrimination in the workplace or losing our jobs—greatly intensify our distress. The key to remember here is that while we may have little or no control over many of these external events, we do have control over how we choose to interpret them. How we do so directly affects how we'll feel emotionally and how we will behave with respect to coping with our illness and efforts to heal.

As stress plays such an important role with respect to health, we must explore the dynamics of how distress and prostress can affect our mind-body health. You'll see that you have the power to largely determine the quality and quantity of stress you experience. Some distressors, such as marital problems, the sudden loss of self-esteem, interpersonal difficulties, and recent loss of a loved one, have been linked with heart disease (Glass 1982) and can also underlie the development of many illnesses, depending on a person's vulnerability, genes, lifestyle, and other propensities. As discussed in *High on Stress*, research suggests the distressors we as women rate as affecting us most strongly occur much more frequently in our lives than the distressors rated by men as affecting them most strongly. If we do experience greater distress overall, this might partially explain the prevalence of ARCs in women.

Stress on the Job

Let's briefly look at "external" sources of distress in our work that can weaken our health. Our jobs often allow us too little of the control and authority that can balance a job's demands. While the situation is slowly changing, men still tend to hold jobs of higher status and greater control, regardless of whether they are white-collar, blue-collar, or clerical positions (LaCroix and Haynes 1987). In the National Institute of Occupational Safety and Health's ranking of the stressfulness of jobs, many of the jobs most highly associated with heart disease, high blood pressure, nervous disorders, and ulcers were those typically occupied by women. Some of these were: secretary, office manager, waitress, health technologist, licensed practical nurse, nurse's aide, registered nurse, dental assistant, social worker, health aide, and teacher's aide (Padus and the Editors of *Prevention* Magazine 1986). These jobs are very distressing because they're physically and/or emotionally demanding, fast-paced, highly repetitive, and offer little room for control and creativity, which could balance out these distressors.

Even in the 1990s, we continue to work in occupations highly segregated by race and gender. The careers we occupy are often more than two-thirds occupied by women. This is one reason men and women face different stressors on the job. The National Institute of Occupational Safety and Health found that women occupying pink-collar jobs that offer less creativity, control, and responsibility have a very high rate of heart disease (Padus and the Editors of *Prevention* Magazine 1986). Many of these women report frustration and anger at "being kept out of the loop," being forced to follow rigid schedules, receiving minimal feedback from male supervisors, and carrying out repetitive work. Of course, what most of you have probably heard is the disturbing fact that even when we occupy the same jobs requiring the same educational preparation as men, we still have less control over other workers and end up doing more support tasks and less decision making and delegating. These jobs are linked with feelings of hopelessness that transfer to other areas in our lives and can be associated with illness.

Do any of the above "female" job characteristics sound familiar? *High on Stress* contains a questionnaire that can help you assess the nature of your job in terms of its negative stressfulness, and also includes techniques to help you increase prostress in the work environment.

The gender wage gap is definitely still around. Estimates these days for women's wages as compared to men's range from seventy-two to ninety-five cents on the dollar. While the gender gap in pay is slowly decreasing, certain obstacles still interfere with equalization. Some of these obstacles involve beliefs about women and their workplace performance that are just plain wrong. For example, one of the most harmful beliefs regarding working women is that we don't progress as far or as rapidly in our careers as men largely by choice, because of our commitments to family. In 1993, M. L. Andersen provided enlightening information: Women are behind men in occupational levels and income *regardless* of whether or not we are married or have children!

One reason for the lower overall salaries for women is the disturbing inequity between men and women in upper management levels. While there have been concerted efforts by a number of organizations to offer equality in hiring and promotion, statistics still show that women have a more difficult time obtaining a certain elevation and status. If you haven't yourself experienced the glass ceiling, you probably know of some friends or relatives who have. In addition, women in powerful positions still experience job-related stress—not only from typical sources, such as deadlines, red tape, and the like—but also from an internal conflict regarding achievement and success in our society. Various studies have shown that even women in the least female-traditional jobs can experience great distress and internal conflict. Women also have a much greater chance of experiencing another negative workplace stressor: sexual harassment. This is yet another workplace element that reflects inequities in power between men and women, and that also contributes to maintaining such inequities.

All Bottled Up

I am constantly surprised by the number of women I come across who have been taught overtly and covertly by society and family that they must be the caretakers, cheerleaders, and "therapists" for others. Most of them don't even question this notion. Since we're supposed to focus on others, the hidden message is that we have to deny, suppress and ignore our feelings and desires in order to satisfy the needs and desires of others. Other women have been taught to avoid expressing certain emotions, like anger, because they aren't "ladylike." Some, while not consciously aware of it, repress and hide their feelings for fear that showing them would anger or disgust their partners and lead to abandonment or abuse. Holding in feelings can cause great psychological and physical damage. Recent studies have shown that communicating feelings and even journaling result in improved immune system functioning.

Your Body Bears the Burden

So that we can understand how negative stress and autoimmune related disorders may be connected, it's important to understand what happens to the body when it is experiencing a negative stress reaction. When you perceive a stressful situation, your body quickly goes through a number of changes. It is truly amazing how our physical bodies prepare for perceived threats by mobilizing and activating physical resources in a well-orchestrated, swift way. We've all experienced this stress response, whether it arises from slamming on our brakes to avoid an accident or from being called on to contribute in a class or meeting. This so-called fight-or-flight response includes the following changes:

1. Heartbeat increases to carry blood throughout the body and provide oxygen and nutrients more quickly to lungs, brain, and major muscles.

2. Blood pressure increases.

3. Breathing becomes shallow and quicker.

4. Muscles tense for action—especially the skeletal muscles of the back, shoulders, arms, jaw, face, thighs, and hips.

5. Blood flow to your extremities—like hands, fingers, and feet—decreases and they become colder.

6. Adrenaline and other hormones are released.

7. Perspiration increases.

8. Immune system is suppressed.

Many of these changes in your body result from activation of a part of your nervous system called the sympathetic nervous system. The sympathetic nervous system and the parasympathetic nervous system together make up the autonomic nervous system. For many years, it was believed that we had no conscious control over the autonomic system. That is, it was believed in our culture that we couldn't voluntarily change our blood pressure, heart rate, body temperature, and the like. Nowadays, there is enough significant evidence negating this that even Western medicine has had to incorporate and devise a number of techniques to cash in on the trend. If you ever listen to the nightly news, you're more than familiar with hearing about how you can plan your diet, take vitamins, and alter your lifestyle to affect bodily functions and improve your health. The truth is that you can actually also directly alter some functions of the "automatic" autonomic system. You'll be reading more about how you can gain control over this system and, importantly, over your body's responses to negative stress through biofeedback, relaxation, meditation, and other techniques. It is thought that such measures will allow the body to regain and refocus its energy appropriately, so that the immune system is properly energized and can work at its maximum efficiency. If we don't disperse the arousal from the stress response, our immune systems will eventually be suppressed. To reach a balanced, harmonious mind-body state, we need to expend the built-up bodily tension or reduce the frequency and impact of distress and increase the frequency of prostress.

It's All in How You Look at It

Recent research shows that it isn't simply the number of such life events you experience that causes distress and illness. Instead, what matters is whether you see these life events and situations in a negative or positive way. Again, I cannot overemphasize this essential discovery . . . it is the *meaning you give* to a situation that determines whether you will perceive it as negative, and consequently whether it will be psychologically or physically damaging. Once you really grasp this realization, you'll gain a tremendous sense of control over your reactions, health, and life. While stress is unavoidable, distress is not!

Another recent discovery is that it isn't only the *major* life events that you interpret negatively that are responsible for the harmful effects of stress. In contrast to what has been touted in stress research, Kanner and his colleagues presented evidence as far back as 1981 that daily minor irritants actually have a greater harmful impact on our health than major life events. These daily stressors, called "hassles," are actually better predictors of psychological and physical symptoms. I'm sure you are all too familiar with a number of hassles in your life. They include everyday distressing events such as driving in traffic; waiting in lines; worrying about your weight; having too many things to do; taking care of your home; losing things; dealing with demands from your children; other family members and friends; and having too much work or ambiguous job responsibilities. How many of you can relate to most, if not all, of the hassles on this list? When you have a chronic illness, the list can expand tremendously. Take some time now to write a list of the hassles that are most disturbing and frequent in your daily life. Also, for the next few days as you go about your daily life, jot down the situations causing you distress. Then reassess all of these situations and determine whether they really justified your body's stress response. If not, these were unhealthy reactions and areas you need to target by perceiving them in a more accurate way.

Uplifts

Fortunately, on the flip side, there are positive, frequently occurring—even daily—events called "uplifts" that can increase the prostress in your life. These include good relations with your spouse, lover, or friends; completing a task; contributing in a meeting; playing a favorite sport; feeling healthy; meeting your responsibilities; eating out; and spending time with your family and friends. The importance of having prostress in your life was clearly and cleverly shown by a study in which some people were told to engage in pleasurable uplifts and others were not. One month later, the people who had engaged in pleasant activities reported a higher quality of life and more pleasure than the people who hadn't been instructed to engage in any particular pleasant events. Another exciting discovery came out of this: The people with the most negative stress before the study who were told to engage in twelve prostress activities reported less psychological distress and greater pleasantness of experiences overall than people who had been dealing with *just as much negative stress before* but who had been told to engage in only two or no prostress activities (Reich and Zautra 1981). The point to remember is that when you're experiencing a great deal of negative stress in your life, the number of prostress experiences you include day to day is more important than ever. Remember that frequently occurring events are central in determining your stress level (distress or prostress). After all, there is a lot more we can do about the minor hassles and uplifts in our lives than about those major, generally unexpected, infrequent life events.

The Downside of Stress

Now that you're well aware of the dual nature of stress, you might wonder how the consequences of distress and prostress differ. Most stress research has remained myopically stuck on studying the association between negative stress and physical and psychological problems. The growing acceptance of the idea that distress harms health through affecting the immune system is seen in the burgeoning field of psychoneuroimmunology. Western medical science is finally taking a serious look at the mind-body link and the associations between emotions and thoughts, the immune system, and the central nervous system.

It's Physical

Your thoughts and emotions, together with your perceptions and experiences of stress, represent complex interactions that impact your immune system and can either hamper or improve your health. This is but one reason it is essential for you to learn how to control your perceptions and responses to distress. You can't afford to expend energy on worrying or other negative actions that do nothing to resolve situations or improve your condition, but only waste your time and energy and interfere with your immune system. The mind-body link is evident in ways beyond the impact of psychological factors on the immune system. Psychological distress also damages other parts of the body, such as the circulatory and hormonal systems.

It's Psychological

Besides the damage distress causes physically, it's also associated with various psychological problems, such as depression, anxiety, eating disorders, and drug and alcohol abuse. Many women use drugs, alcohol, and food as "stress relievers" or as crutches to distance and protect themselves from reality. They feel more outgoing, interesting, and attractive when under the influence of drugs or alcohol, and feel at least illusory control in chaotic lives when they're able to purge after a binge. It's hard for them to stop relying on these external substances, because they give a brief, artificial boost to self-esteem and feelings of control. Imagine being able to eat anything and everything and not gain weight . . . all you must do is tiptoe to the bathroom to vomit, engage in hours of excessive exercise, or take huge quantities of damaging laxatives. Besides being ineffective ways of losing and keeping weight off, these methods are physically and psychologically dangerous. In addition, when the high wears off, so do those feelings of power and control, and the woman is left feeling weaker and more self-loathing than ever. Relying on external substances, objects, or people for self-esteem and to cope with stressful situations ends up increasing feelings of loneliness, anxiety, low self-esteem, and lack of control.

If, added to this, a woman develops a serious ARC, she'll have little energy and at times little hope for the day-to-day struggles, let alone enough to grow or develop in positive ways from the illness! For many of us, our ARC serves as a wake-up call to how we've been passively living our lives. There will be times we can't count on people we could traditionally depend on to help, and the healthiest course will be for us to assume responsibility and control for our lives. If this sounds at all like you, it's essential you have someone you trust that you can talk to during this period, whether it be a friend, a family member, or a therapist. The reason it's so important now is that this enforced reality and realization that you must care for yourself and can't necessarily rely on those we thougt we could can increase emotionality and confusion. I'm not saying the outcome is only negative, as this experience can affect you in positive ways. However, if you feel overwhelmed, incapable, and resentful that this has happened to you, you risk further depression, anxiety, or substance abuse. I recall one of my clients, a delightful, attractive young woman who had a mixed presentation of anorexia and bulimia. Our work was slow and difficult, but we were making good progress. After feeling much more energetic, healthy, and happy, she began feeling sicker and weaker. I advised her to see her physician, and she was finally diagnosed with SLE and FMS. Now she saw her life as completely out of control, and she went back to her old behavior of alternating between starving and bingeing and purging. Her compromised system couldn't handle this, and she wound up in the hospital. With hard work, she realized the real danger of her actions, learned effective coping skills, and gained true self-esteem for the first time in her life.

Does Your Health Care Cause Even More Stress?

Many of these disorders are quite complex and affect several systems; they may present with seemingly ever-changing symptoms. In the chapters dedicated to the particular autoimmune conditions, you will also read about disorders or conditions that may frequently be confused with *your* particular autoimmune disorder. This is one of the biggest challenges when it comes to ARCs; namely, the difficulty in making an accurate, timely diagnosis. This fact, along with the fact that "women's diseases" are vastly underfunded or ignored, contributes to the unfortunate frequency of misdiagnosis. You'll see this confirmed in the interviews I conducted with a number of women afflicted with autoimmune conditions, and, of course, if you yourself have such a disorder, you may be all too familiar with the prolonged time period required for an accurate diagnosis. I hope this book will not only help you deal with the length of time required, but also assist you in being assertive with your doctor or health care professional in moving them along the diagnostic path at an acceptable clip.

Because the numbers of women affected are so staggering, and the patterns and possible causes increasingly clear, it's untenable to continue with the minimizing reaction by medical doctors and others in the medical field. *The American Autoimmune Related Diseases Association estimates that more than 65 percent of individuals with autoimmune disorders had already been labeled as "complainers" or "hypochondriacs" in the early stages of their disorder!* Unfortunately, there remain many stubborn, outdated practitioners who still think in this manner.

I recently re-experienced this just as I was writing this portion of the book. Thanks to the nature of the nonsensical insurance game in our country, which provides me with a never-ending stream of primary care physicians, I was seeing yet another new-to-me general practitioner. After listening to me mention that I had been diagnosed with fibromyalgia some eleven years earlier, he abruptly broke in to respond that fibromyalgia is just a trash basket for symptoms that can't be explained, and that because depression is often seen with this disorder, it's probably just psychological in origin. Fortunately for me and for him, I was able to report to him the findings of a number of different studies indicating that this is a real disorder—and that the depression is now known to be a consequence of living with chronic pain and fatigue, as well as probably part of the disease process, and not the cause for yet another woman's sickness. I dare say that were he living daily with such pain, fatigue, loss of strength, sleep deprivation, cognitive disturbances, and the like, he would probably manifest some depression as well!

Presentation Counts

It may seem odd that we must attend to our clothing, makeup, and demeanor when we are seeking help for an illness. However, these factors do affect our treatment. Let me tell you a short story that is derived from a study exploring these issues. The story involves a woman who plays two very different personalities on a short video screening. The "women" are recorded to play for a sample of doctors who have been divided into two groups. Each group of doctors will see only one woman (i.e., one of the videos).

The hypothetical patient presented for treatment with complaints of chest pains. The first group of doctors watched as a professionally dressed woman discussed her symptoms in an assertive, clear manner. The other group watched a video of the same woman wearing overdone jewelry and dressed in a flashy manner. She also talked about her symptoms in a distressed, emotional tone. Both groups of doctors were presented with the same factors: reports of chest pain, together with the woman's risk factors of cigarette smoking and elevated blood cholesterol levels. Although they had the same information and were aware that these risk factors are associated with heart disease, the second group was apparently so fixated on this woman's emotional presentation and flashy appearance that it seems they "forgot" their years of education and experience. Only half of them said they would pursue cardiac testing and about three-fourths of them would have diagnosed her with anxiety or panic attacks. Shocking, yes, but even more so when compared with data from the first group, who saw the woman playing the role of an assertive, calm professional. With the exception of one doctor, all of them ordered cardiac testing and fewer than one-third even thought about anxiety as a possibility.

This example illustrates the vital importance of being assertive. In order to ensure you're getting the most effective SHOC possible, you must be able to communicate openly and directly. This is one of the most important lessons I hope you will take with you from this book. The way you behave and appear, whether in an assertive, powerful manner or the opposite, can have important implications as you seek assistance from others.

A Word about "Fairness"

In reading literature on this subject, I'm struck by the use of the phrase "It's not fair" in complaints about the gender bias in research and treatment. This isn't surprising, given that it surely isn't fair. However, this very belief is one of the most detrimental and dangerous irrational beliefs we can hold, and it's the very belief that I spend much time working on with my clients. When we operate from a viewpoint that the world is fair and that everything "should" (another dysfunctional concept) be fair, we're bound to be disappointed over and over and over. In addition, people also feel anger, depression, rage, anxiety, frustration, and a whole range of negative feelings stemming from the fact that what happens in reality doesn't match what they believe should happen in a fair world. This world is not a fair one, and the fact remains that sometimes one will be on the winning, favorable, lucky side and sometimes one will be on the losing, unfavorable, displeased side. Later in this book, you'll be learning cognitive techniques that will teach you how to monitor irrational, stress-invoking thoughts so that you can replace them with realistic, positive thoughts, thereby experiencing positive emotions and a more realistic understanding of you, others, and the world.

Thoughts about the Medical System

Many of the issues I've just discussed represent the most negative side of the health professions. I certainly do not want to convey that all members of the medical system are aligned against women, believe they are all malingerers, and are inevitably cold and uncaring. This would be as unjust as someone telling you that your particular illness or symptoms do not exist. There are many, many workers in the medical system who do have the best interests of their clients in their minds. Many have chosen these careers from a true desire to end suffering and to assist in healing. Unfortunately, the current state of the medical system, in which physicians and others must see endless numbers of clients each day, and spend their time on paperwork trying to justify continued treatment rather than being able to spend time with their clients, does not set the conditions for these professionals to form meaningful, healing relationships in which clients feel respected, cared for, listened to, and understood. All of these stressors, in addition to the usual stress of dealing with people who are sick and in pain, tend to cause health professionals to withdraw into themselves and harden themselves against the distress and pain.

Think about how often doctors are described as cold, mechanical, uncommunicative, and uncaring. These perceptions may be partly true, but part may also come from our general anger with the medical profession, our anger at our illnesses, and perhaps our unrealistic beliefs about what our doctors can provide us. I'm not saying, "It's not the doctors' fault, it's society's, and there is nothing we can do about it." I *am* saying that we need to be as understanding as we want our helpers to be. Bringing negative expectations with us tends to ensure the continuation of negative cycles. We need to look at what we can truly expect from these individuals and think about where our anger is really coming from.

Of course, there are spoiled apples in every lot, and if you feel that you've gotten one, you have every right to put it back and select another. Just try to use some thought about your desires, needs, and expectations . . . then you will act from your truest place. Our healers also need to be conscious of what is going on within themselves and their lives. If they see that they aren't able to provide the services they dreamed about when striving to be healers, they will make changes to benefit their clients and themselves. Healing is most often a two-way street.

What You Can Do

Fortunately, there are many things you can do to change your beliefs, attitudes, goals, behavior, relationships, and lifestyle to improve your life quality and mind-body healing. Does this sound like a lot of things to change and a lot of work? It is, and it will continue to be. There is a chance that medical research may one day find the panacea many of us hope for. Until that day, you must make every effort to assume responsibility and control over aspects of your life you can control (thoughts, feelings, and behaviors) and let the rest go. This will be the most difficult work you've ever encountered. While it may not seem like it, you really do have choices and power. You can decide to remain the same person you are and react to the ups and downs of "this thing," or you can exert your free will by deciding just how you'll spend the rest of your life.

By learning about and understanding your illness, you'll be able to cope most effectively. As you build your knowledge about the illness and symptoms, you will more easily accept your body's changes and develop new expectations for yourself. This reduces the distress you feel when it's unclear what is due to your illness and what is due (in your mind) to potential "laziness" or "giving up." As 55-year-old Stacy explained, "When what is going on with me is just like what I have read about or heard about, then I don't put so much pressure on myself to perform the same as or even better than before. I was doing this before to convince myself and everybody else that all was fine with me. Well, everything might not be fine, but I have the choice of who warrants being told and who doesn't. It really lets me ease up a bit on myself." Easing up isn't the same as giving up. Stacy continues to educate herself about her illness, and she integrates conventional and alternative approaches to optimize her healing.

CHAPTER 3

Reclaiming Your Healing Energy

The mind is its own place, and in itself
Can make a heaven of hell, a hell of heaven.

—John Milton, *Paradise Lost*

Out of awareness comes knowledge, and with knowledge comes the potential for power. You must supply the missing ingredient: your energy directed by focused intent. Your body is a self-healing entity. What you and I must do is work together to remove the blockages interfering with your mind-body system's ability to heal. Blockages can be internal or external; regardless, you need to identify them and rid yourself of them.

External Blockages

One external blockage I hear about frequently from clients is their interaction with the medical system. The medical system and health care in this country are powerful forces that reward behavior falling in a very narrow range of the permissible. They don't reward spending quality time with patients, listening to their reports, or offering empathy or sympathy. Instead, in the true business sense, it's a numbers game of dollars and cents that doctors must play if they want to stay in the game. The female experience in this game is summed up beautifully in Nancy Mairs' *Waist-High in the World* (1996). She states, "My disease manifested itself clearly enough so that the doctors didn't dismiss me as an hysteric or malingerer, the lot endured, sometimes for years, by many with MS, especially those with the milder, relapsing-remitting form. I can't say that I'm glad to have the chronic-progressive form instead, because the outlook is bleaker, but at least it spared me the emotional debilitation of being thought, or thinking myself, at least mildly deranged" (28). These words show us her strength in always looking for the positive in her painful, debilitating condition. They also reaffirm the negative impact our "caretakers" can have on us when they're narrow-minded. Even when you come up against this uninformed reception, you don't need to accept it as truth or think yourself even mildly deranged.

If you want to make it through your SHOC in one piece, you'll need to become confident in yourself and question any bad feelings about yourself that arise based on the opinions of others. You'll be learning a variety of ways to do this. You must realize that if you challenge doctors and take matters into your own hands, you'll fare better in remission from illness. Taking an active stance in removing this and other external blockages to healing is key.

Financial and Medical Systems

The reality of autoimmune disorders and related conditions is that they are complex and don't fall neatly within any single category of diagnosis or treatment. Quite often, primary care doctors are unequipped to diagnose the complex diseases and syndromes we are discussing in this book. Of course, this isn't always their fault, as there is only so much that one individual can know. In addition, the medical schools and the board and relevant associations are in charge of ensuring that medical students and residents get sufficient training in a range of disorders. If they don't see a disorder as a true, real, or important one, they're unlikely to ensure that doctors are trained to notice a syndrome and refer the patient appropriately.

If you do get to the point where you are referred to a specialist, the doctor may run some tests, come to some tentative conclusions, and then have the primary care doctor refer you to another specialist. You may not even get any information about the results of the previous doctor's work unless you make a concerted effort to do so. Having to depend upon the primary care doctor to authorize all such treatments adds weeks, or months, to the diagnostic and treatment process. Rarely does the information from each doctor get sent in a timely manner along the same path you are taking. There are so many points along the chain where a particular doctor may not know enough about a disorder or about giving particular diagnostic tests that the march is put to an untimely stop.

You may be uncomfortable making the frequent calls to the primary care doctor, the specialists, and the insurance company that are often required to get any attention and assistance. But you do have to behave in a truly assertive manner; in fact, sometimes your behavior may have to exceed what would typically be defined as assertive.

When you're experiencing a great deal of pain, fatigue, or other symptoms, it's extremely difficult to keep yourself motivated to continue pushing the process along. It's very easy to feel hopeless, worthless, and consequently ready to just give up, but this you absolutely cannot do. Remind yourself what it is that you are risking if you become passive: your chances of reducing your intense pain, getting rid of symptoms, or even prolonging your life. I work on this routinely with my female ARC clients. You may wonder and ask yourself, "I'm paying for this, and these doctors and my insurance company are supposed to be here to serve me. Why *should* I have to be doing all this work? Don't they know I'm sick?" Well, unfortunately, while you're right, this position isn't going to get you whatever it is that you need. If the problem is particularly thorny and you really feel that you can't handle it anymore, then seek the help of relatives, friends or, ultimately, attorneys to assist you. The system is simply and absolutely not "user-friendly"!

Screening Your Doctor: What You Must Know

At the end of this book, you'll find a list of resources for additional information about your illness as well as possible referral names. In addition, a good resource is the *Official ABMS Directory of Board Certified Medical Specialists*, which is published by Marquis Who's Who and is likely to be available at your local library. You want to make sure that you obtain the services of a professional who is highly trained and knowledgeable about your illness. Of course, you also want to hire members for your SHOC committee who are caring, courteous, and dedicated to helping you. While information on training and certification is readily available in the list of resources and through your local hospitals, universities, and medical associations, information on the personal aspect can be found only through word of mouth and your own experience.

Regardless of the referral, you still need to do a good deal of screening yourself. Make sure that the doctor is knowledgeable regarding your illness and ARCs in general. What kind of specialty training and experience does she or he have? How long have they been practicing within the field? and how long have they been working with people with your particular autoimmune-related condition? How many patients does she or he currently treat with your condition? Have they been certified by the American Board of Internal Medicine or by the American Board of Rheumatology? If someone you know offers suggestions, you can get more qualitative information. Ask them how busy the office is. How long do patients have to wait? How much time does the doctor give you? How receptive is she to questions during nonappointment times? Does he return messages? Does she see people as passive patients or does she involve them actively on the team? Most importantly, does she or he believe in your condition? By now, I'm sure you see that this is an essential question.

Do your utmost to ask as many questions as possible before you get started with a health care professional. This won't always be possible, and you may have to allow this person on your SHOC team and hope for the best. However, membership on your committee is not lifelong! If you find that somebody is treating you in a demeaning or dismissive way and find that you keep feeling worse off than ever after seeing or speaking with them, give them the boot! You need to minimize the negative conditions and experiences in your life in order to take the journey toward improved mind-body health. This is just one of many times that you will have to assert yourself and validate your own feelings by paying attention to and acting on them. By choosing to act in a consistent, strong, and healthy manner in this situation, you're increasing the likelihood of behaving similarly in other areas of your life.

One of the things I hope you gain from this book is the ability to make consistent, health-enhancing SHOC decisions and take parallel actions. I am not proposing that you should go around randomly closing the door on people or situations that you just don't like. I am suggesting that you first think about the person or situation and your response. If you see that you are thinking rationally and that your feelings are stemming from an accurate analysis rather than some past hurt, disappointment, personal weakness, or pet peeve, then you'll be putting your energy to a positive rather than negative use by changing the situation.

Don't be worried about hurting other people's feelings when it is your life and yourself that need to be put first in order to grow, heal, and survive. Does this sound like selfishness to you? Yes, you will be giving your "self" top priority, but this is a necessary selfishness if you choose to grow from this experience and indeed, in many cases, just survive. This selfishness, if that is what some choose to call it, will come full circle. By caring for and learning about yourself, you'll be infinitely more able to care for and relate to others. This is but one of the many unexpected gifts of harmonious balance you'll find along the rocky path you'll be carving.

According to Norman Cousins, in *Healers on Healing* (1989), positive emotions and attitudes improve the medical care environment. Patients and their doctors both can use treatment more effectively. In his extensive observations of patient-doctor interactions, Cousins concluded that among the most important is how the physician communicates to the patient: "I cannot think of a single case in which reassurance of the patient is not required or justified. Unless the possibility of something good is attached to . . . treatment, the environment of treatment may be impaired. . . . The patient's hopes are the physician's best ally" (87–90). Certainly, this tells us how important a role a doctor can play in boosting a patient's own health armamentarium, such as her positive attitude, hope, purpose, and thus her own body's defenses, such as her immune system. Now when we combine this fact with what we know (and most likely have experienced) about how medical personnel sometimes treat women with illness, we can truly see how detrimental this piece can be to the healing puzzle.

Fortunately, there are a number of organizations that are humanistically oriented and can be very helpful. In appendix I, you'll find a listing of valuable groups dedicated to women's health and disability.

Internal Blockages

In effect, when we must deal with the external blockage of a disbelieving, cynical medical system, many of us internalize it, as we've done with so many harmful messages our whole lives. The result is that an external blockage is transformed into an internal blockage in which we begin to doubt ourselves or develop feelings of hopelessness, helplessness, depression, anxiety, and other feelings and thoughts based on turning negative energy inward upon ourselves. Internal blockages may be more difficult to contend with than the external, as they effectively distort our ability to accurately perceive the reality of events, situations, other people, and, particularly, our strengths, needs, and mind-body communications.

Let's take a look at some other internal blockages. Much data suggests that more women than men have mental disorders. Females tend to have more internalizing disorders, such as depression, anxiety, and eating disorders, while males more frequently exhibit externalizing disorders, like delinquent and oppositional disorders and school problems. In fact, when disorders typically within the purview of males—such as drug and alcohol abuse and antisocial personality disorder—are considered, the differential rates of mental disorders among women and men become more similar. Before we take the statistics regarding mental disorders in men and women at face value, certain factors must be considered. For instance, social and cultural factors need to be weighed when making such conclusions: women are more likely than men to seek help, admit experiencing psychological difficulties, and be diagnosed by medical and psychological professionals as having psychological problems.

When it comes to physical complaints, studies indicate that doctors label women's problems as psychosomatic (involving psychological factors) more often than men's and so are more likely to prescribe psychotherapy rather than situational or structural changes that might be more relevant. Doctors are also more likely to refer women to therapy than to do thorough medical checkups or search for complex or obscure physical problems that might be present. This discrepancy certainly isn't a modern phenomenon. The very word "hysteria" comes from the Greek word for womb—no "politically correct" terminology here! Hysteria was the term used to describe how women were expected to react to stressors; namely, with histrionic physical or emotional reactions like fainting or becoming ill. It was even said that unfeminine activities were dangerous because they were thought to cause "uterine derangement," which would supposedly lead to mental illness (Swedo and Leonard 1996).

Are We Just More Depressed?

It may be that societal influences lead to the appearance of greater rates of mental disorders in women than in men. That is, as a result of external blockages, we may develop our own self-perpetuating internal blockages. Several recent large-scale studies have tried to clarify if there really is a gender difference in mental disorders given that women are expected to have more psychological difficulties and are more open about admitting problems.

Gender Differences

In 1987, Paul Cleary summarized findings that included 20,000 residents in various cities within the United States. The rates of depression in women and men do indeed vary depending upon type of depression; however, it still seems that women are at least two to three times as likely to have depression as men.

Some experts prefer to focus on how we're socialized to explain the increased depression. A survey of therapists conducted in the 1970s revealed that their descriptions of "healthy personality characteristics" just so happened to be unmistakably equated with the stereotypes of healthy men in those days: active, independent, logical, and competitive. A healthy woman was described as being dependent, emotional, subjective, and easily wounded. Unfortunately, a recent repeat survey showed that even after all of the purported advances made by women, the stereotypes were still quite consistent with those of the previous decade (Ruble 1983). An important fact to note is that the expected so-called healthy female traits are the very characteristics we know increase one's vulnerability to depression. For example, focusing largely on satisfying others—rather than understanding and satisfying our own wishes and needs—is linked with depression. These are the very characteristics which society instills in us so very thoroughly throughout our lives. Let's look at some other factors involved in the development of depression. These are the perception of an emotional loss, the inhibition of anger and aggression, the inhibition of action, and low self-esteem. Again, these are the very characteristics and dynamics women experience more often than men.

Emotional Loss

The emotional loss perceived by a woman can range from a single traumatic loss to frequent losses of emotional connectedness. Because relationships are so important to us, we may often feel let down when all of the energy and efforts we expend are not returned. Emotional losses are harder for many women to bear if they lack the consistent, strong inner sense of self that lasts regardless of the ups and downs of relationships. It's a sad but true fact that many relationships in which one member develops a chronic illness do not last. Unfortunately, when it comes to the disorders discussed in this book, the prevalence is far greater in women than in men. Accordingly, many women dealing with autoimmune-related conditions may lose their life partner or other important people in their lives. In fact, a study conducted by Dr. Alfred Katz at the UCLA School of Public Health examined the effects of chronic illness on lifestyle. It was found that within six months after diagnosis of a chronic autoimmune disease (in this case, systemic lupus erythematosus), 20 percent of the patients experienced divorce or separation due to their partners' disbelief in the sickness and difficulties adapting to new needs and roles (*Head First*, Cousins 1989). Not only is this a trauma upon a trauma, but these women also lose the many health benefits of social support and intimacy.

Suppressed Anger

As little girls, most of us were rewarded for building and keeping relationships and being "sweet and nice." The implied message is that expressing anger or standing up for our desires isn't feminine (just the kind of behavior that leads to uterine derangement!).

Inhibition of Action

Do you frequently find yourself accommodating the wishes and needs of others rather than fulfilling your own desires or acting on your own behalf? Many women with chronic illness realize after they become ill that they have lived their entire lives this way. Eventually, it becomes clear that the mind-body can't continue to live healthfully this way. Turning toward yourself and valuing yourself, even if it's due to an illness that's beyond your choice, is a central area of growth you can attain from being ill.

Low Self-Esteem

Finally, low self-esteem remains a burden for many of us. Rather than having been brought up to value ourselves for the mere fact of our being, or for many of the female elements that are strengths in their own right, we've been taught that to be "good girls," we must make friends and be passive, quiet, attractive, and polite. While there are benefits to some of these elements, such as our ability to develop empathy, form friendships, and help others, there are also negative repercussions. Having to derive self-esteem from external sources and based on external factors (such as beauty, weight, or having a boyfriend or husband) is risky. Your ability to feel good about yourself is necessarily precarious when it depends on the approval of others. This is particularly true when you've developed a chronic illness.

If you've been struggling to project a false image, the onset of a chronic illness can quickly put a giant hole in your balloon. In the long run, it may be the best thing for your development as a mature individual who realizes her own strengths, accepts facts she truly can't change, sees her internal beauty, and acknowledges her importance as a human being. In the short run, it's probably going to hurt . . . a lot. It's also going to be scary for a while. This is because the defenses you've been using to artificially shore up your self-esteem, avoid truly looking at yourself, and suppress painful feelings may have served you quite well for some time. When these are torn apart, you'll have to face these painful feelings, self-doubts, and insecurities.

I hope you'll have true friends and partners in your life who are supportive and value and love you for who you really are, the person beneath the camouflage. In addition, you'll need to be gentle to yourself and stay away from the desire to berate yourself for all of the so-called failures that can no longer be hidden. You'll need to monitor your irrational, negative thinking, and may even have to go back in time to earlier years to explore the origins of such self-defeating patterns, and then confront and modify them into rational, moderate thinking. You may or may not be able to do this on your own. It's very difficult, and you may find it helpful to work with a psychologist or other mental health professional during this challenging period of change.

How Do You Rate?

The internal blockages and depression-linked characteristics discussed above also increase negative stress. Because we often respond to negative stress with depression, we can easily become trapped into a vicious cycle. See how you rate on this National Institute of Mental Health checklist:

1. Do you have a depressed mood most of the day, nearly every day, and has it been present for at least two weeks?

2. Do you have markedly diminished interest in activities most of the day or nearly every day?

3. Have you had significant change in your weight—either loss without dieting or a gain in weight?

4. Have you had insomnia or excessive sleepiness?

5. Have you felt sped up or slowed down?

6. Have you been fatigued or suffered a loss of energy?

7. Have you had feelings of guilt or worthlessness?

8. Have you had trouble making decisions and trouble concentrating?

9. Have you had recurrent thoughts of death or suicide?

If you responded affirmatively to at least five of the nine questions, you could be experiencing depression. This survey is an informal one, and it would be a good idea for you to contact your physician and/or seek assistance from a therapist. Remember that depression is a common companion to chronic illness; you're not alone if you're feeling depressed. Use this measure to get a general baseline, and as you apply the techniques described later, you can retake this survey intermittently to monitor your progress toward a more positive way of thinking and being.

Do You Feel Anxious?

Anxiety follows depression as the most frequent reason women seek professional help. It doesn't take much to figure out why a woman with a chronic illness, whether diagnosed recently or some time ago, would experience a great deal of anxiety about herself and her life. The breakdown of beliefs about yourself and your place in the world can provoke substantial anxiety. Then, there are the other true difficulties of living with an autoimmune disorder, including financial pressures, strained relationships, fears about your future health, the stress of dealing with insurance companies and doctors, and the potential loss of independent transportation or your job. Your anxiety is certainly understandable, but it's another internalized blockage and thus a waste of energy you can't afford. Worrying does nothing to resolve situations. You will learn to take action, do the footwork, and then let go. Don't let external blockages become internal.

One element central to mind-body health is control. There is a difference in the amount of control women and men feel in their lives and in society. It is quite telling that people defined as psychologically normal feel they have a greater sense of control in general than do those with mental disorders. In fact, well-adjusted individuals actually *overestimate* the degree of control they have over situations. They also believe their abilities and talents are greater than they really are. The gender/control link is a very complex and important theme to explore for our purposes, because feeling out of control and helpless has been linked directly with suppressed immune system functioning and the development of physical problems.

What if you're a woman with some form of anxiety? Fortunately, there are both psychological and physiological interventions that you can learn to substantially reduce your distress. You'll need to build control into certain areas of your life (or realize the amount of control you do have) and balance this with accepting lack of control in other areas and letting go. You'll read about a variety of effective techniques to deal with anxiety. I have found these approaches to be very successful with my female clients. Of course, if you have a truly serious problem with anxiety, it is important that you check with your medical doctor and psychotherapist.

Strive for Balance

We have come to a complex crossroads. As you have read and probably experienced, there is no cut-and-dried link between our various roles and whether we feel healthy or unhealthy, distressed or prostressed. The reason for this is typical of our lives as a whole: There are no simple cause-and-effect relations in our lives. Instead, just as we've seen the incredible complexity of the interactions among the body-mind systems, there is a complex, dynamically shifting interrelationship among the different roles, demands, and rewards in our lives. The key to get you through what might often strike you as overly bewildering and complex is the basic essence of life and nature; that is, balance and harmony.

In a moment, we are going to use a powerful tool that my clients typically find extremely useful in observing how far askew their lives are and how much their natural desires urge them toward a balanced life. First, let's look at the possibility that all is not well for us in the workplace in terms of preserving our physical and emotional health. If you are one of the fortunate women who can maintain some type of work schedule while living with the challenge of an autoimmune related disorder, you do owe it to yourself to consider the work environment. Is it such that you can continue to contribute, thrive, derive meaning, and assist the company in attaining its goals? If not, ask yourself if you can make modifications in the work environment to decrease negative stress (possibly through increasing your access to resources and training to meet stringent demands). Can you alter relationships with supervisors or peers to make the human interactions more supportive and pleasurable? Is there a chance for you to engage in extra training to keep you interested, learning, and growing (as well as more marketable)? Is there the possibility for options such as job sharing, part-time work, or telecommuting that might allow you to continue to contribute and find meaning, while not completely taxing you to the point where you can no longer work at all?

If you answered no to all of the above questions, then it may be necessary for you to consider why you still remain in a negatively stressful work environment that you know can detrimentally affect your mind-body health. Perhaps you can find something more in line with your needs and desires. Sure, you'll probably have to give up certain things to gain others; however, this is the way to attain harmonious balance and a new equilibrium. Your finances may decrease, but your ability to work and create may increase. Of course, there are many times when those of us with autoimmune-related disorders simply cannot work. Most of us aren't willing to give in to this so easily, and it only results after a prolonged fight. If you cannot function at a particular level right now, then you are certainly not giving up by choosing to take some time off to recuperate and rebuild your strength. This can work wonders, although you will need to redefine your purpose and meaning and watch out for sabotaging thoughts about being "useless" or "lazy." You'll be working harder than ever on a project more important than ever . . . yourself.

While listening to your mind-body signals, and after giving yourself the opportunity to try in various ways, you may well need to take a break. This isn't failure, and many women find that with proper rest, exploration into new treatments, nutritional changes, or new health care professionals, they can later return to work (whether in the same capacity or in a new business or career altogether) in a much more positive, meaningful, and excited way.

Exercise: Balance Your Life by Slicing Your Pie

Let's look at a simple tool to highlight the discrepancies between your current life and your desired life. Below you will find two circles filled with the activities of a client of mine, Connie, who had always been a high-achieving, self-defined perfectionist. After she'd been diagnosed with rheumatoid arthritis and fibromyalgia, she realized she could no longer keep up her hectic, driven pace. In fact, she was pleased to find the gift from her illnesses: she listened to her body and her true desires and acted accordingly. Look at the differences between her initial circle of how she spent her time and the "ideal" circle for which she decided to aim.

Now, we can turn to examine what it means to us to occupy so many different roles. Roles are positions we fill that come with certain responsibilities, duties, expectations, and rights. As a woman today you probably occupy several or most of the following roles: employee, supervisor, wife, mother, daughter, group leader, friend, social coordinator, coach, mentor, breadwinner, homemaker, and on and on. Is it possible that we are becoming increasingly vulnerable and ill because we're taking on more roles? There is no simple answer; in fact, the truest

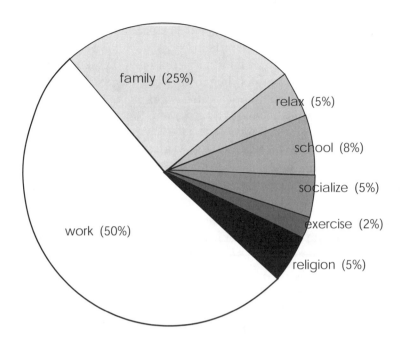

Connie's Current Life Pie

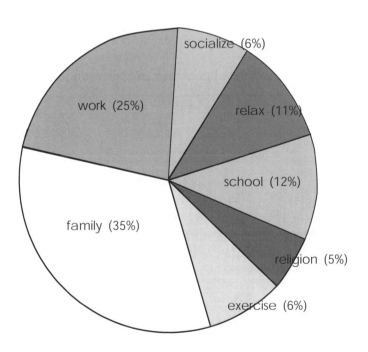

Connie's Ideal Life Pie

response is that "it depends." In your journal, write about your roles and design your current and ideal pie charts.

The shorter lifespan of men has often been blamed on men's involvement in the workplace. When women began to work at greater rates than ever before, it was expected that these gender differences in health would wane and that we would have the same consequences as men. Sure, we could play (to some extent) on the same playground as men, but we'd have to step up and pay the same costs. But the research doesn't show this to be the case. In general, working women have fewer sick days, hospitalizations, acute conditions, and disruptions due to chronic conditions than men. Although various factors—such as the type of job, a spouse's or significant other's support, and one's expectations—make it somewhat difficult to draw a generalized conclusion, overall it seems that women who work outside the home report better well-being and health than housewives (LaCroix and Haynes 1987).

Being involved in multiple roles can improve your health in several ways. These include greater availability of social support, improved self-esteem, financial benefits from working, and improved access to health services. Rewards such as recognition, prestige, improved self-esteem, and financial compensation can make up for some of the costs associated with occupying multiple roles. As I write this, I notice the fit between this theory and my own experience. Staying home several months after having my baby was an enjoyable but tiring and stressful time. I found that when I went back to work, my energy level and overall pleasure in my life, both at work with clients and at home with husband and baby, increased. Yet we can't draw a simple conclusion and say the more roles the better. In order to determine whether carrying out multiple roles is better or worse for our health, we have to examine both the nature of the roles and their interaction. I'll be explaining this important discovery in the discussion that follows and I hope it will prove enlightening and liberating. The mere fact that you may have to occupy several or many roles does not mean, in and of itself, that you must experience increased distress.

Negative and Positive Stress on the Job

If asked, you could probably come up fairly easily with a list of the distressing and exhausting characteristics of your job. But I hope you could also come up with aspects that are exciting and challenging. What are some common elements that can cause distress or prostress for you? In 1979, Robert Karasek presented a model proposing that job strain is determined by the balance between the stressors or physical and psychological demands of a particular job role and the control one has over the work.

Demands and Control

Think about your job for a moment. If it is low in job control and high in job demands, you are more likely to experience effects like exhaustion, depression, anxiety, difficulty awakening, and insomnia. This type of job is also correlated with more sick days and higher rates of drug usage. On the other hand, people with so-called active jobs that offer both high job demands and high job control report the greatest satisfaction. So, you may have a very demanding job, but if these demands are balanced by your ability to exert some control, make decisions, and access resources, your work will be less negatively stressful. In fact, if you have these positive attributes in your job, you can actually experience positive stress and personal and professional growth. This is why it's impossible to say that if you have a chronic illness, you should quit working and conserve energy to focus on yourself. Some women obtain great pleasure, growth, and challenge from their jobs. When this type of situation exists, you can actually increase your overall level of energy, because positive experiences can increase positive energy. However, if you're in one of the low control/high demand jobs, then it might be necessary for you to take time off, refocus your energy on yourself, set new goals, and heal your life.

Exercise: The SAID Technique

Let's look at another valuable technique you can use to assess your current life-style and harmful thoughts, while learning to restructure your life and optimize your SHOC. Take a moment now to check into the thoughts prompted by the above statement. Take note of thoughts such as, "Oh great. Because I'm sick, there is no way I can even have demanding jobs anymore. I can't even apply normal models of behavior to myself." If you're having cognitions like these, it's a great example of how you can sabotage yourself with self-talk. Okay, so maybe you really can't do very demanding or even moderately demanding work at present, but is it really such a terrible, horrifying, catastrophic situation? Also, notice the words "at present." This is to illustrate how pulling your thoughts back into the here-and-now can really make you consider a situation more realistically. Many of women with autoimmune-related conditions have episodic courses. This means that although you may be feeling completely exhausted, pain-ridden, and helpless right now, it doesn't mean this will be the tale of the rest of your life. Now, wait a second. Are you pursuing this unhealthy line of thought?: "Well, my particular case certainly isn't episodic. Or even if it is, my 'good' periods still aren't good, and I certainly can't do a job like the one I've done during those times either." Okay, now what do you do? You use the SAID technique: Stop, Accept, Identify, Determine. Write about your use of the SAID technique in your journal.

- Stop this negative, black-and-white, catastrophic, and forecasting type of thinking.

- Accept the real changes that have occurred within your mind-body and the resulting consequences and need for life changes.

- Identify the strengths, abilities, and benefits you *do* have and stop obsessing about the losses and difficulties. (Because words have such power to create our realities, words like "losses" and "difficulties" themselves are problematic. These occurrences will have less of a negative impact on you if you call them "changes.")

- Determine just what it is that you want to do with your strengths and interests. Set new goals and remember that one of the benefits of going through an experience like yours is that you are being "forced" to dream again, think flexibly, make new plans and grow in new ways.

Money Matters

Now, take a moment to think about one of the greatest sources of negative stress in your life. Without using any powers of ESP, I would feel fairly confident in guessing that a huge number of you thought about money. It is something we worry about endlessly, think about, hope for, pray for, argue about, buy lottery tickets for, marry for, divorce for, and get freedom from having or not having. Money is yet another stressor that is impacting women more strongly today than ever. Thrown together with the fact that our financial income is generally greatly reduced when we develop a chronic illness, finances are likely to be a great concern for most of us reading these pages. I suggest that you consult with financial planners, attorneys, and other professionals within relevant fields to find out just what you do have, what you could be getting, how to get it, and how to maximize it for the future!

Marriage . . . Boon or Bust?

For years, we've faced societal, peer, and family pressures to marry. We were led to believe that, besides having children, marriage was the *piece de resistance* of a woman's life. For you, marriage may well be associated with happiness, security, and social support. A number of studies have shown that married women have higher well-being than unmarried women. Overall, both marriage and working tend to be associated with less distress in women.

While marriage is usually associated with less distress and better health for both sexes, men still benefit in these ways more than women. Why would marriage be more of a stress buffer for men? Simply put, women end up having to give a great deal more social support than they receive in such a relationship (Vanfossen 1986). Take a look at your own relationship. Would you say that you give more support and are more emotionally available to your male partner? If we become ill and don't have the energy to be the family backbone, we experience increased distress if we see this as a failure to live up to expectations. Our partners and other family members might have difficulty adjusting to this change as well. You'll be reading about such family conflict and how to handle it in chapter 14.

The Stress of Being "Mom"

Being a mother is the toughest job in the world. In 1986, Grace Baruch and Rosalind Barnett revealed that motherhood can be associated with psychological distress and isn't predictive of good self-esteem, pleasure, or low levels of depression. There is some evidence, though, that some mothers derive slight health benefits depending on the number and ages of children, employment status, and marital status.

Certainly, being a parent is a source of stress for both men and women. But as with marriage, the strains of this role affect women more strongly. Particular aspects of mothering impact how the role affects us. For example, having young children and having three or more children are both related to higher rates of depression. Women with young children have a greater number of physical problems, such as appetite and sleep disturbances. (If you've gone through this wonderful but taxing experience, you really don't need to rely on research results to understand this!) Caring for young children is more stressful for women of lower income than for others. In 1985, Rosalind Barnett and Grace Baruch found that among the various roles occupied by women these days, only that of being a mother (not that of being a wife or employee) was associated with experiencing role overload and role conflict. So, just what is it about the role of mother that is more distressing than wife or worker? One reason is that the main responsibility for the children's welfare and performance still falls largely on our shoulders. Society's expectations for a mother differ from those for a father, and our identity is often more closely linked with being a mother than is a man's identity as a father. The result is that the demands of parenting are more stringent and stressful for women.

Looking back to the demand/control model, the maternal role is heavily weighted toward the demand end, with little chance of control. Despite the lack of control, we're still expected to produce perfect, well-behaved children. In addition, because our culture expects us to naturally perform this role well, many of us are too ashamed to admit to distress and difficulties with being Mom. Many women who don't naturally perform the mother role "ideally" consider themselves "defective," and may be viewed that way by others. Perhaps knowing that many mothers have anxieties about mothering and that everybody makes mistakes can lessen any overly critical, irrational thoughts you hold.

It's All in the Interaction

As you've probably gathered by now, there's no easy conclusion about whether any particular role you occupy will increase the distress or prostress in your life. The key lies in one of the most important recent discoveries in stress research: To get an accurate understanding of roles and stress, we have to look at the quality and *interaction* of the roles to determine whether you'll experience prostress or distress. Of course, we also have to consider your psychological makeup and changes going on in one or more of your life's spheres.

Not surprisingly, the experience for women who work and mother is greatly affected by their husbands' behavior as fathers. For men, the roles of worker and father typically have some overlap in control, power, and prestige. Often, this same pattern is lacking between the roles of worker and mother. Because of the traditional view of women as homemakers/caretakers and because many of our jobs are still lower in pay and prestige, we have less bargaining power and control over assigning parenting and household responsibilities to our husbands and kids. When working women's husbands do not assist in child care, women don't obtain the usual prostress benefits associated with working (Baruch and Barnett 1986). We see an interesting pattern emerge: The more a wife earns compared to her husband, the greater participation he shows in terms of household responsibilities. The drawback? As men contribute more to child care and home chores, they feel more competent, but they're also more critical of their wives' performance as mothers and of how they manage their time (Barnett and Baruch 1987).

All in all, though, women can benefit greatly from working and, not surprisingly, the more prestigious and powerful a woman's job, the greater the prostress and physical and mental health benefits. In general, the more a husband participates in the housework, the lower is the wife's level of distress and depression. Of course, nothing is ever so clear-cut when it comes to gender and stress, and this is where we can get into a double bind. Those of us with husbands who help with child care experience relief and certain benefits. At the same time, we may end up criticizing ourselves for relying on this help and then end up expressing even greater concern about how working interferes with our maternal role responsibilities. Our old "guilt button" has been pushed because we feel we're not living up to familial or societal expectations.

With chronic illness often comes the reality that we may need more help and support from our partners than we did before. If we can't learn to accept this reality and reestablish equilibrium in other ways, the guilt and loss of healing energy become overwhelming. You aren't completely at the mercy of any particular situation. The danger arises when you feel you must take on more and more and that you must handle it all by yourself. When situations are untenable, you have options such as modifying the situation, getting help, or changing your expectations of how much and how perfectly you "should" be doing everything. As you will read about later in the discussion of Chinese medicine, it is believed that imbalance signifies or underlies illness. While the Chinese may use different words (for example, "yin" and "yang"), the truth of the need for balance is the same. If you want to take care of your physical health, you must learn to listen to your body and say "no" to others—or to more work—when your body tells you to do so.

CHAPTER 4

The Mind-Body Connection

... getting well isn't the main objective. That can set you up for failure. If you set a physical goal, then you may fail, but if you make peace of mind your goal, you can achieve it ...

—Bernie Siegel, *Love, Medicine*
& Miracles

As you've read, illness and health are both psychological and physical. In fact, the division of mind and body is an artificial one imposed by those with difficulty accepting the mind-body unity. This notion of oneness is certainly not new and in fact our culture was more holistically oriented in the 1800s than it has been for most of the 1900s. During this century, most Western health experts have studied physical illness and weaknesses in isolation with little or no attention on psychosocial factors. They searched for particular germs or genes to explain the breakdown of the body while ignoring the impact of the mind. Efforts to treat physical illnesses rarely used the power of one's psychological state and mind to improve physical health and recuperation.

More and more data show that our beliefs and attitudes have an incredibly powerful effect on our physical and emotional states. Dr. Kemeny (1998) instructed Method actors to induce moods of depression, happiness, and neutrality. In those who induced negative moods, the proliferation response (central component of the body's defenses) of the immune system decreased for twenty-five minutes. It took another thirty minutes or so for their systems to return to baseline. Those told to induce a positive mood showed an increased proliferative response. Such results indicate our thoughts and feelings can change our immune system functioning. Even brief positive states increased certain immune functions. Not all reactions to negative states or negative stress represent decreased immune system functioning as negative stress increases natural killer cell activity . . . for a while. Then, as mind-body continues to be suppressed by distress, the natural killer cell activity declines. People who are depressed for a long time period show decreased proliferative responses and numbers and activity of natural killer cells.

Thoughts and hopes can affect your body more strongly than physical elements usually thought to be most important. This was clearly shown in an eighteen-year study (Thomas and Duszynski 1974) of medical students in which more than one hundred initially had high cholesterol but only fourteen eventually got coronary heart disease (CHD). How did the fourteen unfortunates differ? The answer lies largely in their psychological characteristics. Those who eventually developed CHD had, years earlier, reported higher levels of nervous tension, depression, insomnia, and anxiety than their associates. Those with cholesterol levels just as high who didn't develop CHD were calmer and had reported lower stress, anxiety, and depression.

Stress: Not Just Cause or Consequence

The recent literature on ARCs mentions the role of negative stress (distress) in their causation. It isn't known if distress could ever be the sole cause of an ARC, but there is much research linking distress with triggering or worsening many physical problems. The clients with whom I work and those I interviewed varied greatly in their realization of the potent mind-body influence of distress. As they described their lives before the illness or prior to flares or symptom recurrences, I would often be struck by the frequency or severity of their distressors. Some women don't see ties between their experiences or thought patterns and illness, while others accept distress' role in opening the door for or worsening ARC symptoms.

A New Stress Model

Stress is a good example of the mind-body process and its relation to illness, health, and ARCs. What follows is my model of the stress process, showing the reality that your mind, emotions, and behaviors directly affect the type (distress or prostress) and extent of stress you'll experience. You'll find elements that don't appear in many traditional stress models. Some stress models assume that no matter what the stressor, everybody reacts in the same physically aroused, unhealthy way.

However, there is evidence that different people experience very different types of stress responses in their bodies. One woman may be predisposed to a weak heart and may experience heart problems when exposed to distress, while another may have a vulnerable digestive system and experience gastrointestinal distress.

Another outdated notion is that any given stressor is experienced by all people in the same way; for example, that everybody is equally negatively stressed by getting a job, marrying, losing a job, or taking a vacation. In this view, change is always interpreted as a threat, and the result is the fight-or-flight response. Look again at those stressors I just listed. Do you think you would respond to getting married or losing a job in exactly the same way as would your sister, best friend, or employer? Again evidence, if not common sense, reveals this isn't true. For example, marriage for one woman might be wonderful, while another might have had strong doubts about marriage and be quite worried about this new life. People respond in unique ways to the same event, and what is negatively stressful for one person can be positively stressful and challenging—or even neutral—to somebody else. These different experiences are caused by differences in beliefs, expectations, fears, past histories, hopes, physical health, social supports, and so on. As our minds create different views, so do our bodies react differently.

Diagram 4.1   A Stress Model

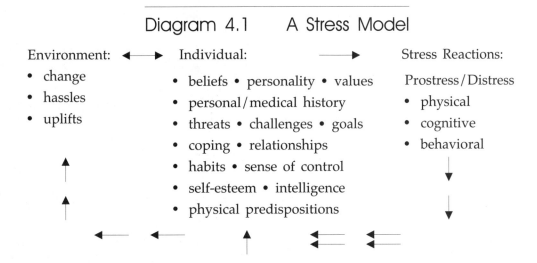

Environment: Individual: Stress Reactions:

- change
- hassles
- uplifts

- beliefs • personality • values
- personal/medical history
- threats • challenges • goals
- coping • relationships
- habits • sense of control
- self-esteem • intelligence
- physical predispositions

Prostress/Distress

- physical
- cognitive
- behavioral

Feedback Loops

As you can see, both the environment and the individual are active, causal forces in a dynamic, complex system. Let's say a potential stressor exists in the environment and may affect you, the individual (arrow from environment to individual). Your individual perceptions and thoughts impact how you see and think about this potential stressor (arrow from individual to environment), that is, whether you see this stressor as a negative stressor, a prostressor, or as relatively unimportant.

Besides being affected by your life experiences, your perceptions and thoughts are affected by your psychological and physical characteristics. The model shows that your stress reactions can 1) feed back to impact your individual coping techniques, beliefs, and habits and 2) feed all the way back to affecting your environment by determining the kinds of situations and stressors you create.

The arrows from individual and stress reactions back to the environment represent important parts of this model. Let's look at an example of the flow from individual to environment/situation. Type As are said to be competitive, irritable, rushed, intense, and time-obsessed; unhealthy Type As see situations as threats or distressors more often than others. (While none of us have Type A characteristics, let's just use this example anyway!) A colleague offers to help Ms. A on a new task, but she sees this as competitive taunting: "You can't finish the job on your own and need my help to do it," or "If I help you, I'll get credit too." (Another woman might perceive this sincere offer for what it is, accept it, and feel relief from the situation rather than more distress. In this case, the feedback arrow would go from stress reactions all the way to environment.) However, Ms. A, even though she feels she is in a stressful environment, wants approval and is intent on showing her perfect abilities. She rejects offers for help, struggles on her own, and by these actions (stress reaction), actively creates more hassles, deadlines, and pressures. The environment is even more stressful because she has alienated her peers.

The stress model also shows how you can change distressors to prostressors and use these in your mind-body self-healing. The feedback loop from stress reactions and individual to environment is seen in people who flourish through challenge. These people put themselves in myriad prostress situations, whether teaching, mountain climbing, performing, writing, or learning.

As you can see, stress isn't inherent in situations—or in you—but instead arises when you appraise things as either threatening and overwhelming or challenging and enhancing. The difference is based on beliefs about control and change, as you'll read later. In terms of chronic illness, you'll face many situations that are tricky and difficult. However, it's often your choice whether you perceive them as distressors with accompanying negative emotions and mind-body damage or as prostressors offering challenge, pride, and enhancement of mind-body health.

Taking Control

Diseases that are mostly or completely genetically or biologically attributable are among the minority. Even with these, thoughts, beliefs, and personality characteristics still have a great impact on course, severity, recovery, life, or death. Think about this: You aren't powerless in the face of your illness. You'll see that I never use the common phrase: "She is a victim of (insert your particular autoimmune disorder here)." I also steer clear of using "She suffers from (autoimmune condition 'x' or symptoms 'x, y')." These phrases are misleading and unhealthy. The word "victim" implies powerlessness, lack of control, and passivity. In addition, "suffering from" suggests a predetermined outcome offering no chance of improvement. I'm not denying that suffering is involved when you have a painful, distressing conditions. However, it doesn't do justice to sum it up as only suffering. True, there is plenty of that, but there can also be growth, happiness, and decisiveness to change your mind-body condition.

You may feel as though your body is betraying you and that you have no control over the distressing changes. While it's truth that you can't wish your illness away or take a pill to make it disappear, that's not the whole truth. You'll be learning how to reduce the severity of your symptoms, the frequency of flares, and the duration of the really bad times. Sometimes you may not be able to do this, but very rarely is life carved in stone with no chance for change. The knowledge that you have some control is liberating and cuts a huge chunk out of your frustration. You can use your thinking to look at situations as challenges rather than terrible threats; you can engage in progressive relaxation to calm your body and regain energy; you can use massage, biofeedback, and physical therapy to reduce the overwhelming pain; and you can try diet changes, vitamin supplements, and herbal remedies to strengthen your immune system and the potent energy force within you.

At the same time, please realize *I am not saying you are wholly responsible for your continued illness and that if you do not vanquish your disease, it is simply because you are lazy, weak, or a failure.* Your mind-body can go far in improving your overall health and well-being, but it won't inevitably take away your disease. You're only responsible for doing what you can to allow for mind-body healing, growth, life satisfaction, and joy.

Positivity

We know that our emotions and thoughts impact our immune system functioning, for better or for worse. Let's look at an example in which a particular type of thinking—illusions—has been found to have health-boosting consequences. Illusions can be adaptive. They allow us to cope in more effective, determined ways; they motivate us to seek our goals; and they play a part in improving our well-being and health. But illusions by themselves don't yield these beneficial changes. Margaret Kemeny (1998) found that positive attitudes predict improved immune processes only when positive expectations cause us to be more involved in our life goals. We may well be optimistic, but if we aren't engaged in our life goals and finding meaning in our lives, we aren't likely to experience any health benefits.

Those Rose-Colored Glasses Really Suit You

This is an important message for those of us with chronic illnesses. You may scoff that with all of your pain and fatigue, it's hard enough to think at all, let alone reduce the negative and go for the optimistic, positive thoughts. Then, beyond that, you're supposed to focus on determining and acting on your life goals? Am I crazy? Well, perhaps. However, the fact remains that these are the lessons we must learn if we're to cope effectively and derive any pleasure or growth from our lives. It can be done, but it's hard as hell. It takes continuous work, day after day, but periods of time will pass in which life flows more smoothly and you are feeling better. Then, the dark times may set in again.

Having meaning and belief in yourself and your life can make these darker times fewer, more brief, and certainly much smoother.

Let's look at another discussion of how your mind, body, and soul are integrated so that changing the nature of any one inevitably affects the others. Many ways of thinking have been found to be associated with slowing illness, easing the burdens, preventing sickness, and even healing against all odds. Some of these include optimism, a challenge orientation, humor, a sense of control, a belief in the meaning of one's life, and a reason to live.

Your Personal Healing Journey

Certainly, healing is a personal journey, and there are as many ways of healing as there are people. Stephen Levine (1987) has a different approach to the question of how to heal. From years of working with many hundreds of chronically ill clients, he now asks, "Where is healing to be found?" The question of where healing is to be found shifts the usual paradigm of exploring this topic. Levine describes healing as a deeper seeing of life and oneself and of the ability to let go of ancient fears, self-hatred, and self-blame. In following this journey into openness, forgiveness, and particularly acceptance of what is at present, Levine has seen some who have ended up beating the odds and living, while others unable to survive have at least faced death in a serene, peaceful, enlightened way. They reported feeling more whole and complete than ever before. Levine saw that those who were able to let go, accept themselves and their illness, and see their fears and pain with compassion actually achieved healing in their body aspect as well as their emotional aspect. Those who "surprisingly" regained their health were actually healthier than before their illness. He came to see the body's healing as coming from the newly attained balance and peace of mind and heart. As he put it, "By investigating the mind, the heart was uncovered, and its light caused so much to come to flower." This is certainly one of the most beautiful, sensitive ways of describing what, on a superficial level, is caught by the term psychoneuroimmunology.

Don't Fight Against Yourself

Of course, we're often dealing with intense physical pain that seems to cast aside our ability to be truly in touch with our emotional pain. We feel we must keep pushing and pushing, do our utmost, let our actions bellow, "See how healthy I am. I can still do this and this and this. . . ." On some level, although we try to deny it, many of us continue to blame ourselves for our illness and pain. We see these unwanted companions as our just rewards, our punishments for being bad. You may have taken up a fighting attitude, with the enemy being your illness, your body, or yourself. In fact, Levine himself talks about those who seemed to heal almost gracefully (not effortlessly) through an ability to accept their condition, think about it, explore it, and be with it. They were ". . . drawing the self-torture out of it by meeting it with tenderness and mercy—'me for me. Me with my pain, with my illness.' It was those who were against themselves [who had the] hardest time and the slowest healing, if healing was present at all" (8–9). These are important words to recall as you think about yourself, your condition, how you view what is happening in your life. Beating your illness in the sense of accepting the challenge offered to your mind-body can be positive; beating down your illness while seeing yourself and your mind-body as bad and sick is not. Jot down Levine's words in your journal as you continue to read through this book. They are words of strength and hope and will help you on this journey.

Pitfalls to Avoid

Now, for the pessimist's half of the cup . . . learning that you can have some control over your physical symptoms, your responses to them, and your life overall can also cause fear and havoc within you. In fact, Caroline Myss, author of *Why People Don't Heal and How They Can* (1997), describes healing as one of the most frightening journeys you can undertake. One of the issues that frequently comes up with my clients is that change can be incredibly scary, depending upon how a person has chosen to use her mind to interpret and act upon it. If you see change as a threat or a negative stressor, then it's only a natural step to avoidance behavior. If, on the other hand, you use your mind to perceive change as a challenge and an opportunity for growth, the situation can provide many mind-body benefits. The fact that new knowledge or new abilities can be perceived as threats might not make immediate sense to you, until you consider that they are likely to change the status quo that your illness has helped to create and maintain. What might initially seem confusing becomes clear when we consider that people can certainly derive benefits from being ill.

Right now, let's take a brief pause. Breathe deeply and slowly, and get in touch with what you're feeling. If you find yourself getting angry or displeased at this point during your reading, it's likely you feel one of your most sensitive buttons being pushed; that is, the one that has been primed by all those skeptics and their mantras: "It's all in your head" or "You're just hysterical, faking, etc." Remember that I'm on your side here and I am *not* saying these accusations are true. If you find it hard to see any benefits from your illness(es)—and this wouldn't be surprising given all of the intense pain and distress—try projecting the role onto somebody else you know, or even a stranger. Try to imagine what reasons they might have for not letting go of the "sick" role.

Let's look at several reasons presented by Caroline Myss. She explains that some people actually get a feeling of physical safety from illness because it gives them the feeling that they can slow down the speed of their lives. Illness accomplishes another goal in that it serves as an excuse or a diversion from truly looking within. For some, illness can be used for this type of avoidance. Women are generally taught to put others' needs, goals, and interests before their own. For many, this allows for the continued avoidance of personal issues that eventually, had they been addressed and changed, would have played an important role in maintaining the flow of healing energy. Myss also suggests a third benefit: the attention and care received during illness.

I've also seen illness work in other ways, including: as a way to get strong dependency needs met; as a tool for avoiding responsibility for important tasks and responsibilities; as a method to avoid developing a strong sense of self or of one's needs, desires, goals or life direction; as a way to forget intense fears or put them into the background; as an emulation of or angry reaction to the behavior of a role model who was chronically ill; and as a way to derive benefits such as financial support, avoidance of trial for illegal behavior, and the like. Please remember that this doesn't mean I think you're faking your illness or even that any of these issues pertain to you. However, in my own personal journey and as an assistant to many other women with health concerns on their journeys, I've found that answering these questions truthfully can allow the destruction of such internal blockages, if present, and thus opens the door to true mind-body healing.

Having Control Doesn't Mean It's Your Fault

After learning of the power and control we can have over certain aspects of illness and recovery, some of us misinterpret this to mean that we've somehow caused our illness. We may even find that others blame us. This is nonsense. While the mind is powerful in healing, and negative stress sometimes plays a role in weakening the body's defenses, there is no evidence that our thoughts or personality can cause biologically-based illnesses, such as autoimmune-related conditions. Negative beliefs, hostility, depression, and other personal characteristics cannot go back in time to determine your genetic predisposition!

While your mind is a vital component of your overall approach to recovery, this isn't the same as saying that all you have to do is think optimistically enough and visualize enough and then you'll be cured.

Building on Prostress

Let's examine how you can modify your ways of thinking and your perceptions so that you can use stress to enhance your mind-body health. Prostress is the growth-promoting stress you want and need in your life. It comes from challenging situations that stimulate positive development. If you feel helpless and out of control in a situation, you'll experience distress. If you believe you can have some control over the situation, you're more likely to experience prostress, the positive psychological state you experience when you perceive a situation as potentially pleasurable and as offering positive consequences, growth, or challenge.

While there is a huge amount of information on the problems caused by stress, there is relatively little on positive stress, positive emotions, and health. In Mihaly Csikszentmihalyi's 1990 book, *Flow: The Psychology of Optimal Experience*, he describes a state similar to prostress that he calls "flow." You may have heard the phrase "being in the zone." These words describe prostress situations in which one experiences challenge, control, skill, and optimal stimulation. These states include a sense of timelessness, accomplishment, joy, and a fading of self-consciousness. Prostress can be associated with activities ranging from work to simple sensual pleasures and play. Artists and athletes alike talk about finding themselves in the zone, at one with the activity, experiencing both calm and arousal. Prostress and distress also differ in that prostress occurs within the stress range in which you feel energizing, pleasurable activation, while distress occurs when there is either too little or too much stress-induced activation. The latter kind of distress, arising from too much arousal, is what most of us think of as stress. Take a minute, though, to recall a situation, maybe another one of those endless waits in the doctor's waiting room, in which you were incredibly bored and had no stimulation. This *lack of arousal* also leads to distress; in the case of the waiting room, you might have become fidgety (trying to increase stimulation), tense, and irritable.

Just as the frequency of negative stress (hassles) influences the amount of harm, the frequency of prostress is central in your mind-body healing. A study of people told to record their moods and levels of happiness at several points throughout the day for six weeks showed that the *frequency* of feeling fairly good, rather than having a few highly intense periods of feeling good, was most important in determining positive mood and happiness (Larsen, Diener, and Cropanzano 1987). The small, frequent pleasures do two important things: They decrease the impact of negative stress *and* contribute to your experience of prostress and happiness. The mere *absence* of enough prostress is associated with mind-body distress and lesser satisfaction with one's life. It might surprise you that the lack of prostress in life can be more strongly related to low life satisfaction than the presence of negative stress in life!

Physical Consequences of Prostress

Unlike negative stress, some of the physical responses of prostress can actually improve your health. After experiencing a prostressor, your immune system actually demonstrates improved functioning. This helps explain why people who develop a minor illness, such as the flu or a cold, often report experiencing an increase in distressors and/or a decrease in prostressors just before getting sick.

How does prostress improve health? While many questions are still unanswered, Jeffrey Edwards and Cary Cooper proposed in 1988 that prostress increases the production of anabolic hormones and HDL—"good"—cholesterol, and also leads to other health-inducing biochemical changes. For example, during prostress, your body experiences a shift in the balance of hormones that can lead to physiological growth, and the epinephrine elevations, which return more rapidly to baseline levels, can protect heart and other muscle tissue.

Deepak Chopra, the well-known doctor who unites the Eastern and Western traditions in his approach to preventing and treating illness, agrees that different emotional states produce different effects on mind and body (Chopra 1993). Love, hate, and excitement activate the body in different directions. We shouldn't scoff at the cliché that laughter is the best medicine. While you're laughing, your body is obviously in an aroused state. Afterward, however, there is an overall healthy net decrease in your body's arousal and blood pressure. The positive state of mind associated with laughing positively affects your immune system by decreasing certain neuroendocrine hormones and stimulating killer cells that prevent and combat disease. Laughter exercises your lungs, relaxes your diaphragm, increases oxygen in your bloodstream, boosts your mood, increases relaxation for more than half an hour . . . and it's cheap! You can't truly laugh and enjoy yourself while feeling anxious and distressed.

Psychological Consequences of Prostress.

Another vitally important way in which prostress contributes to your mind-body health is through increasing your satisfaction and pleasure with life and with social interactions. This then motivates you to maintain or develop your social support circle. Having a strong social support system is touted as a great distress reducer and can be among the most potent of "medications"! Even if we really don't have such a good network, the mere fact that we *believe* we do reduces the negative effects of stress—another example of the amorphous distinction between the mind and body. Most people would classify social ties and their benefits, such as social support, attention, affection, purpose, and responsibility, solidly within the purview of the psychological or of the "mind." However, we see here that this is an artificial distinction because this person-characteristic directly affects the functioning of the systems of the "body." They are linked and share a common currency of energy, neurotransmitters, and neurochemicals in activating the circular system—with no clear beginning or ending. Prostress also reverses the impact of negative stress, reduces depression and anxiety, and improves your ability to cope with stress.

Recall that one of the most important characteristics determining if you'll perceive an event as threatening or challenging is the degree of control you *believe* you have over it. True prostress benefits arise in situations when you feel active, involved, and in control. John Reich and Alex Zautra (1981) pointed out this dynamic beautifully when they compared people engaging in two different types of pleasurable activities: *positive origin events*, in which the person was actively involved in carrying out the pleasant event, and *positive pawn events*, in which the person was only a passive recipient to a positive situation. An example of a positive origin event might be going out and making a new friend or learning a new sport. A positive pawn event might be finding ten dollars on the ground. Those who experienced the positive origin events reported better life quality and rated the events as more pleasurable than those who experienced positive passive events. *In fact, increasing the number of events that were pleasurable and positive, but also passive, did not increase happiness or satisfaction.* As expected, negative events were associated with lower quality of life and with psychological distress.

In order to progress toward healing and growth, you must learn to live life in a more positive, health-enhancing, and enjoyable way every day. Focus on each day—each moment—to derive the greatest possible enjoyment and to avoid the harmful consequences that arise when you continuously look forward, anticipate generally negative events, and ruminate negatively on how your illness will restrict you throughout your life.

Coping: Stacking the Deck in Your Favor

If you've recently developed a chronic illness, coping with your condition and the potentially chronic pain, is unlike anything you've had to do before. There is no way to completely prepare yourself in advance, to avoid the emotional roller coaster, the swings from hope to hopelessness, the comfort of support slipping into the fear of abandonment, the lulling security of feeling like "before" followed by the shock, yet again, of your changed life, and the feelings of grief and loss you must inevitably confront. To move on with your life in a healthy way, you must go *through* these painful feelings and experiences. You'll have little control over their existence and the fact that if you're to live a tolerable, healthy life, you have to accept them. In actuality, you will have the greatest choice of all in terms of your future and your healing. As my client Anita put it, "I was always so healthy. Then, bit by bit, things started going wrong. My body started betraying me. I just attributed it to age but I couldn't hide anymore behind my image of superwoman. My house of cards started to come crashing down."

Find the Middle Ground

You can do some things to stack the cards in your favor. You may no longer be able to ride on the wave of nervous energy and negative stress to function like a "superwoman." In fact, this is one of the worst things you can do. The other is to give up completely. While accepting the reality of your illness and integrating it into your life are essential, they aren't equated with becoming passive or feeling helpless. There are aspects of your illness and health over which you can definitely exert control. How you choose to cope with your diagnosis and your condition directly impacts how you will experience your illness, whether for better or for worse.

Recall that in order to cope most effectively with your condition, you should strive to learn about and understand it, because this knowledge allows you to more easily accept the changes and develop new expectations. This reduces the negative stress you experience when you're unclear as to what is due to your illness and what is due (in your mind) to potential "laziness" or "giving up." Understanding that your limitations and new lifestyles are "normal" in the world of your particular illness lets you stand back and be easier on yourself. Instead, you develop new strengths and find new ways of thinking and being. The last thing you need is to be your harshest critic and own worst enemy. Instead, you must have tremendous faith in yourself and motivate yourself to move forward (albeit sometimes two steps forward and one step back) on your challenging journey. Don't give up; this worsens your mind-body health and contradicts healing.

Banish Hopelessness and Helplessness

By seeking to understand as much as possible about your disease, you're also removing two powerful elements that feed negative stress: hopelessness and helplessness. By learning, researching, and discovering, you're asserting control at a time and in a situation when it's easy to feel as though you've lost control. If you think you have no control, you'll see things as threats, not challenges. This triggers the fight-or-flight response, and the vicious cycle of negative stress commences. While you're ill, there is nothing more harmful to you and your immune system than squandering your mind-body energy on an automatic response that gets you nowhere. On the other hand, sensing control boosts optimism and self-esteem, both of which increase your energy and positive healing forces. These dynamics were clearly evident in the life of one of my clients, Roberta.

For years, Roberta had avoided dealing with her type I diabetes. She didn't educate herself about her illness and simply attributed all of her difficulties and frustrations in life to it. She constantly felt hopeless and helpless, but did nothing about it because in her mind she was powerless to do anything about anything. She certainly didn't follow the SAID path described in chapter 3 (Stop, Accept, Identify, Determine).

She never let go of the word "wrong," because she continued to see herself as a broken or injured person, odd, unable to do the things "normal" people do. As the cognitive behavioral model would predict, her thoughts led to a self-fulfilling prophecy. She never tried to achieve much of anything in her life. Deep in denial, she ignored doctors' warnings about eating unhealthily and not exercising. She had no meaning or purpose in her life, which was probably the most negative element of all. It took a crisis, like it all too frequently does, to force her to stop living in the land of denial. Her cousin, who also had type I diabetes, and who had participated in many escapades of gorging at the ice cream parlor, pizza parlor, and drive-thrus and watching TV endlessly, began to develop side effects of the condition. Before long, she had a heart attack and died.

Roberta tried to live her life as before, but she could no longer keep her worries at bay. Now when she did something not in her best interest, she experienced intense anxiety and paralyzing fear. Finally she agreed to therapy. I had agreed to see her in her house initially because of her paralyzing anxiety. To start, we went back in time while she relived many of her difficult times. Her emotions surfaced and she had to deal with them as never before. Through time, we began leaving her house for brief periods. It took a while to get through the "S" and "A" phases. Her progress sped up as she found that proper nutrition, moderate exercise, herbs, and meditation paid back quickly in increased energy and self-esteem. She realized she did have control over some things in her life, and this belief began to spread to more of her behaviors and different situations. She zoomed through the "I" and "D" phases and came to my office, breezing in, laughingly informing me of her plans to return to school and accept a part-time job in a hospital. These days when she cried, it was in relief and utter joy about her life and how she had turned it around. She planned to go into health care to return the gift of what she had learned. Eventually, she wrote a book on self-care for diabetes. When I opened the book she'd sent to me, it was I who became teary-eyed reading the dedication to her cousin who simply hadn't had a second chance.

Exercise: Your Coping Style

The following coping inventory will give you a clearer picture of just how it is that you tend to cope with difficult situations. Once you're armed with this information, you'll be able to focus on your reactions, their relative benefits or drawbacks, and how you may benefit from modifying them. The stressors listed below differ in terms of severity and duration. Write your honest answers in your SHOC journal without censoring yourself.

1. You had a tentative date to go out with a friend tonight and she hasn't called, although she said she would.

2. You feel very tired but are surrounded by friends who are anxious to stay out.

3. Your boss asks you to do a little project—which you're sure isn't so little—and you're quite busy already.

4. You hear about yet another medicine that might help you. What do you do?

5. You're supposed to go out with a friend who is looking forward to the evening, but you had a very long day and know you're at your limit.

6. You've had to call in sick or arrive late again (to a meeting or work appointment).

7. You have a "friend" whose actions show she doesn't believe you have an illness.

8. You've been asked to dinner with a group of friends at someone's house. This person's cooking is renowned for its taste as well as its sugar and fat.

9. You're waiting once again for at least an hour at your doctor's office.

10. Your doctor gives you about ten minutes and doesn't listen much.

11. You're experiencing great pain and your doctor frowns on pain medication, often talking about it as a weakness or as drug-seeking behavior.

12. Your partner is going out again with his/her friends, and you're feeling a bit tired and wish she/he would stay home for a change and cuddle and relax with you.

13. If you fear losing your partner or friends because of your illness, how often do you express these feelings to them?

14. You've been seeing a psychologist who you feel isn't helping you very much.

15. Your insurance cuts you off from helpful physical therapy after four visits.

16. Your attorney, case manager, or other "service professional" never returns your calls.

Do you actually push yourself forward to get involved, adapt, and make changes in potentially stressful situations? Or are you someone who prefers to avoid conflict, change, and potential stress? Do you hold in your feelings rather than expressing them, possibly hoping that they'll just go away? Do you also tend to avoid difficult situations by shutting down and letting others take control of your decisions and your life? Or, like many women, have you been taught to avoid conflict and give the pretense that all is well, while holding your pain inside or backstabbing to express your anger indirectly and thus "safely"?

It's important that you think about these questions before going on with your reading. You need to know yourself very well, because how you cope directly and indirectly affects your illness, its severity and progression, your physical and emotional health, and whether you will be one who merely survives (I'm not knocking this in and of itself!) or thrives! Those of us who actively pursue information about our illness, follow guidelines provided by health caretakers, search for alternatives, and make necessary changes in our thoughts and behavior tend to fare the best. Remember though: Extremes deviate from balance and are rarely healthy. Approach your situation openly, at your pace, and with love for yourself in your heart. This is one way to ensure you're doing the best you can.

One effective coping technique to address your traditionally distressful and anxiety-producing situations is to practice going through them in your mind. This is a safe place where you won't be at risk of experiencing the array of dreaded consequences (generally unrealistic) that you've conjured up. In chapter 14, you'll be reading about imagery and relaxation. Relaxation and anxiety are opposing reactions; when you're relaxed, you can't experience negative stress. Combining images of what it is that you fear together with the relaxation response also reduces anxiety. Recall the power of your mind and how it directly creates your experienced reality. In many situations, you can design the reality you desire, and through practice, your mind-body will follow through, thus realizing a positive self-fulfilling prophecy.

Coping as a Science?

Different types of coping are best for different types of situations. This secret is essential for those of us with chronic illnesses. For years it has been debated whether men or women cope better. Many have claimed that men are better copers because they seem to use "problem-solving" coping more frequently than women. It is true that this type of coping is healthier in certain situations than being passive. For example, when the issue is one over which you may have some control, when it's in your best interest to educate yourself prior to making a decision, and when specific actions are likelier to solve the problems than others, then a direct problem-solving approach is best. It was also assumed that while men used problem solving, women used less effective, even harmful, emotion-focused coping. This was thought to be a manifestation of women's greater emotionality, lack of strength, and tendency toward avoidance. However, more recent studies have been fruitful in changing such notions.

In studying the very types of stressors and problems women experience compared to men, it appears we're really not less effective copers. This is because women's stressors more often include coping with social interactions and illness or death of those close to them. Men more often report such stressors as financial losses or difficulties and other more tangible happenings. What does this mean? When dealing with the very stressors women more often experience, emotion-focused coping may indeed be most effective. When dealing with stressors men most often face, problem-solving approaches are maximal. Perhaps both sexes use what is most effective for their most typical experiences. Of course, this is a generalization, and some women may use more problem solving than emotion-focused coping and some men may use more emotion-focused coping. So, with respect to chronic illness, consider which of the above characteristics fit the situation. Flexibility in using different coping styles is the healthiest way to move toward mind-body healing.

What Am I Thinking?

On multiple occasions, I've had chronically ill clients tell me with great confusion that one of their health caretakers ordered them to stay off of their feet and "do nothing" while another urged that they "do as much as they can" in exercising. What should they do? The key lies, again, in striving for balance and being mindful of your body. At times, your body will need and demand rest and recovery, perhaps even at a time "inconvenient" for you as you have errands you "must" do or a social event you "have" to attend. On the other hand, you may just not feel like getting your mild or moderate exercise. Is there a TV show you really "have" to watch or a book you "must" finish now? You may realize it would be good for you to get exercise, but you tell yourself that you can always get exercise and the TV show is only on once. Do you recognize this pattern of irrational thinking and tuning out your body's needs to gratify your immediate desires? It's okay to kick back and relax, but it's not in your best interest to ignore your body's needs, particularly when it's a repetitive, long-term pattern. For many, this pattern is one of multiple triggers contributing to illness. As discussed earlier, frequent negative stress, lifestyle, and certain personality characteristics are associated with autoimmune-related conditions. Your irrational, extreme thinking can cause you to do too much exercise or activities, pushing yourself and your body well beyond the point that is healthy for your condition. It can also push aside rational thoughts, allowing you to rationalize a decision to avoid exercise or activities your mind-body desperately needs to counter the stress, pain, and damage of your condition. Whether it's too much activity or too little, the underlying problem is an abdication of control over rational, health-promoting thinking and a refusal to listen to the messages regarding your needs. If you want to optimize your mind-body health while living with an autoimmune condition, you must shift this pattern 180 degrees.

A Few More Words for the Warrior

When you truly grasp the concept of mind-body and realize how much control you have over your response to your illness and thus the course of the illness, you'll feel a liberation and power replacing the feelings of helplessness and passivity. Many empirical studies show that there are both healthy and unhealthy responses to receiving a diagnosis. Those who respond with hope, optimism, and decisions to pursue interests, hobbies, and things they had "always wanted to do but never had time for" are likely to experience less pain, distress, and severity of illness. At the least, they improve their ability to enjoy the life they're leading and to adapt to decreasing mobility, energy, and cognitive functions like memory or concentration. Patients who respond with despair, hopelessness, and other negative reactions interfere with their body's self-healing efforts and certainly with their chances of feeling happiness or joy. Norman Cousins, in *Healers on Healing* (1989), observed that people who respond to their diagnosis with great emotional distress increase the chance of a rapid advance of the disease state. Our expectations about treatment outcomes and our futures are a self-fulfilling prophecy.

We've all had experiences with this dynamic in everyday situations. For example, if you were given a chance to make an important presentation at your job and you were obsessed with failing, letting it slip that you aren't perfect, and other negative, irrational beliefs, you probably wouldn't perform as well as if you'd had positive expectations. How is this relevant to you as you work to grow and combat your illness? In *Getting Well Again*, Carl Simonton, Stephanie Matthews-Simonton, and James Creighton (1978) write of a study directly relevant to your situation. The power of expectancies and thoughts was revealed in a study that rated patients' attitudes toward treatment and their actual responses to treatment. Patients with positive attitudes responded more favorably to treatment than did those with negative attitudes. Out of 152 patients, only two with negative attitudes responded positively to treatment. A positive attitude toward treatment was an even better predictor of response to treatment than was the severity of the disease!

You'll learn many ways to empower yourself in your particular autoimmune condition. The true goal is to help you use your illness and pain to make positive changes in your life, to learn, and to grow. Sound impossible? I wouldn't be surprised to hear a resounding "Yes!" The case studies of women with illnesses like yours will show you that while it's difficult, it isn't impossible. I love the way Bernie Siegel (1989) presents this: ". . . out of pain new love and true healing can occur. One must learn to use one's pain for personal transformation, or longevity will be no gift. The path is difficult but it will lead to moments of great beauty" (3). Remember the discussion of female longevity in chapter 1? Longevity, in and of itself, is not necessarily good or desirable. It can be a painful and horrible thing, depending on your responses to your mind-body health and how you decide to live your life. I hope this book helps you enjoy longevity as the gift it can be. Take a look at what this extra time can mean. Greater longevity gives you more time to spend with your partner or beloved friends, watch your children and grandchildren grow into adults, read more books, learn new hobbies, snuggle in bed with the wind and rain pounding mightily, watch another evanescent sunset, and teach others even a tiny bit of your vast store of knowledge gleaned through tears and laughter. Notice that these experiences don't require unrestricted mobility or tremendous strength. You may have a chronic illness but, if you choose, you can live fully and joyfully. You need not struggle to live meaningfully despite your illness; if you're open, you can learn to live meaningfully because of it.

Maria's Story

I can't help thinking about Maria, a woman referred to me after she received a diagnosis of a serious autoimmune disease, multiple sclerosis. She couldn't accept this diagnosis, and she frustrated her doctors by repeatedly asking them to retest. Her doctors felt she was in for a fall given her "denial" of the diagnosis. Initially, she viewed me with mistrust, as just another doctor trying to "force" her to believe she had this "idiotic sounding disease, multiples le roses." (English not being her first language, Maria wondered how such beautiful words [referring to many roses] could refer to sickness.) I spent much of our initial time together listening to her speak about herself, her children and grandchildren, her move to the U.S., and the two jobs she worked to send money to Peru for the rest of her family.

Slowly, she admitted to increasing fatigue, but she was relentless in her dream to help the rest of her family move here. Perhaps because I listened more than I spoke, she began to trust me. I confirmed what the doctors had told her about her disease but didn't offer her a fixed timeline. I continued to talk with her about her goals and confirmed that her faith in reaching them was among the strongest of "medicines." She agreed to combine Western medical treatment with her home remedies, but her body weakened, her reflexes slowed, and walking became difficult. She finally accepted her illness but continued our weekly visits, always talking up a storm, telling me how much money she'd made that week, and how someday she'd see her family reunited. One week she came in slowly, looking aged and weak. I remember thinking, "No, no! She can't look this sick." I was shocked and saddened by this change and asked if anything unpleasant had happened. Her family in Peru learned of her condition and demanded she stop working her remaining job. This was a powerful blow to her, the hub of the family, the one that would make everything all right again. She felt betrayed by the family, because she took their caring words to mean they'd lost faith in her and her dream. I began to play devil's advocate, knowing her tendency to fight against any hint that her ultimate goal might not be reached. She bolted upright in her chair and her cheeks regained their color. She looked deep into my eyes and yelled at me, telling me I was no better than those other doctors who'd tried to kill her months ago. She fled, but I wondered if that had been a fleeting smile on her face.

Five months later, I heard a great deal of whispering, giggling, and shushing outside my office door. A sharp knocking echoed through the room as I called for the visitors to enter. In came about seven children, ranging from age one to age ten, followed by six adults. I sat confused until in leapt Maria, with a big smile on her face and an unrestrained laugh. She introduced me to everybody as the doctor who'd gotten her so angry I'd cured her. But I know I hadn't had anything to do with the apparent remission of her symptoms. She'd had such a potent dream and goal, such a strong guiding meaning in her life, that when the possibility entered her mind that she might not attain this, she rebelled and removed its power by the incredible force of her mind. She refused to become sicker, because she had too many important things left to do. She did tell me that now she could relax and rest if the symptoms reappeared. She would accept some limitations, but would keep her energy up, especially since her children and grandchildren had learned some bad habits when she wasn't around. She had a lot of work to do to get them back on track. This might take years.

CHAPTER 5

Weighty Words: The Power of the Diagnosis

Don't deny the diagnosis. Try to defy the verdict.

—Norman Cousins, *Head First*

First, let's go over some technical aspects of medical assessment and treatment. It's important to understand "medispeak" and what your doctor is or should be doing. And it's empowering to learn what tools you can use to gain control over your mind-body responses to your illness, and thus to improve your overall well-being. You'll also learn about the processes of illness, mind-body responses to autoimmune-related conditions, effective integration of Eastern and Western techniques and tools, and general mind-body dynamics—all of which you'll use to maximize your ability to beat the odds against your condition. You can't take over the role of your health care professional, but you can learn enough to ensure you're getting the best treatment and to do your part of the healing.

Talk It Through

Much of the information you give your SHOC members will come in the form of historical data and facts about your life and present symptoms. This includes data about your symptom onset; the nature, severity, and frequency of your symptoms; possibly related changes in your body, functioning, or mind; your past history of illnesses; and the physical history of your family members dating back several generations. The best doctors, who understand the inextricability of mind-body functioning, health, and illness, will also ask questions about your emotional health, recent or long-term stressors or changes, your upbringing as a child, the nature of your home life, and your relationships with the central figures in your childhood. A cue to the quality of your caretaker is the thoroughness of this information-gathering process.

Getting Physical

Secondly, the health professional will perform a physical examination. Here you'll also learn much about this person. If all you get is a cold blood pressure cuff, a quick, perfunctory touch here and there, and a "cough and breathe in deeply," you may be satisfying the doctor's tight schedule or his need to watch expenses, but you aren't being treated ethically or in a caring, professional manner. If you have an autoimmune condition, you truly need a thorough examination. Once you have upheld your half of the responsibilities by presenting a thorough reporting of your health history, thoughts, current symptoms, and pain, you should expect a comprehensive exam in which the doctor examines your ears, eyes, nose, throat, and skin; tests your reflexes, coordination, stability, and muscular strength; feels glands such as lymph glands for any swelling; manipulates joints and appendages; measures blood pressure, heart rate, and temperature; and assesses regions and severity of pain. The doctor may be puzzled and unsure as to a diagnosis, particularly if the typical symptoms and signs for your disorder aren't clear. He may first give you the names of several conditions in the form of a differential diagnosis.

Time for Tests

The third step of the diagnostic process is the ordering of tests to help rule out various initial diagnoses. Most of you are probably familiar with the kinds of tests performed by Western doctors, such as X-rays, blood tests, urine tests, cultures, and biopsies. Doctors now have use of powerful instruments such as the noninvasive MRI (magnetic resonance imaging), which uses magnets to yield images of different areas in the body. Fortunately, MRIs can detect certain conditions substantially earlier than X-rays. The difficulty with using these tests to diagnose autoimmune conditions is that you may not yet have the signs for which your doctor has been trained to look. This can perpetuate the "It's all in your head" cycle. It's essential you find a health care professional who is knowledgeable enough to realize this fact and who will perform the tests at the appropriate time (or repeatedly). The doctor should also use other methods, including her or his experience, and should listen to and believe your thoughts and reports of your symptoms.

Getting the Comprehensive Data You Need

The three steps discussed above certainly have their place in diagnosis and must not be left out or ignored. By themselves though, they may be limiting. Recall the importance of your role in actively ensuring that you are obtaining comprehensive services that integrate conventional and alternative methods. Many health professionals still focus exclusively on the medical model, meaning, "Let's look for a physical cause for the onset and continuation of this physical disease." However, as a psychologist who embraces the mind-body perspective, I see the need for a more comprehensive evaluation as just one entry point into a truer way of seeing the person. Traditional Chinese medicine is a good example of an alternative method.

Traditional Chinese Medicine (TCM) Assessment

Some of you may not have experienced this type of assessment and treatment. It's just as important to find the most highly qualified practitioners when it comes to supplementary techniques as it is with conventional treatments. A list of referral sources for alternative treatment methods can be found at the end of the book. Contact these resources to learn more about the requirements, such as licensing or certification. These sources may have referral lists to put you in touch with qualified practitioners in your area. You might ask your physician whether she or he has any links to alternative medicine practitioners. Often you won't find much through this approach. If you have any friends experienced with alternative health techniques, ask them for qualified referrals. Word of mouth is extremely valuable.

We'll use acupuncture as the example. Your first visit includes an assessment phase, just as with your physician. Your physician may hastily take your pulse, but in TCM this is a vital source of comprehensive information. At times, pulse taking will last a few minutes, whereas at other times it might take two hours. An acupuncturist uses three fingers in the exam and makes contact with one wrist at a time. She'll be focusing on the nine pulses—three superficial, three medium, and three deep. Pulses are described in often poetic ways indicating sharpness, softness, and other conditions. The acupuncturist knows many internal and external events affect your pulse at any one time. Some of these are temperature and climate, the pressure, one's gender, and in women, her menstrual cycle phase.

All the information gathered is considered in the typical holistic way so that the acupuncturist gains an idea about the client's qi, or life energy. This indicates the patterns that underlie and are part of the illness, and the nature of the client's illness and symptoms. Your tongue also offers information about your problem and your imbalance of yin and yang. Remember that your body's sympathetic nervous system is activated during the stress response, while the parasympathetic branch calms and returns the body to balance once the threat is over. TCM sees these activating and soothing elements as yin and yang. I recall visiting a very experienced acupuncturist who took one look at my tongue and accurately listed my symptoms (without my having said a word), as well as the nature of my particular imbalance between yin and yang. Imbalance is considered to underlie poor health, which is why it's important to pursue balance not only within your body but also in all of your relationships and among all elements of your life. After these assessment steps, and based on the acupuncturist's knowledge of meridians and acupuncture points, he will commence treatment.

Exercise: Your Self-Evaluation

The following are some questions that are essential to add to those focusing solely on symptoms, pain, bodily systems, and so on. *Right now, take the time to answer these questions.* It may be some time since you received your diagnosis, but given the highly complex and yet malleable personality-illness relationship, you may learn things about yourself to use to improve the current nature of your condition.

- What are your current sources of social support?

- Are you in an intimate relationship and, if so, how healthy is this relationship?

- How would you describe yourself? What are your strengths and areas needing improvement?

- What are your goals and dreams? What are your plans to achieve these?

- What was your family life like? What was your role in the family? (Were you babied, made to be the adult, teased, pressured to achieve, etc.) How was emotional expression looked upon? How was illness treated or talked about?

- What was the emotional and physical health of your primary caretakers and family; do any physical or emotional disturbances run in your family? Any addictions, be they to prescription or recreational drugs, alcohol, food, attention, shopping, sex, or power and control?

- Did you experience any physical, sexual, verbal, or emotional abuse as a child?

- What values or elements were emphasized by your family of origin?

- How is your relationship with your family of origin these days?

- What are the similarities and differences between your current family and your friendships and intimate relationships (healthy and unhealthy)?

- Do you work? Do you enjoy this work? How much control do you have in your job?

- Describe yourself as would one or two of your closest, truest friends.

- How happy/satisfied are you with your life to date?

- What was your life like before the illness in the sense of rapidity of pace, ability to relax vs. the need to do more and more in less and less time (being vs. doing), achievement strivings, healthy or unhealthy lifestyle?

- As a woman, what has been your role in the family, workplace, elsewhere (disciplinarian, caretaker, etc.)? Do you get enough help from your partner or spouse? Do you feel conflict when you rely on her/him for assistance?

- How would you rate yourself (high; average; low) in the following areas?: being in touch with your emotions; being able to express them, whether they're negative or positive; assertiveness; communication skills; self-worth.

- Finish the sentence: My illness lets me/gives me _____.

Consider your answers together with what you have read about health-inducing personality characteristics and behavior. Do you have many of these? Which don't you have? Which do you want to develop?

The Emotional Aftermath of the Diagnosis

We wait and wait and wait for the decisions and pronouncements to come from the holder of our fate that particular week. The prolonged stream of doctors most women with ARCs see prior to obtaining an accurate diagnosis is truly disheartening. What is such an announcement that we spend thousands of dollars for it, often ignore our own rational thoughts to accept it, and perhaps even surrender to it as though it came from a deity? A simple enough word—diagnosis—yet this weighty pronouncement can elicit varied responses based on our history of and knowledge about our condition, previous (mis)diagnoses or demeaning treatment, depth of pain and illness, spirituality, drive to meaning, degree of hope or hopelessness, presence or absence of goals, and our personality characteristics.

When the words do come, the *way* in which they come is incredibly important. There is never a reason for a doctor to deliver the words in a coldly professional way with no offering of hope or care. The extent to which a doctor's manner and delivery of the news can trigger either a decision to fight and maintain hope or a conscious or subconscious decision to give up and let the illness take over is truly incredible. Why is the arrival of the usually so long-awaited diagnosis so powerful? Because it's at this point that you get some validation and are forced or allow yourself to begin making efforts to cope with the reality of your situation. Confusion reigns, and you may be completely baffled about what is happening to your body. You may attempt to deny anything is wrong at all. This lets you minimize the reality of what you may be facing.

Getting It Off Your Chest

Once a diagnosis is made, the relief can be great. This might sound counter-intuitive, as ARCs are often chronic and debilitating. However, at last "it" has a name and you can start taking steps to deal with the illness. I've talked to some patients who, once they've gotten the "label," have taken the time to revisit on paper those many doctors who'd been disbelieving and unsupportive during the painful, extended period of searching for help. For example: "Remember me? I was the one you examined for about five minutes and said nothing was wrong with. You added that just to relieve my anxiety, you would refer me for some testing. When it came back with some deviations but nothing 'major,' you made sure to tell me this was what you'd expected and that I should stop worrying and get more involved in my life and family." Whether or not you actually send a letter, this is a healthy assignment. Try it!

While women often feel guilty, because anger and being opinionated aren't "female" responses, they need not. Anger is an appropriate feeling when one's rights have been violated. In their dismissive attitudes toward female clients or in their reluctance to address certain ailments, many doctors have violated the rights of women as human beings as well as their Hippocratic oaths. Again, recall that there will always be doctors who care intensely about their clients, male and female, and do their utmost to provide the highest quality care possible.

Many Ways to Cope

On the one hand, getting the diagnosis can be liberating and validating. On the other hand, it can be the start of your most difficult period. Each person reacts differently to a diagnosis of something so complex, little understood, and seemingly unnatural as an autoimmune disorder. Nancy Mairs, in her wonderful book, *Waist-High in the World* (1996), describes her particular views on being diagnosed with MS:

> And so, with this diagnosis, what had begun as an uphill struggle turned into a long slow slide downward, actually as well as metaphorically. People disabled traumatically—say, by a spinal cord injury sustained in an auto accident—have told me that they have an advantage because they know the worst from the outset, and any change can only be for the better. Others, congenitally disabled, claim that theirs is the easier lot because, never having known another way of being, they find their lives completely natural. I myself would contend that slow degeneration beginning in adulthood offers one time to grow incrementally into each loss and so more easily retain a modicum of composure throughout the process ... I persist in feeling grateful both that I lived nearly thirty years in the obliviousness of "normalcy" and that I've had

more than two decades to descend step by step (and then lurch by lurch) to the level where I live now. (28–29)

Mairs shows us the indomitable spirit people can have in the face of difficult challenges. She strives throughout her book to find the positives and gives thanks for the wisdom she has learned. Yet, she does a service by remaining honest and clearly communicating the incredible pain such crippling illnesses can cause. She doesn't hide the anguish she has felt from having to trace her course, full of losses and pain.

How Do You Deal with It?

Various models have been proposed for individuals experiencing such loss and change. You may be familiar with the progression proposed by Elisabeth Kubler-Ross when she discusses death or any great loss in her 1969 book, *On Death and Dying*.

The Health and Harm of Denial

Denial is a typical response to being diagnosed with a chronic disease. It's your psyche's way of protecting you from what it believes will be an overwhelming blow to the ego and self. When reality seems overwhelming and threatening, denial screens much of it out. Denial, in its adaptive form, helps you deal with traumatic information at a pace your mind-body can tolerate. With respect to autoimmune disorders, even brief denial can cause problems, because for many of these conditions, the earlier the diagnosis and treatment, the greater the chance of avoiding some harmful aspects. If you use denial for an extended period of time, you greatly increase the risk of many negative problems. A tendency to rely on denial over a long period of time may stem from the belief that illness equals weakness. You may have developed this belief from messages given to you as a child by your family, teachers, and cultures. If you believe this, you won't want to admit your illness to yourself or others because you'll fear being judged negatively.

One of my clients, Mandy, experienced great difficulty in admitting to herself that she was ill. On some level, she knew that if she admitted this to herself, she would have to tell her boyfriend. The intense fear she felt about this was irrational compared to the situation. As we worked together, she recalled a cruel saying her mother often used when she wanted to control her. She would threaten, "If you cause problems for people, they're not going to like you and they'll leave." Subconsciously, this memory led her to erroneously expect that her boyfriend would reject her if he found out she was ill (i.e., less than perfect). We worked on how to tell him of her condition. She was wonderfully surprised when her boyfriend responded with caring, sympathy, and relief. He'd noticed that Mandy had changed and thought her withdrawal reflected a loss of interest in him. He, who loved her dearly, had been crushed and protected himself by withdrawing. Now he told her he didn't care about the illness, it made no difference in his love for her, and he would be with her every step on this difficult journey. Had she continued her self-denial and the result, not talking to him, it's likely she would have lost much more than an outdated, irrational belief.

Solitary Journey

Another reason for the incredible power of the moment of diagnosis and its aftermath is that it can leave you with an overwhelming sense of aloneness or separation from others. Just when you desperately need the soothing, self-esteem, and hope that relationships offer (based on the earliest positive, affirming relationship between infant and maternal figure), you feel isolated from what you now see as everyone else's happy-go-lucky lives. Your insecurity can be intensified by self-blame. Women with whom I've worked have shared their feelings about themselves and their expectations about what others "must" think of them. Sadly, I hear descriptions such as, "broken, infected, disgusting, weak, depressing, too needy, someone others don't want to be around." "Face it," said Denise, a 37-year-old client, "people don't want to be around me or anybody who has major health problems because it reminds them it could so easily be them and that they're getting older anyway and could be living a life just as 'horrible' (their words) as mine."

These feelings can be intensified when it comes to autoimmune conditions. Have you had thoughts like, "Just what did I do in my life that was so wrong or evil that my body is attacking itself? I really must be bad." It's a very uncomfortable position to be furious at your body for letting you down and "attacking you," anxious about its twists of health, and yet thankful for the times when it lets you do something unexpected, something "from before." One woman I interviewed told me of a recent situation she knew revealed her progress since her diagnosis with FMS and CFS. She was angrily getting ready to go to the gym, resentfully changing her clothes at a snail's pace, and telling herself "I'm too tired to do this today. I don't feel like it. I know it's good for me, but . . ." Suddenly, she flashed on the many women in her support group who'd been saying they would give anything to be able to exercise, feel their muscles at work again, and get to that place of peace where pain temporarily disappears and the body feels purified. She quickly replaced her negative self-talk with the chant: "I'm lucky I can do this today. I'm lucky I can do this today." She dressed quickly, looking forward to her chance to help her body, herself. Each repetition of the chant increased her optimism and energy.

Acceptance Is Key

Your reaction to each phase of the grieving process is crucial, and the more positive and optimistic you are, the better. This seems particularly true of the acceptance phase. According to Marcia Van't Land in *Living Well with Chronic Illness* (1994), being able to work through this phase truly distinguishes you from others who may also survive but never get to the point of leading a full, even improved life. She believes a woman reaches this enviable point when she can say, "I accept my chronic condition; now, I'm going to see where I can go from here without letting it run my life." I've noticed that attaining this phase doesn't always mean you'll stay there. There will be times when you'll again be frustrated, depressed, irritable, and ready to give up. Some joyous event may surprise you and help you get out of the hole. Usually, it will require a conscious decision on your part to pull yourself up by the bootstraps. You might say that what you miss most is the degree of freedom you had before your illness. While you may lose certain abilities and freedoms (this distressing turn of events is explored in the coping section), you don't lose what I see as one of the most important human cognitive characteristics: the ability to choose how you'll think about your situation and how you'll react, for better or for worse, in your spiritual, physical, emotional, and cognitive spheres. Remember, certain characteristic ways of coping and reacting to chronic illness indicate a better course of healing. Those who confront their situation, become directly involved in researching and learning about their illness and possible treatments, comply with yet challenge their health caretakers, follow directions from both Western and Eastern professionals, accept their illness yet stretch their supposed limitations to assume some control, have the best chance to grow and heal.

Are These Feelings Normal?

Irene Pollin and Susan Golant (1994) present an alternative way of looking at a person's progression through a chronic illness. They believe there are eight distinct fears that individuals with chronic illness must confront, and that while individual progress through them may vary, there is a specific sequence to these fears. Below is a listing of the fears followed by my commentary about them and, in particular, how they're particularly relevant to us as women.

Fear of Losing Control

As I wrote earlier, one of the most frequent feelings you'll experience is helplessness and a loss of control over your previous activities, energy, work, goals, and mind-body. With so many women these days occupying multiple roles and trying to be the superwomen we thought we could or wanted to be, this comes as a great blow to our desires and independence. These changes lead directly to the second fear. Fortunately, this book offers suggestions and techniques that will help you reassert control over areas, such as your thoughts and behaviors, that can make your life more enjoyable and conducive to healing.

Fear of Losing Self-Image

While most of us try to hide our symptoms and illnesses for as long as possible, often for realistic reasons such as potentially losing our jobs, this often becomes impossible. People begin to notice changes in our energy, appearance, clumsiness, skin and hair, and mental acuity or performance. It's truly unsettling that others notice these changes even when we don't think we're "giving off any signs." You'll also be aware of your internal and external changes. You must watch for thoughts of being a failure, inferior, lazy, a hypochondriac, or even somehow tainted. One troubling aspect for women in particular arises from a society that places great emphasis on beauty and body image. Our socialization is also such that many women still depend extensively on messages from others, beginning with parents and teachers and continuing with peers, supervisors, lovers, and children, in forming their self-image. Our "mirrors" may not remain as positive regarding our appearance or abilities when we're ill, and we must develop the ability to value ourselves for our own being and the qualities we consider important. Most who value us for our selves will be positive and accepting.

Fear of Becoming Dependent

This is a fear most of us share in this day and age. It isn't surprising we feel uncomfortable when placed in a dependent position, because from the moment we're born in this culture, we're taught to become increasingly independent. Even people who are very clearly dependent types don't want to accept that they have these needs. If you lived in a dysfunctional family where you couldn't depend on parents or relatives, this belief may have generalized until your deepest convictions were that you couldn't depend on or trust anyone. For women, this fear may be becoming more potent as time goes by. As we're trying to succeed in a variety of arenas (work, home, politics, athletics), we've come to believe that today's woman must be independent and self-focused. While this is true to a degree, complete independence is neither possible nor desirable. If you have a chronic condition, you'll learn that at certain times, you'll have to depend on others. It can be a difficult battle to wage, which is why some struggle with it for years. I'm not saying you shouldn't do as much for yourself as possible, just that at some point you'll probably need to count on others for help. Remember, you've had people depending on you all of your life, and this will likely continue. You may no longer be always available when a problem pops up, but your wisdom, suggestions, and listening skills will still be there for others. Remember, many people love being needed . . . give them a chance.

Fear of Stigma

This is another fear familiar to all people, and it explains why humans tend to conform. As beings with a strong biological and learned need to belong, the fear of rejection, ridicule, and exclusion ensures we conform. Note that one especially telling definition of "stigma" describes it as an identifying mark, such as a specific diagnostic sign of a disease. We fear the *social* meaning of the word: a mark of shame or disgust. To the extent that we have external physical changes due to our illness, we're even more afraid that others will see something is "wrong" with us. This fear can be hard to fight, as some people may shy away or discriminate against those who appear sick. Socialization and the nature of schools, the workplace, and other institutions already cause many women to have less self-esteem than men. Whether or not you're stigmatized, your very fear of it is enough to cut down your self-esteem even more. You'll have to marshall your resources and focus on accepting yourself rather than requiring external approval or acceptance. Also, keep in mind that not everyone stigmatizes illness.

Fear of Abandonment

This is a basic fear human beings may have from infancy. If we grow up in unstable, chaotic homes, we generally carry into adulthood a deep, often subconscious fear of being abandoned. Our fears of becoming increasingly dependent and of being stigmatized are linked with fear of abandonment. We fear that the changes we may go through when we're chronically ill, such as being more dependent or being seen as different or weak, will lead to our being abandoned by the very people to whom we are closest.

Fear of Expressing Anger

For women, this can be a particularly potent fear as a result of how we've been socialized. We go from childhood with the refrain of "sugar and spice and everything nice" rattling through our brains; to school where we're rewarded for being nice and getting along; to the workplace where a majority of us end up in helping professions or positions similar to men's but in which we don't feel we can delegate, we have less control, and are paid less. Yet, as all of us with chronic illnesses know, there are periods of intense frustration that often cause feelings of extreme anger.

Problems arise when we hold our anger inside or direct it at ourselves. I've worked with many women with depression, anxiety, and other disturbances who have such symptoms in part because they've led lives full of suppressed anger. Also, we don't express anger because of the fear of abandonment described above. We believe that if we show our true natures rather than the artificial, socially accepted ones, others will be so shocked, disgusted, and angered that they will abandon us. Anger generally arises when we feel our mind-bodies are betraying us. In addition, anger is a healthy response when someone violates your rights or belittles you. You must learn to get in touch with your anger, express it appropriately when it arises, and develop a solution to the problem or frustration causing it.

Of course, much of the frustration you'll feel from your illness will be due to situations you can't change. You may not be able to do everything you used to do by yourself: for example, grocery shopping, running with the dog, gardening, taking on more responsibilities at work, housecleaning, and hosting volunteer functions by yourself. Here you change what you can of the situation, but when you get to the parts you can't, you work to accept it. Resetting your personal guideposts and boundaries is essential to living with and appreciating yourself. You'll have to be your greatest fan, as you won't always be the superstar you used to be in so many areas of your life. You can still be the star in those areas you choose to be.

Fear of Isolation

This fear ties in with the fears of abandonment, loss of control, and dependency. While you may sometimes wish for isolation because it seems preferable to dependence, in reality isolation can be very painful. You may have increasing difficulty with mobility and leaving your home. This can increase your sense of social and physical isolation. Being alone can be restful and relaxing or distressing and lonely. The difference lies in how you perceive the situation and your sense of control over it. Obviously, if abandonment is a true possibility, and your control is decreased while your dependency has increased, fear of isolation can seem overwhelming. Fortunately, much of what you experience is under your control. In a later section of the book, I'll be describing techniques you can use to increase your social networks and social support, obtain appropriate resources, and increase your sense of comfort with being on your own.

Fear of Death

While some die of certain autoimmune-related conditions or complications, the majority of these disorders are not deadly. But this may do little to reduce your fear. The truth is that more than we fear death, we fear life. We worry and forecast the worst about how we'll live over time with chronic illness. When you realize the true nature of the fear, you can address it realistically and effectively through planning and decision making.

You need to realize that the stages and phases of the models presented in this chapter are artificial in that humans don't pass cleanly or completely through the steps, one by one. People backslide and find themselves in multiple stages at once. Through time you'll gain practice in dealing with a chronic illness that waxes and wanes. Sometimes you'll feel the lowest ever and think life is no longer worth living. Here you'll need to recall that past episodes have also been incredibly painful but that you've made it through and were able to once again experience enjoyment, satisfaction, and hope. A simple motivating statement, widely applicable to many types of human distress, can help you survive incredibly difficult times: "The only way out is through." Recall that even the worst situations come to an end. And if you're really at rock bottom, then the only way is up. Try to find someone who has a chronic illness, if possible the same one you have, and talk to them. You can learn much from those who are at a different place.

PART II

Specific Autoimmune Disorders

CHAPTER 6

Multiple Sclerosis

Miracles do not happen in contradiction of nature, but in contradiction of what we know about nature.

—Saint Augustine

Multiple Sclerosis (MS) is a chronic inflammatory ARC involving the brain and spinal cord of the central nervous system. According to the National Institutes of Health and the Multiple Sclerosis Society, MS affects between 200,000 and 350,000 people in the U.S. The National Institute of Neurological Disorders and Stroke estimates there are about 200 new cases diagnosed each week. The social, economic, and medical costs of MS are estimated at greater than $2.5 billion annually. Following head trauma, it's the next leading cause of neurologic problems of young adults. One of the most disturbing facts about MS is that it strikes down healthy, primarily young people in the midst of their active lives. People with MS are twenty to forty years old in about 67 percent of cases. As with most ARCs, the prevalence of MS is greater in women than in men, about two to one. Unlike some other ARCs like lupus, MS is more frequently seen in Caucasians than in African Americans and Asians. Caucasians with the greatest chances of developing MS are those with northern European ancestry, such as the English, Irish, and Scandinavians.

As is typical in ARCs, something goes wrong in the immune system that causes it to destroy parts of the body, which are mistakenly seen as foreign invaders. Here, the targeted areas are spinal cord and brain tissues, in particular, the constituents of the myelin sheath, the protective covering of the axons of nerve cells. Axons are long, flexible fibers extending from nerve cell bodies. The inflammation from the immune system's attack destroys parts of the myelin sheaths. This fatty covering, which insulates nerve cell fibers in the brain and spinal cord, underlies the high-speed transmission of electrochemical messages among the body, brain, and spinal cord. Scar tissue, known as plaques, results in destruction of the nerves (sclerosis). The term "multiple" implies the number of places demyelination occurs. As the axons of nerve cells are destroyed, the cells' ability to transmit nervous system signals fails and neurological symptoms arise. For unknown reasons, the inflammation and demyelination stops, perhaps due to suppressor immune cell activity. Remyelination of the plaque and resumed functional abilities may occur, depending on the extent of the inflammatory damage.

If you have MS, you've probably received one of three labels. These three MS types are differentiated based on existence of "flares" and the degree of recovery. (Flares are active phases following periods of remission. They disappear, only to repeat this pattern over and over.) The less severe form is the relapsing-remitting type, which includes repetitive flares lasting days or months, followed by good recovery. Those who don't recover significantly after flares but whose condition doesn't worsen between flares also have relapsing-remitting type. Relapsing-remitting is the most common type of MS, with about 67 percent first having this diagnosis. Later some develop secondary-progressive MS. This differs in that health greatly worsens between flares. The most severe type, primary-progressive, affects 10 percent of people with MS; it includes progressive deficits and no remissions.

What Causes MS?

As with all ARCs, there are many proposed theories of how and why MS develops. The main, most empirically studied hypotheses follow.

Genetics

As with many ARCs, genes are involved in MS onset. No specific MS gene has been identified, and eight or more genes may be involved. People with MS inherit particular locations on individual genes more frequently than people who don't have it. Peter Riskind's article in *On the Brain*, a publication of the Harvard Mahoney Neuroscience Institute, asserts that the most empirically supported link is that with gene locations containing chromosome 6, involved in immune system functioning. This is called the human leukocyte antigen (HLA) or major histocompatibility complex region. These HLAs are proteins, influenced by one's genes, that affect the immune system. People with MS show HLA patterns that differ from those without MS. In fact, in America and northern Europe, 3 HLAs appear more frequently in people with MS. American MS patients manifest these HLAs in groups; namely, they have more than one of the three HLAs more often than the rest of the population. Different HLA groupings are associated with the disease course and severity. The picture is far from simple, as other regions on chromosomes 2, 3, 5, 7, 11, 17, 19, and X have been characterized as possibly having MS-related genes.

One way to assess gene involvement in illness onset is to see whether relatives also develop it. If genes were the whole story, we'd find that identical twins sharing genetic codings would both have the illness. In MS, this isn't the case. When one identical twin has MS, the other has a 30 to 50 percent chance of having it. While some of this difference may be due to different environmental exposure, this doesn't entirely explain the difference. Relatives of people with MS in the first generation have a 30 to 50 times greater risk of getting the disorder as compared to people whose parents didn't have MS (Rose 1993). This supports a genetic role, as the likelihood of developing MS in the population at large is only .1 percent. So, a genetic predisposition, together with triggers like stress, colds, dietary factors, viral infections, malnutrition (poor diet, poor absorption capabilities), food intolerance/allergen (gluten, dairy products), and environmental conditions, set the conditions for developing MS.

Molecular Mimicry and Viral Relations

MS used to be placed in the category of degenerative diseases, a group of diseases in which there is degeneration of one or more parts of the body without a known cause. However, evidence suggests MS is caused by infection or allergy (together with genetic predisposition). One theory of MS is the molecular mimicry theory. According to this view, a normal immune response to certain viruses might react with body tissues by mistake. So a virus like the retrovirus human T-lymphotropic virus (HTLV-1), which is linked with particular blood conditions and diseases affecting the central nervous system, could indirectly trigger an autoimmune response. Studies have shown that people with MS have high levels of antibodies against measles, influenza C, herpes simplex, and other viruses (Carroll and Dorman 1993).

Some studies of mice have provided valuable supportive data. Genetic engineering projects have created mice with immune genes predisposing them to develop an MS-like illness. Riskind explains that the results showed that multiple illnesses related to different viruses were causing the disease. Such results mirror recent studies that suggest gamma-interferon, generated by white blood cells (lymphocytes), may trigger MS flares. It's part of our self-defense against viruses, but what is meant to protect actually turns to destroy our bodies. It is being explored whether the Epstein-Barr virus (EBV), which causes infectious mononucleosis, may cause MS as well. MS patients have low levels of essential fatty acids, as do people who've just had a bout with the EBV.

Hormonal Influences

Hormones have an effect on MS. During the last trimester of pregnancy, women have far fewer MS flares. Unfortunately, after birth, the situation changes, and MS flares can increase for up to nine months. If the reason for the decrease were known, it could be used to reduce flares in general. If you've had children, you know how your hormones are on a roll during and after pregnancy. One hormone that partially explains the increased flares after birth is prolactin. This pituitary hormone is responsible for milk production and is involved with the immune system, which may help explain the increased flares. If you're pregnant (or breastfeeding) and have MS, be cautious with prescription drugs, as they may increase risk of birth defects. Blood and breast milk can transfer these substances.

Allergens & Nutritional Deficits

Another hypothesized cause of MS is food allergies, and many people with MS have such allergies. If you eliminate these toxic substances from your diet, the rate and severity of your disease may lessen. Speak with your SHOC team about common allergens, such as dairy, sugar, yeast, wheat, gluten, corn, ketchup, vinegar, and wine. Candidiasis taxes your body's energy and plays a central role in causing food allergies. At some point, you may have battled the Epstein-Barr virus and been left to fight later infections with a weakened immune system.

As mentioned, many patients have insufficient essential fatty acids, which are required for building the nervous system and brain. Recall that we see higher rates of MS in westernized regions with diets high in dairy, cooking oils, meat, and processed foods (very low in essential fatty acids) than in regions with diets high in essential fatty acids like fruits, oily fish, vegetables, and olive and seed oils (Swank 1950). As is the case with some other ARCs, people with MS can't assimilate all of the nutritional value of their food, which causes nutrient deficiencies. Refer to this chapter's section on Nutritional Enhancement to learn how you can get the healthiest amounts of essential fatty acids.

Environmental Contributors & Toxins

With respect to MS, age interacts with geographic or climatic factors in determining risk. If you moved from a risky temperate to a less risky tropical zone before age fifteen, you'd benefit from the low-risk nature of the tropics. If the opposite pattern existed, you'd have the increased risk of moving to the riskier area. The National Institute of Neurological Disorders and Stroke suggests that if you move after age 15, you keep the risk level of where you initially lived. The patterns may involve climatic elements or a contagious process, or may merely be linked with racial and ethnic vulnerability elements.

A toxin associated with MS (and other ARCs like CFIDS and FMS) is mercury from amalgam fillings. Mercury spreads into surrounding body tissue and may cause MS symptoms. What is disturbing is that the toxic nature of mercury has been known since the 1500s. Mercury attaches to cell DNA, causing changes such that the immune system no longer recognizes these cells as part of the host body, thereby triggering the autoimmune response and the destruction of myelin.

Symptoms and Signs

The symptoms of MS are quite varied. Mild symptoms include tingling, pricking, itching, burning, warmth, and frequent urination. More troublesome are extreme fatigue, paralysis, numb or tingling limbs, great weakness, nystagmus (involuntary eye movements), vision loss or double vision, clumsiness, falling, chronic pain, difficulty with voiding, and speech problems. Symptoms depend partly on the quantity, seriousness, and location of plaques. Initial MS symptoms are blurred or double vision, color distortion, and single-eye blindness. Usually, these problems remit later. Inflammatory problems of the optic nerve, retrobulbar or optic neuritis, affect 53 percent of MS patients and are the first symptoms in about 15 percent. Up to 50 percent have concentration, memory, and judgment difficulties of which they're unaware. Often these come to light only after family or friends notice and intensive cognitive testing is done. MS fatigue can last for months or years or may repeatedly appear and disappear. MS fatigue can be caused by disrupted sleep, changes in brain neurotransmitters, and immune cell cytokines.

Early in the course of MS, the following symptoms appear in a certain percenatge of patients (Rosner and Ross 1992): sensory, 55 percent; ataxia (balance and coordination difficulties), 27 percent; weakness, 21 percent; optic problems, 18 percent; double vision, 18 percent; dizziness, 6 percent; speech pronunciation and rhythm problems, 5 percent; numbness in face, 4 percent; bladder problems, 3 percent; feelings of electricity or burning down back and arms and legs, 2 percent.

The most typical symptoms in order of prevalence occurring throughout the MS course: increased reflexes, 91 percent; ataxia (balance, coordination difficulties), 85 percent; weakness with spasticity, 77 percent; sensory loss, 75 percent; double vision with jerky eye movements, 65 percent; optic neuritis, 53 percent; bladder problems, 45 percent; slurred speech, 33 percent; weakness in gaze, 32 percent; vertigo, 13 percent.

Related Conditions and Look-alikes

As is typical with ARCs, diagnosing MS is plagued by inaccuracies and prolonged periods of testing. Patients typically see at least eight doctors and may wait months to years before receiving an accurate diagnosis. One reason for this is the great disparity in number, type, and severity of symptoms. Some experience mild symptoms and infrequent active periods of illness, while others experience many symptoms affecting multiple body systems and chronic MS bouts.

MS-type symptoms can appear in many disorders, both ARCs and non-ARCs. Because MS shares symptoms with other diseases, the following data can improve your understanding of your case and help to rule out other conditions. This will help you understand why your doctor is ordering certain tests or asking certain questions. You can bring up alternative illness for discussion, perhaps convincing an overworked doctor to order whatever tests or medications represent the best care for your condition.

Lupus (SLE)

In both MS and SLE, actual destructive changes affect systems throughout the body. In SLE, there are harmful changes to the muscles, tendons, joints, and ligaments. Other organs, such as the lungs and kidneys, may also be harmed. The entire body can be hampered by changes in blood vessels resulting from the immune system's self-attack. MS can also involve multiple systems and can cause extensive damage throughout the body. In terms of symptoms, both MS and SLE involve fatigue and lethargy, muscle weakness, hyperventilation or shortness of breath, pain, and inflammation. Another similarity is that both can affect the central nervous system, causing loss of normal sensations and, infrequently, mental disturbances (Isenberg and Morrow 1995).

Lyme Disease (LD)

Many LD symptoms, such as extreme fatigue, muscle weakness, facial paralysis, double or blurry vision, poor balance, shaking, partial paralysis, slurred or slowed speech, pain, and generalized aches, also typify MS. Magnetic resonance imaging (MRI) tests can't distinguish between these two diseases and LD spirochetes can be found in the spinal fluid and tissues of many MS patients. As mentioned, MS occurs more frequently in certain geographic areas and LD seems to be prevalent in the same regions. Such similarities have led researchers to explore whether the LD spirochete can trigger MS or an illness similar to MS (Lang 1997). In the U.S., only Alaska, Arizona, Nebraska, Montana, and Hawaii have no LD cases reported. LD is an international health problem as well. Many countries in Europe, regions in Russia, and parts of China and Japan have high incidence. Two LD vaccines are in final approval stages by the U.S. Food and Drug Administration. The length of efficacy and whether booster sessions will be required are unanswered questions. No serious side-effects are apparent (Gardner 1998).

Neurological Disorders and Other Conditions

When there is spinal cord damage, severe weakness in limbs can arise, as can stiffness called spasticity. When the two types of symptoms appear together, it may suggest MS, though they don't always appear together in MS. If only limb weakness occurs, diagnosis is difficult, as this symptom is linked with many conditions. Your health professional may rule out pinched nerves, slipped disks, diabetic neuritis, thyroid disease, and lead poisoning (Rosner and Ross 1992). Imbalance of the type seen in MS can also arise from inner ear infection, exhaustion, high or low blood pressure, head injury, or drug or alcohol abuse. Problems with coordination may stem from exhaustion, side effects of certain medications, and excessive caffeine or alcohol intake. Likewise, double vision isn't limited to MS and can arise from inner ear infections, head injuries, and drug or alcohol abuse. Optic neuritis is sudden, occurs in one or both eyes, and includes blurriness, depth perception interference, eye movement pain, flashes of light upon eye movement or when it's dark, and highly dilated pupils. Optic neuritis is indicative of MS when all other potential causes are ruled out. However, vitamin deficiency, pernicious anemia, sinus problems, diabetes, alcoholism, immunizations, ARCs affecting the vascular system, birth control pills, and syphilis can also cause it.

It's most difficult to get an accurate diagnosis during the early stages. It's also during this time that you may experience the most confusion and anxiety. What is the meaning of these symptoms, which vary greatly and come and go? Since they often disappear, you may dismiss them as unimportant. The next symptom may be so different that you think it's unrelated. However, as this pattern continues, you become concerned. This difficulty of diagnosis is unfortunate because when MS is caught early enough, it can often be controlled fairly well. When you see your doctor, he may not be able to give you a timely diagnosis in part because you must have at least two symptoms affecting different systems at two different time periods. When you finally get the diagnosis, you may feel an odd mixture of relief and distress. Even when two symptoms are confirmed, your doctor should run tests to ensure the diagnosis is MS and not a look-alike or other autoimmune disorder. You'll read about these tests in the Testing for Multiple Sclerosis section later in this chapter.

The Courses of MS

If you've been diagnosed with MS, recall that descriptions of timeframes and courses are only generalizations. MS has remissions and flares and isn't necessarily progressive. Still, you must educate yourself as much as possible, as this is the starting point of creating your best SHOC. Learn what to expect in general, your options, specialists, the best treatments both Western and Eastern, and what you can do to stretch confines and grow in other ways.

The early signs of MS can rapidly appear, disappear, and reappear. Like many, you may try to explain the changing symptoms as coming from negative stress at work or from a difficult relationship or from trying to balance raising kids, working outside the home, and keeping a good relationship with your partner. Or you may attribute these unexpected changes in your body to the flu or a bout with a virus. (Refer to the earlier description of common first symptoms.) Some of the more frightening early signs can include awakening and being unable to move or finding that you can't rise after sitting on a hot day. Other disturbing early signs include emotional changes like mood swings and depression. As the disease progresses, you may have increased trouble walking, develop a stagger, or have spasticity of movement.

You must make a concerted effort to build your mind-body strength because while 15 to 25 percent of MS patients have fairly mild cases, 33 percent are hit with serious attacks. On a positive note, about one in five have only one attack with no or slight disease progression. Up to two-thirds still walk solo up to twenty-five years after the initial diagnosis, and half still enjoy most activities enjoyed before diagnosis. Some experience paralysis of different degrees and may come to use canes, crutches, and walking aids. Fortunately, MS is rarely fatal, with 93 percent living the average life expectancy of the population. For a very few, MS can result in various life-threatening conditions. Remember that cases vary greatly, and if you're armed with good mind-body tools you can greatly affect the severity of your case by how you choose to respond to it.

MS attacks fall into four patterns; most people have only one pattern and relevant symptoms. The four patterns are: spinal cord attack; brain stem-cerebellar attack; optic nerve attack; and cerebral attack. Most patients have only six to seven of the many potential MS symptoms throughout the course of the disease. No long-term, telltale damage may necessarily occur (Rosner and Ross 1992).

Tina's Story

Tina's bout with MS started abruptly and severely. One morning she awoke, wondering if she'd overslept once again, and looked at her clock. She couldn't make out the numbers and thought something had gotten into her left eye. She rubbed it, but nothing helped; she thought she might have an eye infection from hours spent reading and working. After a day at the law firm, where at thirty-three she was the youngest partner ever, she couldn't pretend all was normal and went to see her eye doctor. Nothing . . . and again nothing when she visited her physician. Her eye cleared up, and she forgot about it until three weeks later, when she wound up at the hospital after being unable to move her legs on a blistering hot day. More doctors and again nothing. A neurologist who did some testing arranged an MRI two weeks later and a spinal tap three weeks after that. The technician who did the tests said nothing, nor did the neurologist.

Six weeks after the spinal tap and four unreturned messages later, she stomped into the office, a nervous, frustrated, fatigued wreck. She couldn't believe that he looked through her as if he had no idea who she was. As he began to walk off, her raised voice caused a stir in the waiting room and he turned around. He coldly told her that he wouldn't speak to her until she'd made an appointment, which wouldn't be for weeks, and besides, he needed time to review the test results. "You've had them for two months already," she thought. In shock, she turned to leave and go back to work.

One month later, when she could no longer make it through another day at work due to fatigue and pain, she visited a neurologist recommended by a friend. More testing, but this time by a caring, patient woman who carefully explained all of the tests and why the diagnosis might be MS. She helpfully answered all of Tina's questions. Tina had now been through so many months of uncertainty, blaming it on herself when the other doctor had been cold and rude, that she felt she couldn't handle this diagnosis.

I worked with Tina for some time and at her request spoke with her wonderful new doctor. I told the doctor how much her optimism and support meant to Tina and how her support of both Eastern and Western treatments greatly helped my work with Tina. Tina moved through the stages of grief, denial, and loss and then moved on to acceptance and revision of her goals. She took it easier when her mind-body needed that, and used medication, herbs, and mind-body work to reduce the frequency and severity of her bouts. She reawakened her earlier passion for classical and jazz music. Her work friends still teased her about the incongruence between her past Type A behavior and her new interests in meditation and visualization. She no longer led the frenetic life but learned how to maintain and build her energy. Importantly to Tina, she kept working as an attorney although she switched fields to represent clients with physical and mental disabilities. She found it much more rewarding than her previous work. These changes helped her adapt in a healthy way to the many mind-body changes that came through time.

Testing for Multiple Sclerosis

There is no single definitive test to show whether you have MS. Someday this may be possible, but at present, your doctor must rely on a variety of information sources: your symptom reports; factors you see related to symptom changes; health-related concerns, illnesses, operations or allergies; medications; mind-body stressors; lifestyle habits (diet, exercise, smoking, drinking, drugs, toxins); social history and childhood experiences related to your current physical health; your family's health history; the doctor's physical exam; records from your other doctors; and a variety of tests. Be as thoroughly prepared with as much information as possible and medical record copies from other doctors, which can save months of wasted time.

Now you'll read about specific tests used to identify MS, changes in course, and to rule out other diagnoses. This knowledge will help you decipher medi-speak (should it sound like a foreign tongue) and will assist you at those times when jargon becomes a necessary communication tool. Being an active, assertive partner in your SHOC increases your sense of control, your immune system functioning, and your chances of improvement.

The physical exam is one of the first steps in diagnosing MS. Your doctor should also take a full history of you and your family as well as your particular symptoms and signs. To diagnose MS, you must have had symptoms in at least two different areas of the nervous system (i.e., brain, spinal cord, optic nerves) over at least two time periods. Keep notes as to your symptoms, how long they last, whether they come and go, and so on.

One of the tests frequently used to diagnose MS is a spinal tap. Cerebrospinal fluid flowing around and inside your brain reveals markers indicative of MS. The fluid is examined to detect an increased number of lymphocytes, part of your immune system that makes the self-attacking antibodies that go after your own nerve myelin covering. The analysis also looks for elevated protein levels, known as myelin basic protein, immunoglobulins, or oligoclonal bands. These increase during acute flares or in relapsing-progressive MS. Typically a local anesthetic prohibits discomfort. Blood tests are taken so your doctor can rule out other conditions causing lack of energy and severe fatigue, such as anemia or thyroid problems.

Noninvasive techniques can determine the presence or extent of damage associated with MS. EEG studies of brain waves and evoked responses tell the speed at which electrical activity proceeds in the nervous system. Multiple lesions can be detected based on whether evoked responses are delayed between points in the brain stem, the brain's visual region, and spinal areas. Another option, the CAT scan, involves an intravenous liquid with special dye, after which an image of your brain is taken. Certain areas of light in the brain can then be used to differentiate MS from conditions like tumors and strokes which also cause areas to light up. More recently, a technique known as magnetic resonance imaging (MRI) is being used in diagnosing MS. MRI scans are useful, as more than 90 percent of people with MS have abnormal brain scans that show darkened areas, indicating tissue destruction. One region damaged by MS inflammation is the blood/brain barrier. This essential area is composed of tissue that protects the brain by blocking harmful substances from passing through. Damage to this tissue allows some harmful substances through and into the brain. Some researchers believe the dissolution of the blood/brain barrier is the first step in the formation of MS lesions. MRI scans are helpful in assisting in the diagnosis of MS, but can't be used alone, as other conditions also produce abnormal brain scans.

What You Can Do

As with so many autoimmune-related disorders, there is no known cause or cure for MS. Thus, treatment traditionally focuses on reducing the pain and disruption of symptoms, controlling the disease process, and educating patients about the disease. Among the greatest single factors relating to the severity of your case is how early it is discovered and treated. It's essential that this disorder be caught and diagnosed early so you have the greatest chances of progress and reduced severity. Also, remember that your mind-body is unique. The last thing in the world you should do is ignore symptoms or distress just because they don't seem to fit with what you've heard or read about the onset and course of MS.

You must be in touch with your body and any changes, and if you suspect something is amiss, you need to see a professional healer/helper as soon as possible. In general, the sooner you determine what is wrong, if anything, the sooner you can form your plan of attack, research the illness and appropriate health professionals, work on your attitudes, and thus decrease the speed of progression or degree of damage. This all fits into your toolbag for maximizing your chances of beating the odds. Secondly, your body's uniqueness means you may need different types of treatments, that you might benefit from treatments infrequently used or even unknown to Western doctors, and that there is no such thing as 100 percent certainty in any doctor's diagnosis or prognosis. You'll have to develop a cohesive mind-body integrity so you can connect with your helpers in a timely way if medications aren't working, if side effects crop up, or if things take an unexpected turn. Just as your body's uniqueness is one reason you'll have an individual experience, the uniqueness of your mind will contribute as well.

Some of you will be open to increasing the width of your SHOC team by adding members who perform acupuncture, prescribe herbal tonics and vitamins and minerals, offer massage, work to balance your yin and yang, etc. In terms of the conventional medicine side, one aspect that is incredibly important is that you develop a trusting, caring relationship with your primary doctor. Given the nature of MS, it's best that you work with a neurologist who is highly knowledgeable about MS and the current testing and treatment. (See appendix I for referrals.) Recall the role your mind, and thus your emotions and behavior, play in improving or worsening symptoms, pain, distress, and prognosis.

Medications

Doctors and health professionals have made great progress in the area of medications for MS. For many, flare-ups are the cruelest part of the disease. Just when you begin to feel physically stronger, return to work or look for work, and resume family duties and sports or hobbies to increase life enjoyment, a flare appears and stands in the way. Flares can be disturbing reminders of repetitive losses, especially if they make you feel you'll never again be able to fully enjoy your life. In addition to cognitive work on reinterpreting your situation, you also now have access to medicines that shorten flare duration and even reduce frequency.

Methyl-prednisolone, an artificial adrenal steroid hormone, acts like cortisone by impacting inflammation and the immune system. While it can't stop the progression of the disorder, it reduces flare duration, thus allowing people to feel physically and emotionally better more of the time. However, it can't be used too often due to negative side effects that occur with frequent usage. Another drug, Copaxone, awaits FDA approval and offers two benefits the drugs just discussed can't: the ability to slow the characteristic decline of MS and reduce recurrence frequency. This drug is most effective for the milder relapsing-remitting type of MS.

Two other drugs, Avonex and Betaseron, types of a natural immune substance, beta-interferon, may reduce relapses by as much as 30 percent among relapser-remitters. The AARDA claims that injections of beta-interferon into the spinal canal may reduce recurrences more along the lines of 50 percent for some. Avonex, like Copaxone, may delay the decline frequently caused by MS. These drugs do something "deeper" than symptom recurrence reduction, as MRIs of Avonex patients show decreased brain aberrances. Some studies suggest that Avonex slows MS progression and associated brain tissue loss. These are important gains in MS treatment, but they're even more important than is immediately evident. Brain tissue loss or "brain atrophy" often occurs before other MS symptoms. Using new technologies like MRIs makes it possible to detect MS much earlier, an essential aspect of reducing MS severity.

One of the most recent, exciting discoveries by Soloman Snyderj and associates at Johns Hopkins and Guilford Pharmaceuticals, Inc., is that *certain drugs can be modified to actually stimulate nerve growth without suppressing the immune system.* This is a major advance in effectively treating neurodegenerative disorders like MS. These new drugs even assist redevelopment of the myelin sheath, an essential neuronal element in regaining use of the nerves.

Other new medications are proving quite helpful in treating MS. One method involves implanting a tiny pump in the abdomen that delivers controlled doses of baclofen (Lioresal) into the spinal cord to reduce MS spasms. The pump contains enough medication for one to three months. When it's delivered this way, the side effects of the pill form don't occur. Another new drug, 4-aminopyridine, helps improve motor skills by increasing the conduction of nerve impulses. Fortunately, this drug is relatively inexpensive and has few side effects. A final treatment, controversial in the U.S. but widely available elsewhere, is hyperbaric oxygen therapy. This treatment involves placing an individual in a special room that delivers pure oxygen at three times the normal atmospheric pressure. While this treatment is used in the U.S. for certain conditions, its use for MS remains limited. People with middle ear infections, spontaneous pneumothorax, or histories of emphysema should avoid this treatment.

Muscle relaxants and anticonvulsants help with muscle spasms. Acetaminophen, aspirin, or antidepressants may be used to combat MS pain. While medications are effective, they can be costly and produce adverse effects. You won't gain the best edge against the odds by relying only on them. The reality for women with MS is now much more optimistic than before, as the chances of leading productive, enjoyable lives are much greater. How do you best fix the odds in your favor?

- New medications

- Surgical techniques

- Tools for protecting the joints

- Sufficient sleep, allocated rest periods

- Education about and the use of appropriate physical therapies and exercise

- Biofeedback, meditation, relaxation, visualization, and pain management techniques

- Nutrition and herbal remedies

- Acupuncture or non-invasive techniques like qi gong, reiki, tai chi chuan

- Psychotherapy and chronic illness counseling

- Assertiveness and proactivity in dealing with your illness and your SHOC team

- Cognitive techniques: thought monitoring/modifying/stopping and coping skills training

- Household and behavioral changes

The key to maximizing your life and moving toward healing and growth lies in combining appropriate types of conventional and alternative treatments. This is akin to the general notion of keeping balance in all areas of your life. It's a key component of your SHOC, because extremes can trigger relapses or a worsening of symptoms. Moderation and balance take work, but they greatly increase your odds of living life to the fullest. Keeping your life balanced is one of the promises of growth if you decide to seek the challenge rather than retreat.

Buyer Beware

Many seeking alternative treatments believe that because they are "natural" they can cause no harm. While these tools can be incredibly effective, you must treat them with caution. As with Western medicine, you should assume an active, responsible role and ensure that you're working with trained professionals with appropriate certification or license (if applicable), training, and experience. Do your best to find one who has worked extensively in and possibly even researched or written about your particular disorder. This should be a basic element in the design and practice of your SHOC. You simply owe it to yourself.

Some chapters later in this book provide an in-depth presentation on various healing methods. Here, we'll explore some management, optimization, and coping techniques most relevant to this chapter on MS. You may read this section first or familiarize yourself with pain management and other techniques by going to subsequent chapters.

Physical Therapy

Physical therapy exercises help women with MS by keeping muscles strong and flexible and by preventing muscle contractions. Massage is also very useful in maintaining muscle tone and function. It's important that you find a physical therapist or masseuse who has experience working on people with MS. Some techniques can worsen your condition. For example, heat is often used in physical therapy and can be very helpful for some conditions, *but not yours*. Heat can trigger severe symptoms, so avoid hot baths, towel wraps, and hot places.

Exercise Do's and Don'ts for MS Patients

This is another essential component of your SHOC. Choose carefully when and how you exercise. If you're feeling very fatigued or are having a bad bout, don't exercise, as you risk injury and worsening your symptoms. This doesn't mean you can't gently move and stretch. Just keep in mind that exercise raises body temperature, and you need to watch out for heat. Your best bet is swimming and strengthening and stretching in cool water, so your body temperature stays down while you benefit from having your body supported by water.

Nutritional Enhancement

Dietary changes can be very useful in treating MS. While I discuss nutrition and its role in illness and health, the discussion is necessarily limited. I'm not providing medical advice; before making any dietary changes, you must consult with your health care professional. In addition, these remedies aren't sufficient as your sole treatment. These suggestions come from my research and the work of others but can't take the place of direct consultation with your medical professional, nutritionist, and other trained health professionals. At the same time, this is an area in which you benefit by keeping an open mind. You need not limit yourself to Western remedies and can gain much from consulting herbalists, holistic nutritional counselors, and the like.

One indication of the role of diet in MS comes from the fact that MS is much more common in the U.S., while it's quite rare in countries like Korea, China, and Japan. Aside from genetics and environment, what could explain such differences? Our diets are replete with cholesterol, saturated fats, and alcohol, which lead to the generation of prostaglandin-2, a hormonelike substance that stimulates the inflammatory response and intensifies negative symptoms of MS. The diets of these other countries have much less fat and more seeds, fruits, and seafood with good amounts of essential fatty acids, such as the omega-3 and omega-6 fatty acids. Fatty acid consumption is one nutritional remedy recommended for ARCs. The two groups of fatty acids, omega-3 and omega-6, are particularly important as they have anti-inflammatory effects and can lessen the effects of joint pain, morning stiffness, and muscle weakness. How do you get sufficient fatty acids? You can take omega-3 fatty acid supplements or you can obtain it the old-fashioned way, by consuming at least two servings a week of the following fish: tuna, salmon, shark, herring, mackerel, and turbot.

Many nutrients that are believed to reduce the impact of ARCs and increase your chances for growth and true healing can't be obtained in sufficient enough amounts through diet. Thus, it may be in your best interest to include nutritional supplements, vitamins, and minerals in your regimen.

One study compared MS patients who ate different diets based on the quantity of saturated fats (Swank and Dugan 1990). Those who ate the least saturated fat showed most improvement. The researchers suggest that people with MS should eat less than the maximum 15 grams/day. It's a good idea to replace saturated fats with polyunsaturated or monounsaturated fats.

Another helpful dietary change is to consume only organically grown foods clean of additives, pesticides, and other chemicals. Build your diet around fruits, eggs, raw seeds and nuts, vegetables, cold-pressed vegetable oils, and gluten-free grains. For those who can manage it, a modified vegetarian diet is a good idea. In addition, as for everyone, drinking at least eight 8-ounce glasses of water daily is important. For people with MS, it helps prevent toxins from collecting in muscles. Lactic acid, found in pickles and sauerkraut, is also important. Try to avoid the following substances: refined sugar; refined foods; wheat; processed, canned, or frozen foods; alcohol; and coffee. Your doctor and nutritionist might add other foods to this list. While not everybody can afford a nutritionist, if it's at all possible, try to consult with one familiar with MS at least once or twice. Make the most of your time by doing research before the appointments, writing down questions, and deciding on your general goals with respect to nutrition and your illness.

Allergies

Recall that a possible cause and trigger of symptoms exacerbation is food allergies. Candidiasis also frequently occurs in MS and other autoimmune disorders. This condition taxes the body's energy resources and is associated with food allergies. The sooner you determine whether and what food allergies you may have, the less nerve damage will occur. Allergy testing is essential, as is removal of elements toxic to you. Speak with your doctor about arranging to have allergy testing and refer to appendix II for more on elements central to *collagen formation and connective tissue repair*, important for people with MS.

While the rapidity of removing these harmful allergens and the foods listed above is important, you don't have to completely and instantly cut out all problematic substances. Many women become resentful after doing this, leading to the return to "forbidden" foods. This practice is perpetuated by self-blame, out-of-control feelings, and anger. You may want to take out one to two foods or elements each week or set up a schedule that works for you. Gradually wean yourself from the food, and you may find that after a time you don't miss that substance at all (or not sufficiently to prove bothersome).

Try to reframe the situation. It's not a punishment, just as having the illness is not a punishment for your being a bad person. You do have a choice, even here. You don't have to change your diet. This element is under your control. When you think through the consequences—and you have in all likelihood already experienced them painfully enough—you'll probably choose to modify your diet to make yourself feel better. Remind yourself that this is something you want to do, for yourself. Try to see it as a challenge, difficult but offering potentially great rewards. Secondly, tell yourself these changes aren't just another thing you have to do because you have MS. These dietary changes are often similar to general recommendations for improved health and well-being. Thirdly, to help yourself see this as a challenge and maintain your motivation, you should create some goals, choose certain rewards, and be creative about your new way of eating. These days there are so many fat-free, sugar-free, and preservative-free foods that your palate won't even be able to discern many of these changes. As you learn about new fruits, vegetables, seasonings, and low-fat cheeses and other protein sources, you can build a sense of mastery and turn this into an enjoyable hobby. Eating is one of the great pleasures of life—to balance other restrictions and losses you feel, live it up here. By using self-talk, reframing and creating prostress by challenging yourself to new menus, you can turn this potential negative into a healing positive.

Supplement Suggestions

As mentioned earlier, people with MS and other autoimmune conditions have trouble extracting and absorbing certain nutrients. MS-related deficiencies can include B12, manganese, B1, B6, folic acid, zinc, calcium, amino acids, and essential fatty acids. To combat deficiencies, use the following information:

- *To help protect myelin sheaths from damage: Choline*, taken as directed. *B12* (preferably sublingual type), 1,000 mcg twice per day. It has been found that individuals with MS have lower than normal levels of B12 in their cerebrospinal fluid. This discovery and many examples of symptom reduction in MS patients given B12 support this nutrient's importance. More physicians are using large injections of B12 intramuscularly with positive results. *L-glycine*, 500 mg twice a day on an empty stomach.

- *To boost immune system functioning: Vitamin B complex* (hypoallergenic type), 100 mg three times per day. *Coenzyme Q10* (liquid type if available), 90 mg per day. *Raw thymus glandular*, 500 mg two times per day. *Vitamin C*, 3,000–5,000 mg per day. *Vitamin B6* (hypoallergenic type), 50 mg three times per day. B6 also helps the nervous system function, stimulates red blood cell production, and a deficiency may be a trigger in genetically susceptible people. Vitamin C, a powerful antioxidant, also increases production of the antiviral substance interferon.

- *To protect against toxic elements: Sulfur*, 500 mg two to three times per day or *Garlic* (a good source of sulfur), two caps three times per day. *Acidophilus* (powder), one teaspoon two times per day on empty stomach.

- *To control symptoms: Fatty acids* from foods listed above or from: *flaxseed* or *primrose oil*, per label three times per day with meals; *gamma-linolenic acid* (GLA), per label three times per day with meals; *omega-3 essential fatty acids*. Many MS patients are GLA deficient.

- *To prevent calcium deficiency, which may be a trigger in genetically susceptible people: Calcium* (chelate form best), 2,000–3,000 mg per day with *magnesium*, 1,000–1,500 mg per day. Take magnesium with calcium to boost calcium absorption; magnesium maintains proper muscle coordination.

- *To maintain enzymatic activity: High potency multimineral supplement. Manganese*, 5 to 10 mg per day taken at a different time of day than calcium. MS patients may have a manganese deficiency.

Herbal Remedies

As with diet, I'm not dispensing medical advice or prescribing any herbs. The suggestions in this book are culled from research and patient reports. You must consult with your SHOC team prior to changing diet or adding supplements or herbs. Again, don't rely solely on herbs, but balance them with treatments prescribed by your doctor if she concurs. There are many herbal supplements with favorable effects. While nutritional books and practitioners may recommend alfalfa sprouts for MS, I can't support this notion, because the AARDA, Inc. suggests there is evidence that they may trigger autoimmune disorders or symptoms in vulnerable individuals.

Balch and Balch (1997) suggest several herbs for detoxifying: dandelion, pau d'arco, red clover, burdock, Saint-John's-wort, sarsaparilla, and yarrow. You may find recommendations for echinacea and goldenseal, but you must take these cautiously if at all. Don't take echinacea for extended periods of time, and avoid taking goldenseal daily for more than one week. You may even want to steer clear of these entirely, as people allergic to ragweed must avoid them, and other people can have bad reactions as well. See the resources in appendix I for places to contact.

Hormones

There are various natural hormones now receiving accolades: melatonin, human growth hormone, and dehydroepiandrosterone (DHEA). These are some of the hormones found in greatest amounts in the body. Talk to your doctor before using melatonin, which shouldn't be used by individuals with certain ARCs. As with the other two hormones, proponents claim DHEA has anti-aging properties. Most of the body's DHEA production occurs up to a person's mid-twenties, after which the amount decreases until only a small percentage remains in one's seventies and eighties. DHEA decrease may be linked to the onset of illnesses, like nerve deterioration, cancer, Parkinson's, and type II diabetes.

This so-called wonder hormone may stimulate bone deposition (thereby avoiding osteoporosis), increase production of the sex hormones estrogen and progesterone, and increase muscle while decreasing body fat. The lower the body's DHEA, the more vulnerable the body's organs and tissues become to weakening and disease. What is important here is evidence suggesting that DHEA supplements may help prevent MS, decrease pain, improve immune system functioning, boost stress tolerance and well-being, and improve body mobility and sleep quality (Balch and Balch 1997). It's also used to treat those with chronic fatigue. However, some say that high DHEA supplementation interferes with the body's ability to generate it, and animal studies have shown liver damage may result. Besides following whatever regimen your health professionals recommend, you should include antioxidants—vitamins C, E, and selenium—to reduce the likelihood of liver damage.

Treatments for Fatigue

Fatigue, a serious complication of MS, can arise when pain disrupts normal sleep cycles. When this occurs, you don't spend enough time in delta sleep, the sleep cycle during which muscle and tissue repair occurs. This causes increased pain, which adds to the difficulty of sleeping, thus creating a vicious cycle. Fatigue also results from cytokines, secretions by the immune cells. Another cause is changes in brain neurotransmitters due to MS. MS patients also can feel negative stress, which interferes with getting a healthy quantity and quality of sleep.

Fatigue is generally handled by the conventional physicians through medications. Approximately 50 percent of MS patients obtain relief from fatigue by taking amantadine, a drug that triggers dopamine release by the brain. What about sleep and herbs? Discuss these options with your health care professionals.

- The body's ability to obtain deep, healing sleep and nervous system relaxation improves when valerian root and skullcap are ingested. Adding hops to this combination may create a synthesis that works particularly well for your sleep and nerve difficulties (Royal 1982).

- Earl Mindell (1985) suggests a regimen that helps sleep and boosts serotonin. Take 1 chelated calcium and magnesium tab three times per day plus three more thirty minutes before bedtime. Take 100 mg of vitamin B6 and 100 mg of niacinamide, which work in conjuction to produce serotonin, essential for sleep.

Steer Clear of These

Various sources list treatments, techniques, and substances that are regarded as potentially harmful to individuals with MS. As toxins may be related to onset or severity of MS, fluoridated and chlorinated water aren't recommended. Since negative stress is a top contender for triggering MS, steer clear of it. Calcium deficiency may open the door to MS. Also, excessive heat, over-exercising and raising body temperature, sunbathing, and staying in hot water too long are linked with worsening or triggering attacks of MS The same consequences arise if you don't listen to your body and push to exhaustion. Besides steering clear of the foods listed above, you should be on the lookout for potential food allergies and get tested early!

Cindy's Story

Cindy, who has MS, exhibits many of the characteristics linked with "beating the odds" and healing growth.

"I'm not denying it sucks . . . it really does. Hey, it's the luck of the draw and this isn't the worst thing that's happened to me. I look around though and see people with cancer or other diseases that hurt all of the time and are worse than mine . . ." Cindy was diagnosed when she was twenty-nine. The first symptom was straightforward—the entire left side of her body went numb. Not easy to miss this. Then, as often occurs, other symptoms came on gradually. She wondered whether these were just extensions of her existing bout with bursitis. Cindy saw an orthopedic doctor, who told her she might have a tumor on the spine. What a way to start! Fortunately, he promptly referred her to a neurologist, who performed an MRI. Lo and behold, she had the MS-characteristic white spots along the spine and in the brain.

Cindy was among the fortunate few who are diagnosed without years of the doctor shuffle. MS wasn't unknown to her, as her uncle had had serious relapsing-remitting MS and died in his early thirties. Her aunt also has this type, and her sister has rheumatoid arthritis. Her doctor said she might go into remission with her particular condition, but next thing she knew she was hospitalized for several weeks and put on prednisone, with what she laughingly called the "dreaded side effects. It helped but I also ate a lot and my face got fat." She doesn't complain much about the drug, as she's sure it has helped her go into several long remissions. Her next big health change began with difficulty urinating. The doctor shuffle began, as she saw neurologists, urologist, and others, with the final outcome being a wire in her spine, an electrode in front of her spine, and a magnet placed outside her body. While less than ideal, it "certainly helps." Then began the bouts of optic neuritis she's had over the years. What she nicknames "the spiderwebs I see" are indicative of the collapse of the vitreous gel. How is she now? "This year has been difficult because I've been out of remission the whole time, the longest time yet. I've fallen a few times and even managed to dislocate my nose." It's clear that she still can smile and keep her positive attitude.

One thing that helps her stay this way is her good relationship with her husband. She told him early in the courtship about her health and potential long-term consequences. His response? "Hey, and I could get hit by a truck tomorrow." He has the best attitude for living and loving someone with a chronic illness! As you may know from experience and will read about later, conflicts and negative feelings are inevitable. However, listening to Cindy's husband gives us an inside scoop on how to reduce the frequency and bitterness of divisive situations. Cindy told me her husband sometimes becomes angry if she doesn't tell him the truth . . . that it's the MS that is causing her to act or react a certain way. Like many of us, she used to jump to negative automatic thoughts (AT) like "If he hears me 'blaming' it on the illness or even mentioning it once more, that will be it. He has got to be as sick and tired of hearing it as I am of talking about it. The more I mention it, the more he'll think about it and the more he'll want to leave me." Then she would withhold information in a misguided effort to hide this particular white elephant. Doesn't it sound a bit irrational though: "If I don't bring it up, he won't see what a big role it plays and won't be angry at me for having it"? Cindy now sees that as long as she doesn't use her illness as an excuse for her mistakes, talking about it can actually improve her family's feelings: "It helps them realize I'm not just hysterical or moody. They also feel good about my being honest and sharing."

Returning to Cindy's ability to stay optimistic for the most part, it's clear that her self-image and self-talk play central roles. She operates according to several important "rules" I've noticed in SHOC winners: she is realistic; she accepts and yet continues to strive; she doesn't give up; she can get out of her own head and take stock of others' lives and conditions; and she is in touch with her feelings.

I asked Cynthia about the meaning, growth, and healing she has developed from her condition. She responded: " I think having these illnesses or conditions is the luck of the draw. I've seen it in my family, so that is involved, of course. How can I smile? Well, this isn't the worst thing that has happened to me in my life. Hey, I'm not denying that it sucks . . . it really does. But I'm also not going to just sit around and say how terrible it is and never smile. People ask me how I can be so positive . . . well, I'm just not going to sit around being negative. I'm not a Pollyanna, but I do and must thank God that I don't have the other more severe type of MS. I also look around at other people with cancer or other diseases . . . people that are in pain all of the time. In terms of meaning and growth, this gives me more patience and makes me appreciate what I do have. I really am so lucky that I can do just about everything, only slower."

One of her best lessons has been about keeping balance in her life and knowing what she can do in a healthy way to increase her energy, unity with others, and the meaning in her life. One example is that she loves volunteering to talk to people who are ill. Unlike before, she now knows she can't overdo it without paying the price: "When I was first hospitalized, I kept trying to hurry and finish my master's degree and—against protests—even had job interviews from my hospital bed." Her growth in understanding balance is clear as she describes healing: "For me, now it's just to walk and not stumble, to see better, and to not be tired all of the time." I wonder what she would have asked for before, in the early days when she lay in her hospital bed exhausting herself with job interviews rather than healing herself. Her growth and balance are clear in her treatment regimen, which combines Western medical treatment, vitamins, whatever exercise she can manage, and her work on acceptance plus growth and reality rather than choosing the role of a negative, passive victim. She certainly hasn't chosen the easy way out—that is where I think we see the "old" Cindy in her new healing and growth-optimizing lifestyle.

CHAPTER 7

Rheumatoid Arthritis

I feel certain that there will come a day when physiologists, poets and philosophers will all speak the same language.

—Claude Bernard, French physiologist

Rheumatoid arthritis (RA) is a widespread illness with an estimated U.S. prevalence of 2.5 to 3 million and a global estimate of 1 percent of the entire population. Women outnumber men with a ratio of about 3 to 1. The onset typically occurs in a person's twenties, thirties, or forties, although this can vary individually. Like most ARCs, RA is a complicated chronic illness with no definitive known cause and thus no definitive treatment. This systemic disease causes widespread symptoms throughout the body. Fortunately, there are things you can do to reduce the distress and pain it can cause in your life.

RA can be hard to diagnose due to the sheer number and similarities among the many joint disorders. Arthritis means joint inflammation though this name also refers to joint disorders without inflammation. RA is an arthritic condition with great inflammation causing joint warmth, swelling, pain, and stiffness, as well as muscle pain, fatigue, fever, and even depression. One way you and your doctors can differentiate RA from similar conditions, such as osteoarthritis, is to study which joints are affected. In RA, joint pain and inflammation occur on both sides of the body in the fingers, wrists, elbows, shoulders, neck, jaw, knees, ankles, hips, and feet. In addition to these areas, osteoarthritis also causes problems in the neck, hips, fingers, and knees, as well as other joints in the lower back, base of thumbs, and toes.

What Causes Rheumatoid Arthritis?

No single etiology of RA has yet been found, but there are certain factors that contribute to the likelihood of its development. For example, genetics seems involved, as a specific genetic marker, HLA-DR4, occurs on the white blood cells of 65 or even 70 percent of people with RA (Shlotzhauer and McGuire 1993). Those with this genetic marker manifest more severe symptoms of RA. However, up to 25 percent of those with this genetic marker don't have RA. To refresh your memory as to HLA and genetic markers, refer back to chapter 1.

Given that genetics isn't the whole story, scientists have followed a traditional route by exploring whether some type of "stressor" triggers RA in genetically vulnerable people. Stressors explored, with little success to date, include viruses, bacteria, and other elements. There appear to be immune system problems in RA patients: the immune response is triggered (by what is still unclear) and the inflammatory response, an important part of fighting the body's "intruders" that generally subsides when this is complete, remains activated. So the body's own immune response, perhaps due to miscommunication among the white cells responsible for ridding the body of infections, remains activated and "betrays" its own home (i.e., the body) by causing pain and damage. The immune response is also self-defeating in RA with respect to antibody production, in that antibodies or proteins that fight the body's invaders are produced in excessive amounts. An antibody you may have in your blood, rheumatoid factor, further intensifies the whole inflammatory process.

Another theory looks at personality characteristics as determinants of disease. As discussed in the introductory section on personality characteristics and illness, a particular relationship has been thought to exist between personality and rheumatoid arthritis. Bernie Siegel (1986) suggests that chronic RA occurs in people with a lifelong pattern of self-denial. RA patients were described as having consciously restricted their own achievements during their lives. It is true that more women than men enact this pattern because we've often been socialized to put our needs and wants after those of others. However, women differ so greatly from one another, and certainly RA also develops in people who aren't this way. While this theory is still being debated, there is evidence substantiating the association between personality factors and certain illnesses, and further research is certainly warranted. Whether or not this theory is accurate, this doesn't negate the fact that your thoughts, behaviors, and characteristics can be used to turn the odds in favor of your health. Also, if you're open to the fact that by modifying characteristics and beliefs, you directly improve your mind-body health and life satisfaction, you'll have very powerful tools along your journey toward reclaiming your life.

Symptoms and Signs

RA strikes only one of the three types of joints in our bodies. These are the freely movable, or synovial, joints, which include: knees, ankles, hips, fingers, elbows, wrists, and shoulders. Joints are complex structures composed of many parts, and RA affects various parts of joints, such as areas of bone beneath cartilage, or the tendons, which connect muscle to bone.

One of the key signs of RA is inflammation. Your white blood cells, central to the immune system, work together to produce poisonous substances that kill invaders and cause inflammation. The key difference between a normal defensive reaction and what occurs in RA inflammation is that in the latter case, the "intruder" is unknown. There may indeed be a virus or other foreign body (antigen) present; however, if so, their precise identity is as of yet unclear. In addition, in a normal immune response, the antigens are destroyed and removed from the body, while it's possible that this process doesn't function adequately in RA. Also, in RA, the body's lymphocytes involved in fighting the intruder remain in a hyperaroused, activated state leading to the continued inflammatory process, which causes the joint damage and arthritic swelling and pain.

Through the course of the illness, other changes arise. Your joints may feel warm while stiffness increases and normal range of joint motion decreases. People with RA often have more severe stiffness in the morning and after sitting for some time. At this time, you may experience increasing fatigue which can be worsened by a condition affecting one-half to two-thirds of RA patients; namely, anemia caused by decreased numbers of the red blood cells that deliver oxygen to tissues. Even at this stage, if you get medical attention, your symptoms can be treated. If not, RA progresses and your body continues to self-destruct. Enzymes called collagenases appear and destroy collagen, the proteins of cartilage; they also create small pockets in the bone. Finally, more enzymes that continue to destroy cartilage and bone are produced, thereby decreasing soft cushioning between the bones of the joints. As cartilage is lost or damaged, smooth joint motion suffers, causing a rough, grating sensation called crepitus when you move your joints. Doctors can find this by touching your joints. At this point, many muscles are weakened and shrunken through lack of use. All of this causes the joints to no longer function properly. Finally, cartilage may be completely destroyed, at which point there is decreased inflammation, and joint structures, completely stretched out, are very unstable and undependable.

There are other symptoms and changes you may experience. Most of these aren't serious but should be watched or brought to your health caretaker's attention in case they indicate a severe RA case. You may develop dry eyes and mouth, which usually aren't too serious but can be uncomfortable. If eyes become too dry, this may preclude contact lens use. Dry mouth can lead to extensive dental decay unless properly handled. (For remedies for these conditions, refer to the Sjogren's syndrome [SS] chapter, chapter 9). If dry eyes are caused by serious but rare conditions, episcleritis and scleritis, you must inform your health expert, who will refer you to an eye care specialist. You may notice small skin bumps, called rheumatoid nodules, developing near joints over areas often bumped or jarred, like knuckles and elbows. These aren't usually serious or painful unless they're infected or located in a place that is frequently hit. Report such nodules to your doctor as they sometimes indicate a more serious type of the disease. Surgery is infrequent; a prescription of a course of medication known as DMARDs (description below) is more usual.

Related Conditions and Look-alikes

As with the other ARCs, you may have waited quite long for your accurate diagnosis of RA. It's less likely you were faced with the "It's all in your head" accusation frequently directed at women with fibromyalgia or chronic fatigue. But as with those disorders, RA can seem to fit the criteria of many different conditions, including the two just mentioned, other ARCs like systemic lupus erythematosus (SLE), and inflammatory and noninflammatory arthritic conditions. Other diagnoses to rule out include ankylosing spondylitis, Reiter's disease, arthritis associated with psoriasis or colitis, gout, and pseudo-gout. As RA patients can have dry eyes and mouth with joint pain and inflammation, doctors may have to rule out Sjogren's syndrome.

One frequent problem in diagnosis is that even the more definitive diagnostic tests don't show the disturbance in the early stages. Often, these tests must be given some time after the disorder's onset so the markers the test is designed to measure have developed. As mentioned earlier, there is no replacement for a medical person's knowledge to retest and use various tests. Commitment to truly listening to your story and reported symptoms is also crucial.

Because of the complexities of diagnosis, the following list will help you in your exploration and improved understanding of your particular case. In addition, it will enable you to be an informed member of your very own SHOC team.

Arthritis Related to Colitis

Colitis is one of the bowel diseases collectively known as irritable bowel syndrome (IBS). The most common complication of IBS is joint involvement, with 25 percent having joint problems, though not all are arthritic conditions. The most prevalent joint complaint among people with IBS is arthralgia or joint achiness. Arthritis differs as it involves inflammation and joint tenderness and redness. Several forms of arthritis are linked with IBS, the most frequent, monoarthritis, in which one joint, knees or ankles, are affected at a time. Even more likely to be confused with RA is the IBS arthritis, polyarthritis, which moves among several joints. This type of migrating arthritis can look like RA, although the IBS-related arthritis types don't cause permanent joint damage and can be less serious than RA. The proper diagnosis is essential as the treatments differ. Treatment of the latter focuses on the bowel disorder with prednisone or sulfasalazine prescribed to control diarrhea and bleeding. Prednisone robs the body of vitamins C and B6, and zinc and potassium. Use appropriate supplements if you're on prednisone for some time. Another IBS-related arthritis is sacroileitis, which is fairly minor and affects the lower spine and pelvis. However, IBS is also related to a severe rare form of arthritis and autoimmune condition, ankylosing spondylitis, which attacks the spine and sometimes the shoulders, hips, and knees.

Anemia

A detailed look at anemia is essential because it may arise from various causes in RA, including one that is potentially dangerous. Anemia, the loss of significant numbers of red blood cells, can occur whenever inflammation is present for an extended period. This type is called anemia of chronic disease. Anemia may also be a side effect of medicines used to reduce inflammation (nonsteroidal anti-inflammatory drugs, also known as NSAIDs).

Felty's Syndrome

While rare, affecting less than 1 percent of RA patients, Felty's syndrome can be dangerous and warrants mention. The anemia resulting from Felty's syndrome contributes to the fatigue and weakness experienced by people with RA. Equal to red blood cell loss from Felty's syndrome is the perilous loss of white blood cells central to the body's ability to withstand infections. Another harmful loss in the blood from Felty's syndrome is the decrease of platelets, which allow your blood to clot. If you have fewer platelets and are injured, you risk excessive blood loss.

Ankylosing Spondylitis

This disorder goes by a variety of names: ankylosing spondylitis, strumpell-marie, marie-strumpell, bekhterev-strumpell, and spondyloarthritis. This is one of the arthritic conditions that occurs in conjunction with IBS. It's a chronic, progressive autoimmune disease that shares some symptoms with RA. It's very painful and involves inflammation, arthritis, ultimate immobility of various joints, and sometimes fusing of the spine and pelvis. In general, onset occurs between 15 and 35 years of age. This autoimmune disease is notable in that it's more prevalent in men, by a three to one ratio. When women develop this disorder, it's typically milder.

Sjogren's Syndrome

Because people with RA may experience dry eyes, dry mouth, joint pain, stiffness, muscle aches, and inflammation, all symptoms of SS, doctors may need to rule out this syndrome.

Gout and Pseudo-Gout

Fortunately, RA is fairly easily distinguished from both gout and pseudo-gout through particular tests. Doctors draw samples of the fluid from affected joints, and if crystals are detected within the fluid, it's likely the patient has gout or pseudo-gout. To differentiate between these two, a doctor discerns the makeup of these crystals. If uric acid is detected, the diagnosis would be gout, whereas if calcium is detected, the diagnosis would be pseudo-gout. Women's hormones, thought by some to cause ARCs and other illnesses, actually seem protective against gout. It appears that estrogen prevents the accumulation of uric acid until menopause, whereas this process is a continuous one from puberty onwards in men. However, this protection is not absolute. There is a genetic process in gout; if it runs in your family, you have a chance of developing it. Other causes of gout in women include being overweight, taking anticancer or blood pressure medications, and having high levels of triglycerides in the blood.

Osteoarthritis

RA is sometimes confused with osteoarthritis, also called degenerative joint disease. The most common type of arthritis, osteoarthritis affects about 16 million Americans. While the two share some of the same affected joints, the overall patterns differ: rheumatoid arthritis affects feet, ankles, knees, hips, fingers, wrists, elbows, shoulders, neck, jaw, and sternoclavicular joints; osteoarthritis affects toes, knees, hips, fingers, base of thumbs, lower back, and neck

Lyme Disease

From forty-eight cases when the numbers were first tallied in 1983 to the currently wide disparity in estimated number of cases, which ranges from 11,250 to 400,000 (Lang 1997), this disease is the most common U.S. illness caused by ticks. Lyme disease represents a serious international health problem as well. In Germany, the illness has hit epidemic proportions, with an estimated 5 to 10 percent of the entire population being infected. Many other countries in Europe, regions in Russia, and portions of China and Japan also have high rates of incidence. The area of infection is often called a bull's-eye rash because the center may clear up while the infection spreads outwards in a circular pattern. Other symptoms include muscle weakness, fever, rashes, facial paralysis, inability to sleep, fatigue, flulike symptoms, neck and back pain, general achiness, headaches, nausea and vomiting, enlargement of the spleen and lymph glands, enlargement of the heart muscle, abnormal heart rhythm, joint pains attacking the knees, pain and swelling in other joints, and even degenerative muscle disease. Some of the symptoms shared with RA include swelling and pain in the joints, fever, fatigue, muscle weakness, pains, and achiness.

Chlamydia and Silicone Breast Implants

Chlamydia is an organism associated with the onset of urethritis. It also seems to be linked with the onset of a type of arthritis appearing in young women. Over the last decade, there has been an uproar on the part of many women who seem to be experiencing myriad negative health consequences associated with silicone breast implants, including symptoms linked with arthritis, such as fever, joint inflammation, pain, and severe fatigue. Also, some with silicone breast implants have elevated levels of antibodies that target collagen. The presence of silicone in the body has also been assoicated with the presence of other autoimmune disorders, such as scleroderma and lupus. Some product manufacturers are finally beginning to partially compensate these women financially.

A True Story of Diagnostic Confusion

Thirty-eight-year-old Janis now knows she has both RA and fibromyalgia syndrome (FMS). From the section about diagnostic confusion, you understand part of why she didn't come by this knowledge easily. In fact, it took ten years of severe pain in her shoulders before she thought something might really be wrong. This pain was worsened by her job of lifting clothes to place on display. She continued to think, as many women do early on, that her symptoms were just a sign of getting older or having a mild injury . . . something that would pass with time. However, over the last ten years, she has experienced many strange symptoms. As her feet and ankles became increasingly painful, she couldn't find any bearable shoes: "I thought everyone had problems like these." She also had an increasing number of sinus infections and bouts of fatigue. Again, as many of us do, she waited. As is typical of autoimmune conditions, the symptoms were diverse and didn't point to any particular disease entity.

Finally, her symptoms became so severe that she went for help. The saddest fact is that she'd actually seen a doctor eight years ago who had found rheumatoid factor in her blood. Despite knowing that her father, his mother, and others in her family had RA, he downplayed it and sent her back to a life of pain and confusion. Fortunately, she found a rheumatologist who was, in her words, "great." He was also able to diagnose her FMS. His treatment approach has been wholly patient oriented. He hasn't denied prescriptions for things like therapeutic massage, nor does he have an "I know it all" attitude. While he bases his decisions on knowledge and experience, he combines this with respect for her abilities and intellect. She has used various pain medications, including Tylenol with codeine, Darvocet, Ultram, oxycontin, and methadone. Methadone is most helpful in reducing pain, but she wonders, as most of us do, about long-term consequences of such drugs. Thus, she doesn't rely solely on drugs, but integrates them with alternative methods like meditation, prayer, and diet. The FMS pain is worse for her, particularly given its frequency, while the RA joint pain is intermittent and manageable. She uses Celebrex and Zoloft for cognitive functioning and sleep.

She is careful to maintain an active, involved life. Her husband and child help get her out of her head and focus on others—an extremely effective tool! Janis endorses the importance of family and how potent others can be in healing: "If it weren't for my child, I often wouldn't get out of bed!" Janis has some characteristics many women with autoimmune conditions have. She's a striver, an achiever, and her earlier overwork, overextension, and resulting stress and fatigue may have partly triggered her conditions. Particularly with FMS and CFIDS, patients are often self-admitted perfectionists, overworkers, achievers, and doers.

Janis' condition deteriorated such that she and her SHOC team decided she ought to stop working and work instead on herself. When I asked her about the meaning of healing and what she had gained from these experiences, she answered with thought and optimism: "I see healing not only as 'getting better,' but as exploring and healing problems in my life. Now I try to do everything in the proper way (i.e., meditation, prayer, exercise, rest). Of course, I could eat more vegetables! I've learned to live every day to the very best, not to take things for granted, and to enjoy everything, even walking down the street!" Any advice for fellow women? "Keep their heads up, don't get depressed, try to keep moving in your life and literally as well. Listen to your body and slow down when you need to. When I can't exercise, at least I stretch. Listen to your body for once and do any good things for it you can. That's the way."

The Courses of Rheumatoid Arthritis

If you've been diagnosed with RA, remember that descriptions of time frames and courses are only generalizations. Your individual case can vary greatly. Still, you must educate yourself as much as possible as this is the starting point of your creating your self- and health-optimization course (SHOC). Learn what to expect in general, your options, the specialists in your area, the best modalities, both Western and Eastern, and what you can do to stretch any confines of your condition and grow in other ways.

RA symptoms usually begin in one or more joints on both sides of the body. You may feel stiffness, pain, and fatigue and may not notice inflammation for several months. A gradual onset, symmetrical symptoms, and continuous progression are typical. However, you could just as well experience sudden strong pain, inflammation, and stiffness followed by a repetitive disappearance and then resurgence of symptoms. Or, you might feel a general malaise and achiness rather than specific painful joints and stiffness. On a positive note, as many as 20 percent of RA patients experience spontaneous remission at some point during the illness. This doesn't mean a magical cure, as 50 percent again develop RA symptoms. Your job is to work at beating these odds or at least decrease the severity of RA and increase your life satisfaction and fulfillment.

Testing for Rheumatoid Arthritis

As of today, no single test can definitively diagnose or rule out RA. Someday this may be possible. At present, your doctor should rely on a variety of information sources: your reports of current and past symptoms; factors you see as related to symptom changes; symptom onset; previous health-related concerns, illnesses, operations, or allergies; medications taken (even if some time ago); mind-body stressors (past or ongoing); lifestyle habits (diet, exercise, smoking, drinking, drugs, exposure to other toxins); social history and childhood experiences possibly related to your current physical health; your family's physical health history; the doctor's physical exam; records from your other doctors; observations of your illness' course; and a variety of tests. Be thoroughly prepared with as much information as possible, as many associated dates as you can recall or have in writing, and names of hospitals or treatment centers. Always get your medical record copies, because taking them to the next doctor can save months of wasted time.

Now you'll read about testing to identify RA, detect changes in the course, and rule out differential diagnoses. This knowledge helps you decipher medi-speak (should it sound like a foreign tongue) and assists you in using the jargon if necessary when asking questions and stating preferences. Remember, being an active, assertive partner in the treatment phase of your SHOC increases your sense of control, your immune system functioning, and your chances of improvement.

As with a number of autoimmune-related conditions, it can be risky to diagnose RA based solely upon test results. When it comes to diagnosis, our medical system's traditional emphasis on the outcomes of tests as the only "real" data to consider is problematic. More holistic approaches to health, which consider the extensive information listed above, can be superior for diagnosing complex disorders, such as autoimmune-related conditions. RA tests may even contribute to misdiagnosis and poor treatment. During the early phases of RA, blood tests and X-rays may appear normal, leading to the conclusion that treatment is unnecessary. However, RA's early phases are also when intervention can be most effective. You'll now be aware that a comprehensive approach is essential, and if your health care professional relies only on limited informational sources, no matter how cutting-edge, you need to assume responsibility and exert control over the aspects you can control, namely, discussing testing options and, if you feel shutdown, considering whether you'd be better served by a different doctor.

X-rays are often used to diagnose and track changes, although they may not be very telling during early RA. They're used to spot decreasing cartilage between bones (on the X-ray, this looks like bones moving closer together) and the small pockets in bones described earlier. More advanced tests, like magnetic resonance imaging (MRI) and computed tomography scan (CAT scan), are helpful in showing soft tissue, muscle, cartilage, and joints in addition to bone. X-rays can also be used to rule out other illnesses that cause similar symptoms to RA.

Blood tests help diagnose RA, provided their limitations are considered. One blood test tracks the rate at which red blood cells settle in a test tube (sedimentation), which indicates the amount of inflammation. The faster the settling, the more inflammation, although this doesn't necessarily indicate RA. A test that's superior in pinpointing RA examines the number of white blood cells (neutrophils) in fluid removed from a swollen, painful joint. The more neutrophils, the more likely RA is the culprit. A blood test that illustrates the similarities among ARCs is the antinuclear antibody blood test. This may indicate RA when abnormal results are obtained; however, similar results can also suggest systemic lupus erythematosus, Sjogren's syndrome, scleroderma, and connective tissue disease. Briefly, antinuclear antibodies (ANA) differ from the usual antibodies in that they don't only seek invaders or foreign antigens to destroy. Instead, ANA indiscriminately react to the nuclear material or proteins from cells. To antinuclear antibodies, these are the bad guys, or antigens, and many harmful physical consequences to the human body can result from this error.

Biopsies in which your doctor removes a bit of tissue from a joint are often used to test for RA. If you hear your doctor mention arthroscopic biopsy, don't panic. It's like traditional biopsies but gives a view of the inside of your joint. Neither type is very painful.

As referred to earlier in the discussion on potential causes of RA, a specific genetic marker, HLA-DR4, can be found on the white blood cells of about 65 percent of people with RA and suggests susceptibility to developing it. Thus, a blood test is useful, though it can't be used alone as a valid measure because about 25 percent of those with the genetic marker don't have RA.

What You Can Do

Remember, your body is unique. The last thing in the world you should do is ignore symptoms or distress because they just don't seem to fit descriptions you've read or heard about. You must be in touch with your body and its changes. If you suspect something is amiss, even though it doesn't follow any rigid description, see a professional. The sooner you determine whether something is wrong and what it is, the sooner you can begin forming your plan of attack, researching the illness and good health professionals, working on your attitudes, and thus reducing the speed of progression or degree of damage. This all fits into your toolbag for beating the odds. Secondly, your body's uniqueness means that you may need different treatments, including alternative types, or that you may do better integrating the services of different types of health care helpers. Remember, there is no such thing as 100 percent certainty in any doctor's diagnosis or prognosis. You'll have to develop mind-body integrity so as you travel along your unique path, you connect with your SHOC team in a timely way if medications aren't working, if side effects crop up, or if things take an unexpected turn. Just as your body's uniqueness is one reason you'll have an individual experience, so, too, the uniqueness of your mind will contribute to disparities in your particular situation. Don't forget the role your mind, emotions, and behavior play in either improving or worsening your own particular symptoms, pain, distress, and prognosis.

Cutting-Edge Medications

When it comes to treating RA, the most widely used method is medication. At this writing, wonderful things were happening with medications. A new medication, etanercept or Enbrel, the first genetically engineered protein to combat RA, was touted as the newest RA treatment. The improvements from this medication seem rapid, appearing in as little as two weeks and continuing as long as six months. With a higher, 25 mg dosage after six months, patients' average tender points decreased by 56 percent. Subjects receiving 10 mg dosages had tender points decrease by 44 percent! At this time, it's still unknown if the drug can stop disease progression in the crucial early years. In addition, there was significant initial excitement going at research centers, schools, and hospitals about the discovery of the first new agent designed for treating RA in particular in over ten years. The new drug, leflunomide, will be known as Arava. This drug reduces RA's symptoms and actually *slows the deterioration* of joints and structural damage. Because this structural damage can develop as early as the first year or two of RA, timely diagnosis and intervention with Arava can be critical.

Nonsteroidal Anti-inflammatory Drugs (NSAIDs)

These medications have been among the mainstays of RA treatment and are often used early in the course and during flare-ups. Given the frequency of their use and the number of potential negative side effects, I've focused on them so you can educate yourself sufficiently. These drugs come under a variety of names: aspirin (acetylsalicylic acid), naproxen (Naprosyn), ibuprofen (Advil, Motrin, Nuprin), piroxicam (Feldene), and indomethacine (Indocin). While they're from different chemical categories, they all work like aspirin. They differ from acetaminophen (Tylenol being the most recognized brand) in that they reduce swelling and decrease pain. These drugs quickly reduce inflammation, joint and muscle pain, fever, and sometimes fatigue. Sound like miracle drugs? Unfortunately, one of the biggest problems with NSAIDs is adverse side effects, some of which are fatal. According to the U.S. FDA, as many as 10,000 to 20,000 annual fatalities stem from NSAIDs, which can cause liver damage, stomach ulcers, kidney problems, and gastrointestinal (GI) bleeding. Some of these effects occur because NSAIDs target prostaglandins, which may cause unwanted inflammation but also protect against irritation of the stomach lining.

You must be cautious when taking NSAIDs; if you have stomach pain, heartburn, nausea, vomiting, or bloody stools, it's essential you contact your SHOC team immediately. For those who use NSAIDs over the long term, there are some other medications that can reduce the chances of such damage. Misoprostol (Cytotec) actually helps increase stomach prostaglandins, thereby reducing chances of GI damage. Medications that protect against ulcers by interfering with stomach acid production, such as antacids (e.g., Maalox) or H2-receptor blockers (e.g., Tagamet, Zantac) may be helpful. Carafate functions differently by creating a "new" layer of stomach protection. Another option is misoprostol, which may proactively prevent GI damage. However, if you're considering having children or are currently pregnant, steer clear of this drug as it can lead to miscarriage. Inform your doctor immediately so she or he can prescribe a different medication. If you don't fit into this category but are a smoker or have had GI problems, misoprostol may be your best bet. Many people can tolerate NSAIDs well; however, if you've had previous ulcers or GI bleeding, are over sixty-five years of age, or have any kidney or liver problems, you must be cautious.

If you're taking NSAIDs, you must stay in close contact with your SHOC team, so that if any signs of adverse effects, such as bloody stools, decreased blood flow, or liver toxicity are detected, testing and alternative treatment plans can be put into place. Also, since some NSAIDs cause bleeding problems, if you have surgery or a dental appointment, stop your medicine several days (or in the case of aspirin, at least 2 weeks) in advance.

COX-2 Inhibitors

Quite recently, there was much celebration in the scientific community, among drug companies, and within the media of a drug called Celebrex. This was the first of a class of drugs called COX-2 inhibitors, which had been effective in treating both osteoarthritis and RA. The main reason for their fame was that pre-liminary studies suggested that these drugs didn't produce the harmful side effects of NSAIDs, such as ulcers and GI disturbances. One month later, though, press reports appeared stating that the future of these drugs wasn't as rosy as first thought. Evidence seemed to suggest that the drugs might have their own host of negative side effects, including heart attacks, strokes, and cardiovascular problems. At the time of this writing, the debate was heating up as to this drug's safety. By the time you read this, more information will have been revealed. Make sure you and your doctor have the most recent information regarding its safety.

Whereas NSAIDs don't truly impact RA's underlying disease state or pro-gression, other medicines called disease-modifying antirheumatic drugs (DMARDs) are used to jump-start a remission. If you're having more periods of increased symptoms and pain, or if they're long-term and increasingly disruptive, then it's probably wise to introduce these drugs into your toolbag. As mentioned above, DMARDs are often used in patients who have developed rheumatic nod-ules, which may indicate a more serious disease process. Due to potential adverse effects, you and your doctor may wait and see if symptom remission occurs by itself or with NSAIDs. However, since DMARDs are most effective if used early, and since they may take weeks or months to work, DMARDs may be an option when remission is unlikely or joint damage is occurring. If your disease has a rapid onset and deteriorating course, DMARDs may be best to slow or stop this rapid progression. Today's medications can be quite effective, and efforts con-tinue to discover more effective medicines. No cures have yet been found, so it's in your best interest to search for various ways to ease your pain and distress.

While medicines can be effective, you won't gain the best edge against the odds by relying solely on them. People with RA these days have much greater chances of beating the odds and leading more productive, full, enjoyable lives. It's almost certain that your experience with RA will not be as negative, frightening, or disruptive as it would have been even a decade ago.

Mind-Body Techniques

• Keeping up on new medications

• Surgical techniques and tools for protecting the joints

- Education about and the use of appropriate physical therapies

- Nutrition, vitamins and minerals, herbs

- Biofeedback, meditation, relaxation, visualization, and pain management techniques

- Acupuncture, acupressure, and other noninvasive techniques

- Psychotherapy and chronic illness counseling

- Assertiveness and proactivity in dealing with the illness and your SHOC team

- Cognitive techniques: thought monitoring, modifying, stopping

- Coping skills training and socializing

The key to maximizing your life and movement toward healing and growth lies in combining appropriate types of conventional and alternative treatments. This is akin to the general notion of keeping balance in all areas of your life. It's a key component of your SHOC. Extremes can trigger relapses or a worsening of symptoms. Moderation and balance take work, but they greatly increase your odds of living life to the fullest. Keeping your life balanced is one of the promises of growth if you choose to seek the challenge rather than retreat.

Buyer Beware

Many seeking alternative treatments believe that because they are "natural," they can cause no harm. While these tools can be incredibly effective, you do need to treat them with caution. Just as with conventional medicine, you must assume an active, responsible role and ensure you're working with trained professionals with appropriate certification or license (if applicable), training, and experience. Do your best to find one who has worked extensively in and possibly even researched or written about your particular disorder. This should be a basic element in the design and practice of your SHOC. You simply owe it to yourself.

There is actually a well-known program that incorporates various elements from the above list and has been found effective in treating RA. Theodore Pincus, in an excellent article appearing in the 1993 *Mind/Body Medicine*, describes the Arthritis Self-Help Course, which includes education, coping, communication, relaxation training, and nutritional suggestions. People who have followed this program report a 15 to 20 percent reduction in pain, less depression, fewer doctor's visits, and more active, social lives. Check appendix I for the Arthritis Foundation listing.

As with the other conditions in this book, you can refer to later chapters on general coping, and will find here management, optimizing, and coping tools most relevant to RA.

The Power of Human Touch

While medicines remain as primary treatments, they don't always ease pain. There is also the chance that long-term or high-dosage analgesic usage may produce liver or renal failure. Medications have their uses, but why don't we consider how we can use our mind-body resources to ease our own pain? Such was the question posed by a study comparing therapeutic touch to progressive muscle relaxation to reduce chronic arthritis pain (Peck 1997). Pain and distress levels from the study's start to the end showed significant decreases for both techniques. Integrating these alternative treatments is a humane, effective action that must be taken.

Fresh Air and Exercise

These very words conjure up images of health and vitality. With so many warnings about exposing ourselves to the sun, it's important to know that people with RA derive benefits from the sun's warming rays. The sun assists synthesis of vitamin D, which is essential in proper bone development. However, if you also have lupus, you must discuss the risks of sun exposure with your health professional. The issue of exercise is tricky when it comes to autoimmune-related disorders because the intensity and type of exercise affects different conditions differently, at times intensifying symptoms. When it comes to RA, it's important to strive for regular moderate exercise while avoiding extreme exhaustion and activities that place excessive stress on joints, muscles, and bones. Good exercises for RA include swimming, moderately paced walking, and other low-impact exercises. Exercising in water is a component of hydrotherapy, a technique that uses heated water and body movements to treat a range of physical disorders. Hydrotherapy increases muscle strength and joint flexibility while protecting the body from gravity's impact.

Acupuncture, Acupressure, and Massage

Here, we'll briefly explore how these techniques work and how they can be applied to RA. Many of my patients and associates have said that these methods significantly reduce their pain and stiffness, improve their sleep, and increase their energy. Studies, including the theapeutic touch research cited above, corroborate these reports. The connection established through touch with another human being offers you somatic, or physical, healing. Not only is touch physically healing, but it also improves your emotional state, an obvious conclusion given the notion of mind-body unity upon which this book is based. A variety of techniques based on touch can achieve specific goals, such as reducing pain, increasing flexibility, opening blockages, realignment, and reestablishing body balance. Massage is one of these; it can be very useful for RA patients whose movement is limited. When you're experiencing a bout of severe RA, the manipulation, movement, and stretching act as a type of exercise, albeit a more passive version. Massage, though, offers mind-body benefits at all times, as you can read about in appendix II, which discusses specific types of massage. Acupuncture and acupressure are also helpful in reducing pain and stiffness for many people with RA. A detailed exploration appears in appendix II and referrals are listed in appendix I.

As of this writing, there was growing excitement about a potential treatment for RA known as pulsed signal therapy (PST). It works on painful, inflamed joints linked with chronic neck and back pain, as well as arthritis, by sending a biological signal through a magnetic field. The signals are sent on programmed frequencies to specific areas of connective tissue and cartilage to boost the body's own healing process by increasing the metabolic rate of cartilage cells. There are reports of successful treatment of arthritis and other painful chronic conditions. Treatments last for one to two months, are painless, and haven't yet been found to produce side effects. At the time of this writing, the treatment has been approved in England, Italy, Germany, Canada, and France, and it's pending for the U.S. Because this treatment is new and hasn't been sufficiently studied, you should check with your SHOC team before trying PST.

Hot or Cold? Dry or Wet?

These four conditions have been used to treat illnesses and ailments for centuries. However, debates remain as to which of the four should be used to treat particular conditions. For example, one doctor may tell you to apply ice packs to reduce pain, while another may tell you to use heating pads. One expert may tell you only moist heat will do, while another says this is nonsense. All in all, find out what works best for you. Some people swear by icing, while others shudder at the mere thought. With respect to RA, most people report benefits from using heat and moist heat. Interestingly enough, immersing the body in a neutral temperature bath (95 degrees F.) for about two hours can reduce the joint inflammation of RA (Burton Goldberg Group 1997). If you don't have the two hours suggested, the use of hot compresses, saunas, or warm baths and showers is effective in reducing pain, relaxing your muscles, and releasing significant, widespread tension in your body. The newest findings also point to balance in the manner of yin and yang in that alternating heat and cold seems most effective in reducing pain.

Nutritional Enhancement

While this book discusses nutrition and its role in illness and health, it shouldn't be your sole source of information on this subject. Don't use herbs, nutritionals supplements, or other substances without consulting your doctor or as your only treatment. The suggestions presented here cannot and should not take the place of direct consultation with your medical professional, nutritionist, or other trained health professional. At the same time, this is an area in which you can benefit greatly by consulting herbalists, holistic nutritional counselors, and the like.

RA is associated with malnutrition, but not the sort of which we usually think. This type of malnutrition exists even in the face of abundant food and liquid, because many people with RA cannot extract valuable vitamins, minerals, and other substances from food they consume. Also, food allergies can be linked with RA, as you'll read about later.

Melvyn Werbach (1993) states that many RA patients have low levels of pantothenic acid and vitamin C. He describes a study in which giving pantothenic acid led to significant declines in pain and in the duration of morning stiffness. If you have RA, your body may not be absorbing or using enough vitamin C even if you eat healthfully. Frequent bruising and skin hemorrhaging is helped by vitamin C. Vitamins C, B6, E, and zinc seem to improve connective tissue repair and collagen generation, which produces cartilage in your body. Red berries and cherries may also boost collagen production. Good juices include carrot and cucumber, lemon juice before meals, and when symptoms are severe, one pint to one quart of celery juice daily. Try to avoid tomato juice (Burton Goldberg Group 1997).

Two factors that deplete vitamin C and call for increased consumption are cigarette smoking and frequent use of aspirin. Vitamin C is also present in a variety of herbs and foods, including cayenne, dandelion, garlic, horseradish, kelp, plantain, papaya, raspberry, rose hips, strawberry, and watercress. While alfalfa contains C, you should know that excessive use of alfalfa may be linked with the onset of autoimmune symptoms in vulnerable individuals. If you're a tea drinker, you may be in luck, as anecdotal claims say that Kombucha tea is rife with health-promoting nutrients and has been very effective for some in reducing RA stiffness and pain.

You've probably heard of melatonin, which has received an incredible amount of press. It has been touted as the cure for insomnia, jet lag, cancer, aging, and chronic pain. There is some corroboration for expecting relief in some of these areas. However, melatonin is not recommended for people with ARCs, such as RA and lupus (Rosenfeld 1996).

Iron is usually a healthy nutrient; however, with arthritis it can intensify pain, joint damage, and inflammation. Try to stick with iron from foods (i.e., broccoli, cauliflower, fish, peas, lima beans) rather than taking iron supplements or vitamins with iron.

Collagen Formation and Connective Tissue Repair

Some experts believe that foods from the nightshade family contain alkaloids that interfere with collagen formation. These foods also contain solanine, a substance to which people with arthritis are often vulnerable. It causes pain by interfering with enzyme functioning and formation in the muscles. Just as time is required to rule out allergens, it may also take time to find out if members of the nightshade family affect your condition negatively. If so, you don't have to banish these foods entirely, but you will have to greatly reduce the frequency and quantity of consumption. This is important to know, as some of these foods, like eggplants, peppers, tomatoes, and potatoes, may play a big role in your diet. It may turn out that you aren't affected by nightshade plants and so can reintroduce them into your diet.

Much attention has also been given to glucosamine sulfate, which may help in collagen generation and cartilage repair. Researchers believe glucosamine thickens the synovial fluid that bathes the joints, thereby protecting and lubricating them, and reducing pain. Most of these studies have been done on people with osteoarthritis rather than RA (Rosenfeld 1996). More research for RA is needed, though findings to date seem positive. Another newly released product, Collastin, works as an immune system modulator inhibiting leukotriene B4 generation, which reduces some of RA's immune system dysregulation. This product seems to be most effective when taken with zinc, vitamin C, glucosamine, and manganese.

L-Cysteine, a detoxifying amino acid central to immune functioning, is also an element of collagenous tissue. Take 500 mg twice per day on an empty stomach with water or juice (not milk); its best when taken with 50 mg vitamin B6 and 100 mg vitamin C (Balch and Balch 1997).

Other substances involved in essential connective tissue repair, strengthening, and rebuilding include: silica (supplying silicon); copper (taken in conjunction with 2,000 mg per day of calcium and 1,000 mg per day of magnesium); 60 mg per day of coenzyme Q10; free-form amino acid complex; multivitamin complex with 10,000 I.U. vitamin A per day; 15,000 I.U. per day of natural beta-carotene; and pycnogenol or grape seed extract (Balch and Balch 1997). I also suggest taking MSM daily to provide sulfur, or at least eating onions, eggs, and garlic, which contain sulfur.

All Fats Are Not Created Equal

Among experts, there is some consensus about general amounts and types of nutrients you should have. The common component among different viewpoints is that low-fat, low-protein diets are health-enhancing if you have an autoimmune-related condition. Please recall that your needs are unique; you should work early on with a nutritionist, physician or other health care professional trained in nutrition and knowledgeable about your particular autoimmune-related condition. Some experts claim vegetarian diets are best. This doesn't mean strict vegetarianism, as some fish and the fat they provide are essential for you. Didn't I just say that many experts favor low-fat diets? Yes, but the fact is that not all fats are created equal. You'll want to decrease some fats and increase others. Greatly reducing polyunsaturated vegetable oils and partially hydrogenated fats while increasing amounts of omega-3 fatty acids is the healthy way to go. The two groups of essential fatty acids (EFA), omega-3 and omega-6, are important for autoimmune conditions because they have anti-inflammatory effects and reduce joint pain, morning stiffness, and muscle weakness.

Anti-Inflammatories

Given the damage of inflammation, nutrients with anti-inflammatory properties, such as those listed below, are essential in reducing disturbing symptoms including pain, swelling, and stiffness.

- *Vitamin B complex* daily with *primrose oil*, an *omega-6 EFA*; also seeds, nuts, beans

- *Omega-3 fatty acids* by supplement or eating at least 2 servings per week of tuna, salmon, shark, herring, and mackerel. Deep sea fish also helps reduce fatigue and painful joints due to anti-inflammatory properties. Other omega-3 are vegetable oils, canola and flaxseed, which should be consumed in supplement or natural forms. Don't expose these oils to heat.

- *Grape seed extract* and *shark cartilage*

- *Vitamin C*: 3,000 to 10,000 mg per day in several doses with bioflavonoids, 500 mg per day, which increase vitamin C's potency (Balch and Balch 1997)

- Fresh *pineapple* containing the anti-inflammatory enzyme bromelain

- *Anti-TGF-B* injections reduce joint inflammation by 75 percent (Balch and Balch 1997)

- Bee venom (may also boost immune system functioning)

Sweet and Gooey: What a Pain

It's convenient and tasty to start the day off with some donuts and coffee. A few hours later, when you're feeling lethargic and low, it's time for that candy bar and cola. When lunch hour rolls around and you're off to do some errands, you may have just enough time to hit the drive-thru, pick up a greaseburger, fries, and shake, and gobble it down while rushing back to the office or home. When the inevitable four o'clock slump arrives, you pray that vending machine selling candy or chips down the hall is working or that you have some sugary or fatty snacks at home. Dinner . . . well, you get the picture; don't forget that late night snack attack! Maybe it's a different scenario for you. Exhausted, stiff, and in pain, you barely manage to get out of bed or off the couch at times. You certainly don't feel up to making a fresh, healthy meal or cutting up crisp fruit and veggies for a snack. Maybe you can toss some frozen food into the microwave and get the fatty, bland stuff down. Maybe that is still too hard and you're feeling depressed, so a nice bag of cookies or chips sounds like the perfect prescription.

Whatever the cause, it's so easy to fall into unhealthy eating habits these days. Sugar, fat, and caffeine are real trouble, particularly if you have an ARC like RA and have severe pain and stiffness. These substances may give you a rush or surge in energy. As you probably know, this peak is temporary and soon you crash. What is harmful about these elements? In effect, they trigger your body's fight-or-flight stress response. Most of us have too much unnecessary stress in our bodies and don't need any more from our food! Results of prolonged distress, like decreased cortisol, blood vessel constriction, and tightened muscles and tendons, increase RA's inflammation, pain, and stiffness. Refined, fatty carbohydrates (cookies, pastries, chocolate, etc.) and other fats (lunch meats, whole-milk dairy foods, red meat, palm and coconut oils, etc.) worsen RA pain by making us gain weight. Additional weight, unless you're underweight, further stresses your body by putting your joints under more pressure and making your muscles work overtime! Fat contains twice as many calories per gram as protein or complex carbs. What you want to strive for with food, as in all areas of your life, is balance. Include plenty of fresh fruits and vegetables (primarily nonacidic fruits), whole grains, brown rice, complex carbs, fish, and other low-fat proteins in your diet. Minimize sugary foods, unhealthy fats, white bread, caffeine, alcohol, red meat, and dairy products.

Antioxidants

Antioxidants, one of today's health buzzwords, include natural substances in our bodies, vitamins, minerals, and enzymes. They protect you against free radicals that damage your cells and immune system and are linked with infection, disease, and aging. Some free radicals arise as a result of exposure to chemicals, cigarette smoke, radiation, excessive sun exposure, and natural body processes. In the body's wisdom, there are free-radical scavengers whose job is to neutralize the free radicals threatening your body's internal integrity. These enzymes are assisted by vitamins, herbs, minerals, and hormones with antioxidant properties.

Elements with antioxidant properties are important in combating RA. The multitalented nutrient, garlic (Kyolic), interferes with the free-radical development that causes joint damage. The suggested dosage is two caps three times daily with meals (Balch and Balch 1997). Grape seed extract, germanium, vitamin C, vitamin A (beta carotene), and selenium are potent free-radical scavengers that reduce the inflammation and pain of RA.

When Jewelry Is More Than Decorative

For generations, copper has been suggested as a means to ease arthritis pain and swelling. A 1976 study by Walker and Keats seems to support this notion. Subjects were given two bracelets, a pseudo-copper bracelet and a true copper bracelet, in either order to wear. They did not know if they were wearing the true or pseudo-copper at any given period. When differences in symptoms were reported, the true copper bracelet was more effective in reducing symptoms. Also, those who'd worn the true copper bracelets at onset reported a worsening of symptoms when wearing the pseudo-copper bracelets. In addition, the copper in the bracelets decreased after they had been worn. Perhaps subjects absorbed copper into their bodies.

If you decide to take copper supplements, take with zinc as well, since copper reduces zinc absorption. Werbach (1993) suggests the following:

- 60 mg of copper salicylate once or twice per day. Alternative: 2 to 4 mg of copper amino acid-chelate per day. Take the copper salicylate with meals and fluids. Trial period: ten days.

- 220 mg of zinc sulfate three times per day. Take with meals. Trial period: six weeks.

This issue disturbs many as it includes shades of gray, disagreement, and conflict. The above view supports increasing copper in the body to treat RA while an equally powerful theory is that people with RA already have elevated copper levels. This camp recommends ways to reduce copper in the body, such as taking the amino acid histidine, which purportedly rids the body of excess levels of metals. They suggest that those with arthritic conditions consume foods with this amino acid, such as rice, rye, and wheat (Balch and Balch 1997). Obviously, there is no single "right" thing you can do to guarantee decreased pain and distress and improved health. This situation is, in fact, much more representative of the state of affairs with respect to illness and healing than is the illusion that there is a single method of prevention, treatment, or healing applicable to every individual with disorders as complex as the autoimmune-related conditions. Now you have some facts, and it's up to you to do research and confer with your SHOC team to make the treatment decision that's most suitable for you.

Homeopathic Remedies

Here, too, you want to locate remedies that target pain and inflammation. Recall that the longer mind-body pain exists, the more likely it is to become entrenched into the brain and body. You want to stop this vicious cycle. Remedies like Aconitum 12x (severe pain, arthritis pain), Arnica 6x (acute pain), Chamomilla 3x (chronic pain), and Pulsatilla 6x are useful. In addition, Apix 12x has anti-inflammatory properties. Some women have found both Rhus toxicodendron and Bryonia effective in reducing pain and stiffness. Find a homeopathic professional with training and experience in RA before taking any such remedies (appendix I). A professional can also advise you about adverse interactions, such as camphor blocking the benefits of arnica.

Herbal Remedies

Penny Royal (1982) recommends two herbal formulas to treat arthritic conditions like RA. One synthesis includes black cohosh, bromelain, burdock, cayenne, centaury, chaparral, comfrey, lobelia, yarrow, and yucca. Another includes black cohosh, black walnut, brigham tea, burdock, cayenne, chaparral, hydrangea, lobelia, sarsaparilla, skullcap, valerian, wild lettuce, wormwood, and yucca. These two formulas are said to have beneficial effects on arthritis, bursitis, gout, inflammation, rheumatism, and general swelling. You may notice that cayenne is a component of both formulas. This herb greatly benefits the digestive and circulatory systems and, when taken with herbs in the above formulas, it produces a synergistic effect and increases their efficacy. Cayenne (capsicum) is a good pain reliever because it contains capsaicin, which interferes with substance P production, our pain neurotransmitter. You can take cayenne alone in pill form, or you can ask a knowledgeable alternative health care expert to combine cayenne powder with wintergreen oil and apply it directly to the skin.

Black cohosh, an herb that's said to alleviate an array of female problems, is a natural estrogen source. If you get a headache from the black cohosh, it means your body may have enough estrogen, and the extra would be eliminated. You can substitute it with herbs containing progesterone, like sarsaparilla or ginseng.

If you're pregnant or nursing, avoid both black cohosh and the latter two herbs due to hormonal effects on the body. Also, if you have diabetes, avoid these herbs, as they contain lobelia. Primrose oil, cat's claw, feverfew, and ginger are all useful in reducing the pain and stiffness of RA. *If you're pregnant, do not take cat's claw or feverfew.* Chinese herbal products Du Huo Ji Sheng Wan and Yunnan Pai-yao (inflammatory pain) are both helpful in reducing RA pain.

Aromatherapy may help people with RA. Try cypress, fennel, and lemon as a detoxification combination. Massaging painful joints with benzoin, chamomile, camphor, juniper, and lavender is effective in reducing pain (Burton Goldberg Group 1997).

Allergies

Food sensitivities and allergies are another nutritional culprit and possible trigger of ARC. Some frequent allergens are nuts, eggs, dairy products, grains, and various meats. It is a good idea for you to work with an allergy specialist. Testing can be lengthy as different foods are added or removed from your diet. If an allergy is present, managing it is central to your SHOC.

CHAPTER 8

Systemic Lupus Erythematosus (SLE)

Health is a precious thing, and the only one, in truth, meriting that a man should lay out, not only his time, sweat, and labor and goods, but also his life itself to obtain it.

—Montaigne, *Essays*

There are actually four different types of the autoimmune disease called lupus. These include discoid lupus, systemic lupus erythematosus, drug-induced lupus, and neonatal lupus. Lupus is a rheumatic disease, meaning it causes aches, pain, and stiffness in the joints, bones, and muscles. This chapter discusses systemic lupus erythematosus (SLE), which is the condition usually referred to as lupus. I follow this tradition. The word systemic refers to the fact that this illness can affect different systems and thus many different parts of the body. Discoid lupus generally affects only the skin and manifests as a red rash on areas like the face and scalp. These rashes may last from days to years and may come and go. It's fairly infrequent that this develops into SLE. Neonatal lupus is also infrequent and may appear in babies of women with lupus or other immune-related disorders. Fortunately, progress has been made so that many of these potential cases can be identified early and treated immediately at birth. Effects on the baby range from a rash or abnormal blood counts, to heart or liver problems.

In 1851, a French doctor named Cazenave observed that the classic butterfly-shaped facial rash developed by some with lupus looked like the bite of an animal. This fellow had quite an imagination, and based on the fear of wolves in his day, he attributed these facial "bites" to the lupus, "lupus" being the Latin word for "wolf". SLE, like some other ARCs, involves problems with connective tissue. The connective tissue, made up of the protein called collagen together with fibers and other tissues, connects the cells and tissues of our bodies together. It was thought that collagen was the target of the body's antibodies, although now it appears that people with SLE don't often make antibodies to collagen. The name you may still hear associated with lupus, collagen disease, isn't accurate (Lahita and Phillips 1998). In SLE, destructive changes to the muscles, tendons, joints, and ligaments, and even the entire body, can occur. This was discovered in the late 1950s, when it was observed that some SLE patients had antibodies binding to their DNA. Accordingly, SLE is termed a generalized autoimmune disease.

Until fairly recently, SLE was considered fatal. Robin Dibner and Carol Colman (1994) provide enlightening statistics: In the 1950s, less than 50 percent of all patients with lupus survived even four years after diagnosis; today figures range from 75 to 90 percent of patients living ten years or more after diagnosis. New statistics estimate that lupus affects over 500,000 Americans. However, these studies only include people who have been hospitalized, and most with lupus haven't. The Lupus Foundation of America suggests the number closer to 2 to 2.5 million. Lupus is one of the ARCs with the highest female to male ratios: nine to one. The mean age at onset is about twenty-nine to thirty, and the range generally falls between the teen years and the forties. The gender difference isn't the only difference: Lupus prevalence in Caucasians is about one in four hundred women; in African-American women, one in 250; and in Latinos, one in 500 (Lahita and Phillips 1998). It also appears to be more frequent in Asian women than in Caucasian women. These statistics are important given the importance of obtaining consistent, good health care and the association between better health and greater income and educational levels. Women who are more likely to be affected by SLE often can't get good health care and don't have benefits of education and money.

What Causes Lupus?

Theories about the etiology of lupus include those typically proposed to explain ARCs. That is, researchers have looked for genetic underpinnings, hormonal influences, viral or bacterial attacks, and the like. When the scientific literature is looked at as a whole, it seems SLE may result from a complex interaction between hormones, genes, and the environment. Hormonal explanations are sought due to the extreme prevalence of SLE in women and because lupus often affects women during the years between menarche and menopause. After age fifty-five, the difference in prevalence between women and men drops from nine to one to about two to one. As most women never develop SLE, researchers wonder whether women with SLE have very high levels of estrogen or whether men who develop it have very low levels of androgen (the proposition being that male hormones, androgens, protect men). Results of studies focusing only on amounts of estrogen and androgens in affected individuals haven't been conclusive.

However, when certain hormonal processes were broken down and studied, some interesting findings arose. Sheldon Paul Blau and Dodi Schultz (1984) reported a study in which sex hormones were injected into male and female lupus patients and male and female healthy subjects. The sex hormones were broken down differently and different proportions of metabolites were excreted. It's thought that people with SLE may convert more testosterone to estrogen and then convert the estrogen into a disruptive metabolite. Why these hormones are processed differently in SLE patients versus healthy individuals may be genetically based but is as yet unclear. Another example supporting the role of hormones in lupus comes from studying women with polycystic ovary disease. These women don't have lupus but do have autoantibodies and joint pain that occurs when their estrogen levels are elevated. SLE patients do tend to have more ovarian cysts, and most findings of lupus occur when estrogen is quite high (Lahita and Phillips 1998).

There is definitely a genetic predisposition toward developing lupus, as with other ARCs discussed in this book. The genetic link isn't completely clear and simple. For example, the chance that a person with SLE will have a close relative (sibling or parent) with the disorder is about 10 percent, but only 5 percent of children born to a parent with SLE develop the illness. People with certain types of genetic tissue, called human leukocyte antigen or HLA types, are more likely to develop SLE than are people with other genetic tissue types. The genetic role is also supported by the fact that when one identical twin has lupus, the other twin has a bit less than 30 percent chance of developing it, whereas when one fraternal twin (not sharing the same genetic material) has SLE, the other twin has a lower chance of 5 to 15 percent. Blau and Schultz (1984) discuss an interesting study of two identical twins, only one of whom had lupus despite their sharing the identical genetic inheritance. While one twin with SLE tested positive on certain blood tests for lupus and her unaffected sister did not, both showed typical false-positive results typical to lupus on another test and both had very high levels of immunoglobulin. The most interesting finding was that the non-SLE twin had had her ovaries and uterus removed earlier. So, clearly, genes are one part of the puzzle, while hormonal activity is another.

Genetics and hormones don't explain the whole story. It has been found that there is a higher rate of SLE in members of the same household, even when they're unrelated (Dibner and Colman 1994). Other environmental conditions must factor into the development of SLE as well. People in the same house may be exposed to certain viruses, toxins, chemicals, or perhaps even severe emotional stressors sufficient to trigger lupus in household members already genetically predisposed to develop SLE. Sunlight is another possible trigger.

Tissue damage arises in two ways. Antibodies fighting a host tissue can damage it directly, for example, if antibodies are fighting red blood cells and destroy them. The second way is the typical way of autoimmune disorders, through inflammation. When the antibodies go after the body's own tissue, the usual antibody-antigen complex is formed. In healthy people, the immune system's mechanisms remove the destroyed complex. In people with SLE, the immune complex remains trapped throughout the body, causing inflammation that can destroy cells, tissues, and organs. Women with SLE do tend to have hyperactive immune systems.

No specific "lupus" gene has yet been identified, and several genes may be associated with a susceptibility to developing lupus. It's been discovered that a mutant mouse strain that develops a lupuslike illness has defective genes that control apoptosis, or programmed cell death. Apoptosis lets the body get rid of damaged, potentially harmful cells. If the process doesn't work smoothly, these damaged or harmful cells stay in the body and cause problems to the body's tissues. Scientists have been able to replace the bad genes with good ones in mice, who then did not manifest the lupuslike disease. It is hoped that similar discoveries and techniques will be relevant to human cases.

Symptoms and Signs

As with other ARCs, lupus presents with a wide array of symptoms. This is one of the reasons you may have to play the circus wheel of doctor visits typical of most ARCs. Robin Dibner and Carol Colman (1994) discuss other reasons for the rampant misdiagnosis of SLE. Firstly, lupus doesn't get much attention in traditional medical educational formats. Fortunately, the American College of Rheumatology has attempted to design courses with more attention focused on rheumatology in medical schools. Secondly, lupus lacks the media interest that AIDS and now breast cancer receive. Because it isn't known how lupus develops, but the condition is believed to be noncontagious, the media and other groups don't feel the urgent need to cover this disease.

Discoid lupus is characterized by rashes on the skin that can appear on the scalp, neck, face, and inside the ears. It doesn't affect internal organs and isn't truly serious. However, the results can be distressing, because if it's left untreated, the rash can leave scars and baldness. In addition, about 10 percent of those with discoid lupus will go on to develop SLE, usually a fairly mild form. The lupus discussed in this book is the most severe type, SLE, which involves connective tissue, such as the skin, tendons, and joints. Previously, lupus and related disorders that involve muscles, tendon, and bones were called connective tissue diseases. This term is still sometimes used, and you may hear it from your doctors or come across it in your reading. It's also referred to as a collagen vascular disease, because inflammation of the blood vessels, or vasculitis, commonly occurs. Often this inflammation isn't serious, so it may not require treatment.

One frequent symptom you can probably relate to is fatigue, not the ordinary run-of-the-mill fatigue, but a severe fatigue in which doing any activity is difficult and normal daily activities can be greatly restricted. You may also be in pain, ranging from a general achiness throughout your body to areas of specific pain and swelling in your hand and foot joints. Pain is often worse upon morning awakening and may wane during the day.

Your skin can be very sensitive, and you may experience a variety of rashes, most frequently the aforementioned red facial rash called malar, or butterfly rash. In addition, your skin can be very sun sensitive and after sun exposure you may even have fevers, pain, or an increase in rashes. Another frequent symptom is a prolonged elevated temperature of about 100 degrees, or episodic high fevers that may increase at night. The tendency toward hair loss is also very disturbing. In discoid lupus, scarring of the scalp may lead to permanent hair loss, though this doesn't necessarily occur in SLE. Other symptoms you may have are cold hands and feet (possibly Raynaud's syndrome), depression, swelling of the legs, ankles, or the area around the eyes, a tendency to bruise easily, and very dry eyes and mouth. Finally, due to the hormonal connection, your symptoms may intensify right before your period.

SLE also sometimes involves other body organs. For example, chest pain can occur as a result of the swelling of the lining of the heart and lungs. Kidney disease can also arise from lupus; an early indication of its presence is often an increase in swelling. As with other ARCs, SLE is chronic with no definitive cure, though the prognosis is much less threatening than it was just several decades ago.

Lupus and Pregnancy

Many health professionals believe people with SLE shouldn't use birth control pills, as they've been associated with flare-ups. Until fairly recently, they were warned against pregnancy, based upon the increased number of miscarriages and lupus flare-ups during or after pregnancy. If you have SLE and are planning to have children, you need to know some facts. While there are some drawbacks to becoming pregnant, advances in research and treatment have greatly decreased the risks you and your baby face. If you become pregnant, it will still be considered a high-risk pregnancy, although the majority of SLE patients have fairly normal pregnancies and healthy babies. In general, the risk of miscarriage is about 10 to 15 percent, while in women with lupus, the risk is about 20 to 25 percent. While about 8 percent of all births are premature, the figure is around 25 percent when the mother has SLE (Sheldon Paul Blau and Dodi Schultz 1984).

When you become pregnant, it's important that you're not having a flare or active phase and that you've been off most of your medications for at least six months. The possible complications of an SLE pregnancy, like miscarriage or flare-up, are associated with the woman's health up to six month prior to conception. If you have kidney disease or any other major organ impairment, you really must think carefully about pregnancy given the great strain it puts on your body and the apparently greater chance for postpartum illness. The greatest risk of miscarriage or worsening of the mother's health is associated with an active disease state at the time of conception. This brings new meaning to the words "planned pregnancy," so do your utmost in timing your baby's conception. Contraceptives and lupus are discussed below.

Blood tests taken early in pregnancy are an integral part of early pregnancy health care. Make certain that your obstetrician draws your blood for the requisite blood tests. If a woman has had a previous miscarriage and certain antibodies are detected, she'll probably be prescribed baby aspirin or heparin to use throughout her pregnancy. In a smaller number of women, antibodies called anti-Ro (SSA) and anti-La (SSB) will be found. These women can give birth to babies with certain lupus symptoms such as low blood count, rash, or heartbeat irregularities. This isn't SLE, is usually of a short-term nature (six to twelve months), and often doesn't need treatment.

Although severe flare-ups are possible during pregnancy or after giving birth, they don't happen to everyone. There may be an increased chance of serious flare-ups after birth, when the ratio of progesterone to estrogen drops. Other problems that can arise include high blood pressure, diabetes, high blood sugar, and kidney problems. You must thoroughly educate yourself about pregnancy in general and about lupus pregnancies in particular, and must maintain regular contact with a doctor you trust, feel comfortable with, and who is very knowledgeable about lupus pregnancies.

Related Conditions and Diagnostic Criteria

SLE is among the most troublesome ARCs to diagnose. It's been called the "great imitator," so you might partially understand why it can take an estimated eight years to be diagnosed correctly (Phillips 1984). While you may understand this intellectually, it doesn't necessarily help allay the frustration and pain you experience as you go from doctor to doctor and test to test. You may have also been sent to one or more mental health workers by doctors who, because they aren't sure as to your condition and because you are a woman, may believe it's all in your head. Like other ARCs, SLE shares symptoms and signs with various autoimmune-related disorders, which also explains some diagnosis delay. For example, the pain in the joint areas can make it seem as though you are battling RA. When the pain is the diffuse aching type that is worse in the morning, or if it focuses on certain areas, this can make it seem as if you have fibromyalgia syndrome (FMS). In fact, up to one-half of SLE affected individuals may also have FMS.

Let's look at the established criteria for diagnosing SLE. In 1982, the American College of Rheumatology developed the Revised Criteria for the Classification of Lupus. This list contains eleven indicators most highly related to SLE. Your doctor should be using this list, together with other information, in making your diagnosis. In general, if you have four or more of the following criteria, not necessarily experienced concurrently, you can be diagnosed with SLE. Familiarize yourself with this list so that when you speak to your doctor you can make certain he is familiar with SLE. Remember, those who are active and involved in their understanding and treatment of their illness fare best in terms of their health!

Rash (Malar)

This is made up of red, raised bumps that can take the form of a butterfly, covering your cheeks and the bridge of your nose. This area can be tender and hot. It's possible that the development of this rash is linked with another criterion, photosensitivity. An autoimmune response seems active given the discovery of two telling signs: the typical inflammatory response in the blood vessels and an excessive number of antibodies in the area of affected skin. Fortunately, the rash can be treated and does not leave scars.

Discoid Rash

While 50 percent of SLE patients develop malar rash, only half as many develop this rash. This is fortunate, as the consequences are more severe. Discoid rashes are small, round areas that usually appear on the face but also may occur on the scalp, ears, back, and arms. A doctor might initially think you have psoriasis. The telling difference is that beneath the discoid rash are a number of small points that look like blackheads. (Beneath the psoriasis rash there is just red skin.) If you develop a discoid rash, seek treatment immediately. If these areas aren't treated, the chances are high that scarring will result. If you develop the discoid rash on your scalp, the scarring may cause permanent hair loss. This type of rash is worsened by exposure to sun, giving you further reason to avoid sunlight. Your doctor may need to distinguish discoid lupus, in which this is the only "lupus" symptom, from the discoid rash appearing with SLE. These are separate diseases, though about 10 percent of those with discoid lupus can develop SLE.

Photosensitivity

Most people with SLE are sensitive to sunlight and other types of light. Exposure to sunlight may cause rashes, fever, pain, fatigue, and even kidney disease! The need to avoid excessive exposure to sunlight (UVA and UVB rays) is incredibly important, and you must also watch out for halogen lamps (UVA) and fluorescent lights (UVB). Suggestions will be provided in the What You Can Do section below. While we're still largely in the dark about this sensitivity to light (pun intended), one explanation is that sunlight damages the skin's DNA and makes it appear "foreign" to the body's immune system. As you know, this triggers the immune response and sends out self-harming antibodies to destroy the DNA. This destructive autoimmunity results in inflammation and damage to the body's own tissues and cells.

Ulcers

About 40 percent of SLE patients develop these, which are caused by inflammation and aren't often painful. These ulcers are like small cold sores and may appear in the hard palate of the mouth, the nose, or the throat. Obviously, most people have mouth sores at some point, but the distinguishing characteristic is the frequency.

Arthritic Symptoms

As you know, joint and ligament inflammation and pain are common. In SLE, two or more joints must be affected and no noticeable or marked deformity of the joint(s) should exist. This often waxes and wanes and fortunately doesn't generally cause damage to your body's bones.

Pleuritis or Pericarditis

About 50 percent of people with SLE experience this inflammatory response, which affects the linings of the heart, lungs, or abdominal region. When lungs are affected, it's called pleuritis, which you experience as chest pain and difficulty inhaling. You'll also have similar chest pain if you develop pericarditis, or tissue swelling around your heart. To diagnose this, your doctor will use noninvasive electrocardiograms (EKG), chest X-rays, or echocardiograms. EKGs measure your heart's electrical activity, and echocardiograms bounce sound waves off your heart, creating a physical picture. Physical exams are useful in detecting pericarditis, as your health care worker may hear sounds that indicate inflammation and/or fluid buildup. Less frequently, SLE patients have inflammation of the abdominal region's lining or peritonitis. This is quite painful and can resemble appendicitis.

Kidney Problems

While many people with SLE develop kidney problems at some point, only about 50 percent of those who do will have permanent harm to the kidneys. Inflammation is again key in underlying and detecting this symptom. The kidneys act as filters for the body, and if you have SLE, your body will try to eliminate the autoantibody/self-antigen complexes with the help of the kidneys. However, in SLE patients, the complexes often can't be removed, and those that remain trapped in areas such as the kidneys can damage that tissue. Most people with SLE who develop kidney problems aren't even aware of it. If you work with a knowledgeable, proactive health professional, she'll probably conduct a urine analysis. If not, ask for one. If the urine analysis indicates very high protein levels or the presence of white or red cells (all indications of inflammation), it's likely you have a kidney disorder.

Neurological Disorder

About 50 percent of SLE patients develop neurological problems related to the central nervous system. As with many SLE-related symptoms, neurological abnormalities range from mild to severe. You could experience anything from mild memory loss to dangerous seizures or even psychotic behavior associated with severe depression or schizophrenia-like disturbances in perceptions (visual, auditory, or tactile hallucinations), cognitive functioning, and behavior. Given that up to 25 percent of people with SLE initially present with neurological problems, your SHOC should include a thorough mental status exam, including questions exploring your memory, attention, concentration, mood, perceptual accuracy, and thought processes.

Blood Changes

Four blood cell disturbances may occur, though as usual, they also occur in other conditions. Having one or more of the following counts as one of eleven criteria. These are caused by the attack of various blood cells by antibodies (i.e., autoantibodies).

In hemolytic anemia, your body produces antibodies that target your own red blood cells. This can occur in the liver or spleen and can be dangerous, calling for immediate treatment. About 15 percent of SLE patients have thrombocytopenia, or a low number of platelets or clotting cells. Autoantibodies are again at work, attacking the body's own platelets in the spleen. Leukopenia means you have a very low number of white blood cells. Not too serious in itself, it can mean your lupus is active or becoming so. Lymphocytopenia means your lymphocytes are low, though not too serious. Your red blood cell sedimentation rate (ESR), or the sinking rate of your red blood cells, is often examined when diagnosing SLE. While many people with SLE have elevated rates, so do people with RA, infections, or tumors. The test isn't very specific for diagnosing SLE.

Immunologic Abnormalities

When found in conjunction with some of the other criteria, four antibodies in the blood suggest SLE. If one or more of the following are found in the bloodstream, it indicates a positive on this particular criteria: anti-DNA antibodies; lupus erythematosus cell preparation (present in those with active SLE about 90 percent of the time, unfortunately also found in Sjogren's syndrome, RA, and scleroderma); Smith antibodies (a more accurate predictor of SLE); antibodies resembling those that fight off syphilis.

ANA Tests

These are used to discern the presence of autoantibodies targeting the nuclear material of proteins liberated from your own healthy cells (ANA = antinuclear antibodies). Up to 95 percent of SLE patients score positive, though so do people with other ARCs, unrelated diseases, or even no apparent physical problems. As with the other tests, this can't be used alone to diagnose SLE.

More Important Facts on Testing for SLE

Blood tests can also be used as an indication of how well your kidneys are functioning. Remember that kidney problems are one of the criteria for determining the diagnosis of SLE. How well your kidneys are performing their blood purification tasks can be partly determined by looking at creatinine, serum albumin, and blood urea nitrogen levels. Abnormal levels indicate possible kidney damage. Protein found in your urine also suggests kidney problems.

Much has been said about SLE and RA similarities. The rheumatoid factor (RF) test helps distinguish between the two, as about 75 percent of RA patients test positive, while only 20 percent of SLE patients test positive. If you have SLE and test positive for RF, you'll probably have a less severe case (Dibner and Colman 1994).

People with SLE may have multiple symptoms also appearing in AIDS: low white blood cell count, skin rashes, ulcers of the mouth, loss of hair, protein in the urine, and inflammation of various lymph nodes. As with the syphilis test, many SLE patients can erroneously score positive on an HIV test. Those who score positive for HIV must also take an HIV test called the Western blot blood test. This is more tightly delineated for HIV and helps clarify if HIV does exist. The reasons for detecting HIV are obvious; however, it's particularly important if one has an autoimmune disorder, as immunosuppressive medications prescribed for SLE do the opposite of what the body needs to combat AIDS and could increase the disease progression.

People with SLE can also score false positive for Lyme disease on the ELISA (enzyme-linked immunosorbent assay). When this occurs, it's important to use the more specialized Western blood blot test. There are additional, complex tests more specific to SLE than those discussed so far and you should be familiar with these whether or not your doctor seems to be having difficulty with your diagnosis. You may want these tests to ensure the utmost accuracy in your diagnosis. You've nothing to lose by maximizing your information about your case; that is, nothing but the expense your managed care or HMO company may gripe about. However, having the knowledge and information gained here can be useful should you need to prove the need for the tests. Regardless of the problems arising from the overlap among autoimmune-related conditions and our lack of knowledge, these tests are an improvement and should be used until we have more specific tests available.

RNA testing can be done to determine the presence of particular antibodies that go after ribonuclear protein. While these antibodies are found in lupus, they can also be found in related conditions. In particular, there is a condition fairly recently labeled "mixed connective tissue disease" which would appear to be an amalgamation of lupus, scleroderma, and polymyositis and which has, as its only consistent characteristic, the presence of such antibodies for ribonuclear protein. Besides mixed connective tissue disease, a woman with similar symptoms and test results might be told she has overlap syndrome or undifferentiated connective tissue disease. Fortunately, an anti-DNA test that can more conclusively indicate the presence of lupus involves looking for antibodies attacking the body's own DNA. This test is positive in about 70 percent of lupus cases and is rarely positive in other illnesses. SLE-afflicted people who do score positively on this measure tend to have a currently active disease state or some type of kidney disease. In addition, testing positive for antibodies targeting certain proteins in the nuclei of the body's cells, known as anti-SM antibodies, is highly specific to SLE.

A major problem with diagnosis is that diagnostic tests don't always detect early stages of the disturbance. Tests must often be given after onset so the markers have developed. Having an experienced doctor is essential as he should know about this delay, and will (hopefully) redo the tests or use other tests. There is no substitute for a medical person's experience and commitment to really listening to you.

SLE, the "great imitator," can cause a vast array of symptoms, many of which come and go. If you have SLE, you might be experiencing just the arthritis and muscle pain, and visiting a doctor at this point might result in a diagnosis of RA or connective tissue disease. On the other hand, you might only be experiencing the severe fatigue and elevated temperature, which might lead a doctor to diagnose chronic fatigue immune dysfunction syndrome. Fibromyalgia syndrome might also be mistaken for SLE, as could infectious diseases, such as Lyme disease, syphilis, or tuberculosis. Other conditions confused with SLE are blood disorders, such as lymphoma, neurologic disorders, such as MS, and psychiatric disorders, like depression or schizophrenia.

Because of the symptoms SLE shares with other diseases, the following list will improve your understanding of your particular case and help in ruling out other conditions. You'll be an informed member of your own SHOC. You'll understand why your doctor is ordering certain tests or asking certain questions and you can bring up alternative illnesses for discussion, perhaps convincing an overworked doctor to order whatever tests or medications represent the best care for your condition.

A Closer Look

RA

Confusion between RA and SLE arises in part from shared symptoms of joint pain and inflammation. Tests also confuse these two. Unlike in RA (primarily untreated cases), SLE arthritis shouldn't include noticeable deformity of affected joints or bone damage. Diagnosis is made more difficult by shared joint involvement: ankles, feet, knees, hips, wrists, elbows, shoulders, and lower jaws.

MS

Like SLE, MS can involve destructive changes to body systems and joint pain and diffuse pain, including harm to muscles, tendons, joints and ligaments, respiratory system, kidneys, and blood vessels throughout the body. Both MS and SLE involve fatigue and lethargy, muscle weakness, hyperventilation or shortness of breath, and inflammation. Both can also affect the central nervous system leading to loss of normal sensations and, rarely, mental disturbances.

FMS and CFIDS

These share elements of SLE, such as localized joint pain, general diffuse pain, fatigue and other symptoms. SLE patients can also have one or both of these disorders. Up to 50 percent may have FMS as well.

SS

This chronic autoimmune inflammatory disease can occur by itself (Sjogren's disease) or with another illness (Sjogren's syndrome). Many people with SLE develop SS, so it's necessary to detect the primary disease. SLE can affect the eyes in many ways and while the causes may differ from those of SS, the resulting symptoms—dry, irritated, and red eyes—look similar. Some tests can help determine whether SD or SS is present.

Raynaud's Phenomenon

Confusion between SLE and this disorder arises because about 20 percent of people with SLE develop mild to severe degrees of cold hands and feet. If your toes and fingers are cold-sensitive even in moderate surroundings and your fingers turn white and blue when cold and then red as they regain warmth, you have this condition. Stress also triggers Raynaud's. As it occurs in various connective tissue disorders, it can't be used to diagnose SLE.

Endometriosis

This condition appears at greater rates in SLE patients. Endometriosis occurs when your uterine cells, typically shed and eliminated during your period, stay and grow like a benign tumor. Such cells can be destroyed by taking male hormones, Danacrine (danazol) or Lupron (leuprolide acetate), which stop the pituitary gland from stimulating hormone metabolism. Endometriosis can be confused with SLE because it can also cause rheumatic problems. Tests increase confusion if you also have autoantibodies or positive ANAs.

Lyme Disease

From forty-eight cases when numbers were first tallied in 1983 to the current disparity in estimated numbers, from 11,250 to 400,000 (Lang 1997), this is the most common illness caused by ticks in the U.S. Symptoms can include muscle weakness; fever; rashes; facial paralysis; inability to sleep; fatigue; flulike symptoms; neck and back pain; joint pain and swelling; achiness; headaches; nausea and vomiting; enlargement of the spleen, lymph glands, and heart muscle; abnormal heart rhythm; and even degenerative muscle disease. Symptom overlap with SLE and other autoimmune conditions explains diagnostic confusion.

The Courses of Lupus

If you've been diagnosed with SLE, remember that descriptions of time frames and courses are only generalizations. Your individual case can differ greatly. Still, you must educate yourself as much as possible, because this is the starting point of creating your self and health-optimization course (SHOC). Learn what to expect in general, your options, the specialists in your area, the best treatments, both conventional and alternative, and what you can do to stretch any confines of your condition and grow in other ways. Lupus is tricky due to the great symptom variety and the extended period of time over which the disease can manifest. Your SLE is likely to be least severe if diagnosis is early, you and your doctor(s) take a proactive role in tests and treatment, you follow your health professionals' guidelines, you actively devise and follow your SHOC, and you develop acceptance balanced by the willingness to fight back and derive meaning and growth from this experience. The ideal balance is to have experts in both the conventional medical tradition as well as the alternative, complementary schools of thought and practice. You can often gain synergistic benefits from the two traditions.

Early symptoms resemble those of arthritis, with pain and inflammation in various joints. Sometimes SLE appears quickly and includes a high fever. You may be fortunate and have only a mild case with long remissions, mild to moderate fatigue, and infrequent skin rashes. On the other hand, you may have long bouts of fatigue, severe joint pain, depression, headaches, sun sensitivity, and frequent malar rashes. If you're lucky, you may have one body system, such as your skin or your joints, affected. On the other hand, you might develop kidney inflammation, hair loss, and central nervous system symptom such as memory problems, behavioral changes, dizziness; and vision changes. About 50 percent of people with SLE develop nephritis or kidney inflammation.

Testing for SLE

As with other ARCs, there is no single definitive test to unerringly diagnose SLE. At present, your doctor must rely on various information sources: your reports of current and past symptoms; factors that you see are related to symptom changes; previous health-related concerns, illnesses, operations, or allergies; medications (past/present); physical or emotional stressors (past/ongoing); lifestyle habits (diet, exercise, smoking, drinking, drugs, toxin exposure); social history and childhood experiences related to your physical health; your family's physical history; your doctor's examinations and data; and various tests. Be prepared with as much information as possible when you visit your health caretaker.

What You Can Do

As is the norm with autoimmune-related diseases, individual SLE cases don't follow any norms. You must grasp the fact that your body is unlike anybody else's. The last thing in the world you should do is ignore symptoms and distress because they don't seem to fit descriptions you've heard or read about. It's important to be in touch with your body and any changes. If you suspect something is amiss, even though it doesn't fit any particular examples you've seen, heard, or read about, go see a professional as soon as possible. The sooner you determine what is wrong, the sooner you can form your SHOC, research the illness, contact appropriate health professionals, work on your attitudes, and thus slow down the illness' speed of progression or degree of damage. This all fits into your toolbag for beating the odds. Your mind-body's uniqueness means you may benefit from integrating conventional and alternative treatments. Your uniqueness also means that you can use your mind to impact the course of your condition, to steer toward healing and beating the odds with a sense of control that is balanced by acceptance of those things that are out of your control. You'll see how true this is when you read Susan's story at the end of this chapter.

Step one in dealing with SLE is ensuring you have the right members on your SHOC team. Through reading, calling, talking, and asking many questions, you'll find healers with whom you feel comfortable. Because of the many bodily systems affected by SLE, you may have an array of team members over time, from a family doctor, to a neurologist, ophthalmologist, psychologist, dermatologist, hematologist (specializing in blood disorders), or nephrologist (specializing in kidney disease)! Depending on your beliefs, the span of your SHOC team may widen to include acupuncturists, herbalists, chiropractors, osteopaths, and massage therapists. The most important thing is that you feel comfortable with your team members, and their level of knowledge and expertise in your condition. You may not develop deep, empathetic relationships with all or even most, but you should feel respected and important. If you realize that a member is demeaning or unhelpful and that your reaction isn't misplaced anger at yourself or your illness, or some other personal peeve that you'll benefit from working on, kick them off of your SHOC team! It will be one of many times you assume control, make decisions, and take action in the process of healing and optimal mind-body health and growth.

Medications

Several types of medications are used to treat SLE. The particular ones depend on your symptoms and other personal factors.

Nonsteroidal Anti-inflammatory Drugs (NSAIDs)

For swelling and joint pain, nonsteroidal anti-inflammatory drugs (NSAIDs) are used. While you can buy some NSAIDs over the counter, you need a prescription for others. Work closely with your doctor, as the dosages for SLE may differ from those listed on the package insert. Also, drugs may interact negatively, and your doctor, who should be aware of all of the medications and herbal remedies you are using, can inform you about such interactions. What follows is the National Institutes of Health's (NIH) list of NSAIDs often used to treat SLE. Aspirin, or acetylsalicylic acid, is the most well-known and probably most frequently used NSAID. Below, you'll find the generic name given first, followed in parentheses by a brand name or two. The brand names are only examples and aren't necessarily recommended by the NIH.

NSAIDs Used to Treat SLE

Ibuprofen (Motrin, Advil)	Naproxen (Naprosyn, Aleve)	Sulindac (Clinoril)
Diclofenac (Voltaren)	Piroxicam (Feldene)	Ketoprofen (Orudis)
Diflunisal (Dolobid)	Nabumetone (Relafen)	Etodolac (Lodine)
Oxaprozin (Daypro)	Indomethacin (Indocin)	

Given the frequency of their use and the number of potential adverse effects, it's important to educate yourself about NSAIDs. The list contains commonly used NSAIDs that, while from different chemical categories, all function like aspirin. They differ from drugs like acetaminophen (e.g., Tylenol) in that they reduce swelling in addition to decreasing pain. These drugs work quickly (in days or weeks) to reduce inflammation, joint and muscle pain, fever, and sometimes fatigue. Sound like miracle drugs? Unfortunately, one of the biggest problems with NSAIDs is the presence of adverse effects, including heartburn, fluid retention, diarrhea, stomach ulcers, kidney problems, gastrointestinal (GI) bleeding, and liver and/or kidney inflammation. Some of these effects can be fatal. According to the U.S. FDA, as many as 10,000 to 20,000 fatalities occur annually from the use of NSAIDs.

The prostaglandins affected by NSAIDs cause unwanted inflammation at times, but they are also important in protecting against stomach lining irritation. Thus, users can experience anything from gastritis (mild to moderate stomach disturbances) to GI bleeding. If you have stomach pain, heartburn, nausea and/or vomiting, or bloody stools or vomit, contact your health professional immediately. There are some medications you can take to reduce the chances of such damage. Misoprostol (Cytotec) actually helps increase stomach prostaglandins and reduces the chances of GI damage. Some medications help reduce the chances of developing ulcers. Antacids (e.g., Maalox) and H2-receptor blockers (e.g., Tagamet, Zantac) interfere with stomach acid production. Carafate functions differently by creating a "new" layer of stomach protection. Misoprostol can proactively prevent GI damage, but if you're considering having children or are pregnant, steer clear of this drug, which can lead to miscarriage. If you fit this category, inform your doctor immediately so she can prescribe a new medication. If you don't fit into this category but are a smoker or have had GI problems, misoprostol may be your best bet. Fortunately, there are many people who can tolerate NSAIDs without any problem; however, be cautious if you have had ulcers or GI bleeding, are over 65, or have had any type of kidney or liver problems.

For any of you who take NSAIDs as part of your SLE treatment, you must stay in close contact with your health care team so any signs of adverse effects are detected immediately, appropriate testing is done, and an alternative treatment plan, if necessary, can be put into place. Have your stool checked intermittently to detect whether it contains any blood, which could indicate GI bleeding and would necessitate medication changes. Another side effect of NSAIDs is a decrease in blood flow to the kidneys. In general, this isn't problematic, but if you've had kidney damage or kidney disease, you should be cautious with NSAIDs. Your doctor should conduct intermittent examinations of your renal function. Liver function must also be checked due to the possibility of developing liver toxicity from NSAIDs. Finally, some NSAIDs cause bleeding problems, making certain precautions necessary. For example, if you have a surgery or dental appointment coming up, stop taking your medicine at least several days (in the case of aspirin, at least two weeks) in advance. NSAIDs, unlike the drugs discussed next, aren't likely to have any true beneficial impact on the underlying disease state or progression of SLE.

Antimalarials

Interestingly enough, drugs initially used to treat malaria are effective in treating SLE as well. Antimalarials may work by suppressing parts of the immune response. Some of these drugs are hydrochloroquine (Plaquenil), chloroquine (Aralen), and quinacrine (Atabrine). They are particularly effective for fatigue, joint pain, skin rashes (including discoid lupus), mouth ulcers, arthritis, and lung inflammation. In addition, if taken continuously, they may reduce recurrent flares. These drugs take some time to work, and SLE patients who take taking them don't usually experience many adverse effects. Some potential side effects include stomach upset and, rarely, retinal damage called retinopathy.

When taking antimalarials, be active in your SHOC and ensure you have regular eye exams every three to six months. Your eye doctor (who must be familiar with SLE) may give you tools for home use. You may be given some paper like simple graph paper that you'll use to discern whether you're experiencing any peripheral vision loss. If you note any changes in what the paper looks like, you must immediately contact your doctor. A second home self-management tool is a simple red swab or piece of paper. You'll regularly look at the sample to see if it begins to look any lighter or darker. If it does, contact your ophthalmologist immediately. Finally, because retinopathy is worsened through UV exposure, ensure you buy and wear appropriate UV-protective sunglasses. Rarely, people on these medications may develop nerve damage or peripheral neuropathy. Your doctor should test for reflexes and changes in muscular strength that might, though not necessarily, indicate such a condition.

Corticosteroids

These hormones, which work quickly by suppressing inflammation, are often used to treat SLE. These include prednisone (Deltasone), hydrocortisone, methylprednisolone (Medrol), and dexamethasone (Decadron, Hexadrol). Your doctor may prescribe these if your symptoms don't improve with NSAIDs or antimalarials. Prednisone can deplete your body of vitamins C and B6, zinc, and potassium, so add to your supplements accordingly. SLE patients who experience painful arthritis, inflammation, muscle and joint pain, kidney disease, pleuritis, pericarditis or great fatigue may benefit greatly from corticosteroids which also assist in suppressing the immune system. Corticosteroids have allowed many people with SLE to dramatically improve their physical and thus emotional states. These substances are related to cortisol, an anti-inflammatory hormone produced by your body. You can read more about cortisol by referring back to the section on negative stress and how it impacts your immune system. Your doctor may prescribe these in the form of skin creams, injections, or oral formulas. You may have unpleasant but generally short-term side effects like weight gain, increased appetite, swelling, and emotional changes. These usually disappear when the medication is stopped.

There are two issues to look out for and incorporate into your SHOC. Firstly, because these drugs work well and often quickly, some women subscribe to the "more is better" illusion. This is why it's essential you have a close relationship with your health caretaker so you feel safe and open to discussing such a problem. If you're fortunate and persistent, you'll have found a caring, wise doctor who knows your judgment and whether to give a green light to increase your dosage slightly when your pain increases. You must be honest with yourself, though, if "slightly" turns into something of a greater quantity or frequency. The second issue to be added to your SHOC knowledge base is that you must not suddenly stop taking this medication. Be a proactive self-manager to ensure that you don't run out of medication before the weekend or a trip, or that you don't just forget to take it for a few days now and again. These medications must be tapered slowly and in concert with your doctor's advice and guidance, or you risk severe consequences such as a severe SLE flare-up or adrenal insufficiency, involving fever, inability to eat, GI pain, great fatigue, and dizziness. The goal of tapering is a good one; namely, to get down to the lowest amount of medication you need. While tapering may involve discomfort like fever, joint and muscle pain, and fatigue, self-talk that reminds you that this is a temporary condition can help tremendously, as can supportive friends and family.

Your doctors may give you a large amount of corticosteroids by vein ("bolus" or "pulse" treatment), which reduces side effects and makes slow tapering unnecessary. However, there are also longer-term effects of these substances, including high blood sugar, infections, cataracts, high blood pressure, increased hair growth, and damage to the bones and arteries. The higher the dose and the longer the drugs are taken, the higher the chances of these side effects. So, as with other SLE drugs, keep in close contact with your doctor when using them. Ensure she is using the lowest possible effective dose, or considers using a higher dose but only on alternate days, or using lesser amounts of these in conjunction with other, less potentially harmful drugs. Remember to get sufficient supplemental calcium and vitamin D to reduce the risk of developing the weak, fragile bones that characterize osteoporosis.

Immunosuppressives

If you have kidney or central nervous system disturbances, your doctor may prescribe an immunosuppressive. These work to slow overactive immune systems by stopping production or weakening the action of various immune cells. You may be given these drugs by mouth or infusion. As with corticosteroids, the chance of side effects is related to how long you take the drugs. Potential side effects include bladder problems, hair loss, vomiting, nausea, fertility problems, and increased chance of infection and cancer. Methotrexate (Folex, Mexate, Rheumatrex) is an immunosuppressive given to those who are unable to tolerate corticosteroids. SLE patients with multiple system involvement may be given intravenous gamma globulin (Gammagard, Gammar, Gamine), a blood protein that helps fight infection and boost immunity.

One of the cutting-edge areas in SLE research includes developing ways to selectively block parts of the immune system by using drugs based on naturally occurring compounds in the body. An obvious benefit is that the chances of side effects are lessened. Efforts are also being made to reconstruct the immune system by bone marrow transplantation. Further research is needed.

Analgesics

Unlike NSAIDs, which can reduce pain due to inflammation, analgesics reduce pain by numbing the sensations. Some typical analgesics include acetaminophen (Tylenol) and propoxyphene hydrochloride (Darvon), while for severe pain, narcotics like oxycodone (Percocet), meperidine hydrochloride (Demerol), and morphine sulfate are used. Some people are frightened when they hear the names of these drugs, because they've heard that they're addictive. There is great debate about using such drugs in treating chronic pain, and many doctors under-prescribe such medications. People with chronic pain who don't have previous histories of addiction rarely become addicted to their pain medicines. They typically don't experience the euphoria, or high; instead their bodies use the substances to alleviate pain.

Mind-Body Techniques

People with SLE today have much greater chances of beating the odds with respect to their illness and leading more productive, enjoyable lives. It's almost certain that your SLE experience won't be as negative, frightening, or disruptive as it would have been even twenty years ago. After you read this list of general tools, you'll learn specifics of how best to treat and cope with SLE-related symptoms.

- New medications
- Tools for protecting the joints
- Education about and use of appropriate physical therapies
- Sufficient sleep and rest periods; getting whatever exercise is possible
- Recognizing warning signs (fatigue, rashes, headaches, dizziness, fevers, and stomach upset)
- Nutritional remedies including nutrients, supplements, and herbs

- Biofeedback, meditation, relaxation, visualization, and pain management techniques

- Acupuncture and non-invasive techniques: qi gong, acupressure, reiki, tai chi chuan

- Psychotherapy and chronic illness counseling

- Assertiveness and proactivity in dealing with your illness and your SHOC team

- Cognitive techniques: thought monitoring, modifying, stopping

- Coping skills training; creating meaning whether from work, hobbies, volunteering, etc.

The key lies in combining appropriate conventional treatments with appropriate alternative, complementary measures. This combination is akin to the general notion of keeping balance in all areas of your life, a key component of your SHOC. Extremes can trigger relapses or the worsening of symptoms. Moderation and balance take work, but they greatly increase your odds of living your life to the fullest, obtaining the most satisfaction, and even growing and thriving. Keeping your life balanced is one of the promises of growth if you choose to seek the challenge rather than retreat.

Buyer Beware

Many seeking alternative treatments believe that because they are "natural," they cause no harm. While these tools can be incredibly effective, you do need to treat them with caution. Just as with conventional medicine, you must assume an active, responsible role and ensure you're working with trained professionals with appropriate certification or license (if applicable), training, and experience. Do your best to find someone with extensive experience in your particular condition. This is something you owe yourself and a basic element in your SHOC.

Symptoms and Self-Management

Pain is one of the few symptoms appearing consistently among people with SLE. It stems from the immune complexes and the secretion of inflammatory substances like serotonin and histamine, coming from cells reacting to what your immune system mistakenly sees as invaders. Another aspect of SLE that contributes to pain is disturbed sleep, common across ARCs. If you don't get enough deep, uninterrupted sleep, your body can't repair muscles, tissues, and joints. Another element that increases pain is inactivity, which interferes with the release of sufficient helpful endorphins, as well as leaving empty time to focus on pain. See chapter 17 for a discussion about sleep.

Physical Therapy

Physical therapy deserves a note as it's very helpful in treating SLE. If you have severe SLE and must stay in bed for periods of time, physical therapy is important in keeping muscles flexible, strong, and relaxed. However, physical therapy should not be used during acute phases of illness, as it may worsen your condition. Physical therapy can also help women with joint damage, osteoporosis, or neurological impairment from SLE. When possible, physical therapy should include aerobic exercise, which offers benefits such as increased energy, improved sleep and relaxation, excretion of toxins through perspiration and deep breathing, decreased depression, and improved cardiovascular functioning and overall well-being. Physical therapists often use heat and cold in their work, which may reduce pain but won't reduce your SLE-related inflammation.

Nutritional Enhancement

While this book discusses nutrition and its role in illness and health, it isn't meant to be taken as a sole source of information on this subject. Check with your physician and health professionals before making changes or modifications to your current diet. At the same time, you can benefit much by keeping an open mind here and need not limit yourself to conventional remedies. You can gain much from herbalists, holistic nutritional counselors, and the like. Depending on your healer's orientation, you may hear very different stories about the efficacy of diet modification in treating SLE. Many conventional professionals don't believe that what you eat can greatly affect SLE's course, beyond the need to maintain a balanced, nutritious diet. However, if kidney disease develops, these health professionals might recommend reducing both protein and salt. Protein should be limited because the products of protein metabolism generate toxic chemicals, such as uric acid, urea nitrogen, and potassium. If your kidneys can't perform their job of filtering efficiently, these substances can stay in your body in amounts that can cause harm. Salt should be restricted if high blood pressure and edema are experienced.

Healers from alternative schools see dietary changes as having a great impact on illness. Many suggest your diet be low in fat and high in vegetables. Evidence suggests that cruciferous vegetables, like cabbage, kale, and brussels sprouts, contain a chemical called indole-e-carbinol that may be central in combating SLE and maintaining health.

Some SLE patients become overweight and have higher fat levels due to steroids. Those who develop kidney disease also have higher blood fat levels. As we know, high cholesterol is associated with increased risk for cardiac disease, so it's important for people with SLE to reduce dietary fat. Overall, there is support for a diet low in fat, animal protein, and salt. For one, this combination is easy for kidneys to tolerate. As discussed in the segment on RA, all fats are not equal and must be treated differently. Go for olive oil or canola oil and avoid other types of oils. The essential fatty acids (omega-3) provided by oily fish, such as sardines, are helpful for those with SLE and other ARCs.

As with RA, sulfur is a necessity for SLE, as it repairs and rebuilds connective tissue, cartilage, and bone and helps with the absorption of calcium. Sulfur is found in foods such as garlic, onions, eggs, and asparagus or in the supplement MSM. In planning your diet, include foods listed in the RA section: brown rice, green leafy vegetables, fish, fresh fruits (non-acidic), whole grains, and high-fiber foods. Don't forget fresh pineapple, which contains bromelain, an enzyme central in reducing inflammation. Avoid nightshade vegetables (eggplants, peppers, tomatoes, and white potatoes) which contain solanine, a compound that increases pain and swelling. Also steer clear of red meat, dairy products, caffeine, acidic fruits, tobacco, salt, and especially sugar. With respect to iron, you may want to consult with your SHOC team. Some people can benefit from taking iron supplements if their diet is lacking. However, for those with SLE, the ingestion of iron in supplementary form may actually backfire by increasing pain, inflammation, and the destruction of joints.

In the RA chapter, there were suggestions regarding the inclusion of alfalfa. However, I also mentioned that some regard the usage of significant amounts of alfalfa as risky, because alfalfa may trigger ARCs or symptoms in susceptible people. With respect to SLE, the warning focuses on alfalfa sprouts. Alfalfa sprouts contain canavain, which can be toxic and must be avoided by those with SLE. However, the issue is debatable, and if you decide to use alfalfa, do so only after discussing it with your SHOC team professionals who are familiar with SLE and nutrition.

Vitamins, Minerals, and Supplements

Certain vitamins, minerals, and supplements may decrease SLE symptoms and improve mind-body well-being. Two of the most important for SLE are essential fatty acids (EFAs) and glucosamine sulfate. The EFAs, both omega-3, found in fish oil and vegetable oils, such as flaxseed and canola (consumed as supplements or pure liquid and not heated to avoid harmful free radicals) and omega-6, found in seeds, beans, grape seed and primrose oils, are helpful for various ARCs and may reduce the chances of arthritis. You can take these in food or as supplements. Much supportive research on glucosamine in treating osteoarthritis has been publicized. If you have SLE, glucosamine sulfate helps maintain healthy skin, bones and connective tissue. Skin cells are also protected by consuming EFAs, like primrose oil, and L-cysteine and L-methionine (with water or juice, not with milk).

Any substances thought to boost immune system functioning are critical. Garlic has been touted for hundreds of years as a health aid; it improves immune system functioning and protects important enzyme system functioning. It's best to disperse ingestion several times during the day. Vitamin C (3,000 to 8,000 mg per day) and zinc (maximum of 100 mg per day) help your immune system and healing. Talk to your doctor about raw thymus and raw spleen glandulars, which help immune processes of the spleen and thymus. N-acetylglucosamine may help prevent SLE (Balch and Balch 1997). With other suggested nutrients, it's wise to take a comprehensive multivitamin/mineral complex. Some ARC patients may need liquid formulas.

Two behaviors that deplete your levels of vitamin C and call for increased consumption are cigarette smoking and frequent aspirin use. Recall that vitamin C is found in a variety of herbs and foods including catnip, cayenne, dandelion, garlic, horseradish, kelp, plantain, papaya, raspberry, rose hips, strawberry, and watercress.

Anti-Inflammatory Nutrients

Nutrients with anti-inflammatory properties are of obvious import to people with SLE and are central in reducing disturbing symptoms like pain, swelling, and stiffness: vitamin B complex daily; primrose oil (boosts the generation of prostaglandins with anti-inflammatory properties and reduces pain); omega-3 fatty acids in fish oils; grape seed extract; shark cartilage; vitamin C; and fresh pineapple containing the enzyme bromelain. SLE patients should discuss iron with their SHOC docs as it can increase inflammation, pain, and joint damage in those with arthritis. You may want to avoid supplements or multivitamins with iron and instead obtain some of this substance through foods (broccoli, cauliflower, fish, peas, and lima beans are a few sources).

Our bodies produce TGF-B, which is involved with the inflammation process. About 75 percent of people injected with the protein anti-TGF-B experience a great reduction in inflammation (Balch and Balch 1997). You may want to discuss this with a SHOC member well-versed in SLE; if she or he refuses such alternative treatments, it may be time to move on. A natural substance with increasing attention paid to it, honeybee venom, is being used to treat CFIDS and FMS. It seems to have anti-inflammatory properties and has successfully been used to treat arthritis and other symptoms. Make certain you get allergy tests prior to using this treatment. For further information, refer to the American Apitherapy Society (see appendix I).

Sweet and Gooey: What a Pain

It sure is convenient and tasty to start the day off with one or two donuts and some hot coffee. A few hours later, when you're lethargic and low, it's time for that candy bar and cola. When lunch hour rolls around and you're zooming off to get some errands done, you have just enough time to quickly stop at the drive-thru, pick up a greaseburger, fries, and a sticky sweet milkshake, and gobble it down while rushing back to the office or home. When the inevitable four o'clock slump arrives, you're lucky that vending machine selling candy or chips is just down the hall, or maybe you'll dig into your stash of sugary or fatty snacks at home. Dinner . . . well, you get the picture. Exhausted, stiff, and in pain, you barely manage to get out of bed or off the couch at times. You're not up to fixing a fresh, healthy meal. You meant to have some crisp fruits and veggies cut up, but you didn't, so you easily toss some frozen food into the microwave and get the fatty, bland stuff down. Maybe even that is too hard and you're feeling depressed, so a nice bag of cookies or chips sounds like the perfect prescription.

Whatever the cause, it's too easy to fall into unhealthy eating habits these days. Sugar, fat, and caffeine are a real troublesome trio, particularly if you have

SLE and its pain and stiffness. When you consume any of the trio, you may feel a rush or surge in energy. This peak is brief and is soon replaced by the crash. What's harmful about these substances? In effect, they trigger the fight-or-flight stress response in your body—and you certainly don't need any additional stress from your food. Elements of prolonged, frequent distress (in long-term stress), blood vessel constriction, and tightened muscles and tendons increase inflammation, pain, and stiffness. Refined, fatty carbohydrates (cookies, cakes, pastries, chocolate, etc.) and other fats (lunch meats, whole-milk dairy foods, red meat, palm and coconut oils) worsen SLE pain by making us gain weight. Many women with SLE are already battling extra weight associated with the onset of their illness. Unless you're underweight, more weight further stresses your body, because your joints are under more pressure and your muscles must work overtime! A gram of fat contains twice as many calories as a gram of complex carbohydrates or protein. What you want to strive for in your foods, as throughout your life, is balance. Follow the dietary suggestions given above and minimize sugar, fats, white bread, caffeine, alcohol, red meat, and dairy products.

Antioxidants

Antioxidants are a current health buzzword . . . but what are they and why do they matter? Antioxidants include naturally occurring substances in our bodies, as well as vitamins, minerals, and enzymes. They're essential in protecting against free radicals that damage our cells and immune systems and are linked with infection, disease, and aging. Some free radicals occur in the body from exposure to chemicals, cigarette smoke, radiation, excessive sun, and natural body processes. However, in the body's wisdom, we also have free-radical scavengers whose job is to neutralize the free radicals. These enzymes are helped by vitamins, herbs, minerals, and hormones with antioxidant properties.

Many elements with antioxidant properties are useful in combating SLE. For example, grape seed extract, vitamins E and C, and garlic are antioxidants and free-radical scavengers that also help reduce inflammation. Beta carotene (vitamin A) is an important antioxidant; you may want to include both vitamin A and natural beta carotene. If you're pregnant, don't take more than 10,000 IU per day.

Herbal Remedies

Several herbs have been recommended particularly for treating lupus. These include red clover, echinacea, feverfew, and pau d'arco. The last three of the four have been receiving a significant amount of press as of late. (A note of warning: If you're pregnant, avoid feverfew.) Herbs also help in treating SLE symptoms through topical application. For example, for mouth sores, one of the most distressing aspects of SLE, take a medical-type gauze and saturate it with (nonalcoholic) goldenseal extract. Place this on the sores overnight while you sleep or during the day if you'll be resting. This reduces irritation and speeds up the healing process. (To prevent the development of mouth sores in the first place, try taking the amino acid L-lysine. Another benefit of this nutrient is that it helps the immune system defend against viral infections.)

Again, you can't rely only on herbal remedies to deal with SLE. The idea of balance is central to building and maintaining health. In this case, you'll gain maximum benefits by using a balanced approach through seeking guidance from conventional doctors and alternative experts, like holistic nutritionists and herbalists. Visit your local natural foods market, health foods store, or even supermarket to stock up on important herbs, vitamins, and minerals.

Hormone Supplements

Melatonin, one of today's biggest supplement sellers, is actually a natural hormone produced in our brains. These days, its primarily used to help reduce sleeping problems. As mentioned, poor, insufficient sleep is often involved in SLE. However, melatonin is not recommended for people with ARCs, such as rheumatoid arthritis and lupus (Rosenfeld 1996). Check with your doctor prior to taking melatonin or any hormones or supplements.

DHEA is another hormone that's been receiving great attention recently. As with melatonin, DHEA is touted as having anti-aging properties. DHEA is produced by the adrenal glands, with the majority of production occurring up to the mid-twenties, after which the amount in the body decreases until a small percentage remains (late seventies and eighties). The decline in DHEA may be associated with the onset of illnesses, such as cancer, Parkinson's, type II diabetes, and so on.

Just what are the many claims about this wonder hormone? It is thought to stimulate bone deposition (reducing osteoporosis), increase production of the sex hormones estrogen and progesterone, and increase muscle while decreasing body fat. The less DHEA in the body, the more vulnerable the body's organs and tissues are to weakening and disease. What is important here is evidence suggesting that DHEA supplements can help treat SLE, improve immune system functioning, decrease pain, improve stress tolerance, and increase mobility and sleep quality (Balch and Balch 1997). Before taking this or any supplement, consult with your doctor and health care professionals. Some believe high DHEA doses interfere with the body's own ability to generate DHEA, and animal studies have shown that liver damage may result. Make sure to take antioxidants like vitamins C and E, and selenium to reduce the chances of liver damage.

Fighting Photosensitivity

The simplest way to avoid problems with sunlight is to limit your sun exposure. When you go outside, hats, scarves, umbrellas, and maximum clothes coverage are wise. Also, schedule your appointments and outings for when the sun isn't at its peak hours. Sunscreens that are both UVA and UVB protective—the higher the SPF the better—should become second nature. It's not only outdoors that you need to protect yourself. Some indoor lights are damaging, such as fluorescent bulbs, which emit UVB rays, and halogen bulbs, which emit UVA rays. Do a walk-through of your home and office and replace these types of bulbs with alternatives.

Dealing with Digestive Problems

Some people with SLE experience gastric disease with dyspepsia (gastric irritation), pain, burping, nausea, and vomiting. These symptoms are common and often result from the various medicines being used. Pain relievers and cortisone are common sources of gastritis or gastric ulcers which you'll feel as abdominal pain. Other possible lupus-related digestive system symptoms include diarrhea, constipation, colitis, rectal bleeding, and problems swallowing and moving food down the esophagus. Doctors might diagnose these problems by viewing affected areas with their instruments or by examining levels of various substances in your blood. Treatment of these conditions is limited but may include antacids or acid receptor blockers for the heartburn. There are also medications that relax the muscle separating the esophagus and stomach, reducing heartburn and the sensation that food has become lodged in the throat.

Handling Hair Loss

Unfortunately, our society doesn't teach us to view baldness in women as equivalent to baldness in men. Bald men may be seen as sophisticated, attractive, sportsmanlike, and possessing other characteristics linked to a positive, ego-enhancing self-image. There are very few bald women who are comfortable, and far fewer who derive any positive self-esteem in showing their natural state. If it's a choice, it's usually done as an act of rebellion, whether against the gender rules, the church, or society in general. This is one of the times in which you'll have to work hard to keep the views and comments of other people in perspective and feel good about yourself because of who you are inside.

As a result of one of my many autoimmune-related infections, I have spent extended periods of time graced with much less than a full head of hair. Although I'd flirted with the idea of shaving off my hair in my youthful, defiant days (and settled instead with a very short haircut and bleached white hair), the actuality was initially painful. I developed a variety of ways of wearing my hair to hide the large barren patches until I had to purchase a wig. Now when the painful infection appears, I work to accept it and do what I can to heal.

For women with hair loss, there is a huge network of women who've gone through the experience, often as a result of chemotherapy, and are willing to give emotional support and useful information. You can use hats, wigs, big bows, whatever. How a woman deals with this female "no-no" often says a lot about that woman. One of my clients, Julianna, had an artistic bent and, among other things, was a jewelry designer. She enjoyed shopping for interesting hats and scarves, and also designed her own head coverings, for which she was always complimented. What a way to pursue the path toward acceptance and growth rather than resigning herself to a "hopeless, uncontrollable" situation. She strove to change the latter into an opportunity for self-expression, self-acceptance, and as a way to derive a sense of control where others often feel only increased depression, helplessness, and self-loathing. There are many wigs and hair pieces that are deceptively natural if you choose to go this route. You may be able to get reimbursed by your insurance company. The American Cancer Society has brochures in which you can view and order wigs and flattering, cheerful head coverings.

Treating Mouth Sores

SLE oral lesions most often appear on the roof of the mouth and may be very painful or painless. They seem to be linked with vasculitis, or inflammation of small blood vessels. In fact, many patients rely on the appearance of lesions as a signal of a flare onset. When lesions are painful, you may have difficulty eating or drinking. From my experience and that of my clients, this can be one of the most bothersome, disruptive experiences associated with SLE. Several prescription mouth rinses, like Lidocaine rinse, can be used to temporarily alleviate some pain.

Anemia

Anemia is the most frequent blood-related problem in SLE. Anemia may result from an insufficient number of red blood cells or the inability of the red blood cells to carry enough oxygen due to insufficient iron or vitamins. Also the inability to process or effectively use the right nutrients can lead to such an insufficiency as well. If you're experiencing typical anemia brought on for the above reasons, you may benefit from iron-rich foods and must consult your doctor or nutritionist. However, if you have the rare hemolytic anemia (which occurs in only 2 percent of SLE patients), your body is making antibodies that destroy the oxygen-carrying red blood cells. This is serious, and you must obtain prompt treatment. You may be given prednisone, cortisone, or cytotoxic agents (in dire cases), all of which decrease the destructive antibody and allow a return to healthy amounts of red blood cells. If you have SLE, you'll probably develop the chronic anemia associated with it, but you can work on this with your SHOC team.

Eye Care

SLE can affect the eyes in a variety of different ways. In addition, if Sjogren's syndrome is present, measures should be taken to ease distress and reduce the chances of eye damage. Eye dryness is more than just uncomfortable—it can lead to corneal injury or eye infection. Dry, stinging, and gritty eyes can be soothed and moistened with artificial liquid tear formulas, steroid drops, or steroid formulas, all of which decrease swelling and replace tear supplies. Lubricating formulas may be used before sleep but should be minimized during daytime, as they cause blurring. Lacrisert releases liquid into the eyes over time and can be used once daily. Anticoagulants and even chemotherapy may be used to treat SLE-related eye problems.

Combating Fatigue

Fatigue, the most frequent complaint of people with SLE, may be ignored by conventional medical professionals who focus on other, more apparent symptoms. One reason is that we still lack medications to reduce fatigue consistently across people or even in the same person over time. Researchers are working on the development of some substances that seem promising. One of these includes male hormones, which seem to work by inhibiting particular cytokines, thereby reducing fatigue. Some people find relief with corticosteroids, while others find anabolic steroids beneficial (Lahita and Phillips 1998). This is an area in which you'll have to try various remedies to find what works for you. Of course, medicines aren't the only way to combat low energy and exhaustion. Vitamin and mineral supplements, exercise, relaxation, breathing exercises, and herbal remedies can be extremely helpful as well.

To Work or Not to Work?

As SLE varies greatly in different women, no two experiences are the same. You may be unable to work or carry your former responsibilities for brief or extended periods, depending also on the use of appropriate medications and alternative treatments. Or you may be able to carry on with your current job, modify it, or find a new one. If you can continue as a productive employee, it will help keep you focused and feeling useful, and can be a source of meaning in your life. Refer to chapter 14 for more on chronic illness and work. For referrals and resources, refer to appendix II.

Susan's Story

Just thirty-two years old, Susan has now been living with lupus for seventeen years. She was diagnosed with SLE at the age of fifteen. In our country, most girls of this age are contending with their bodies, boys, parental rules, curfew, acne, idolizing actors or musicians, and school grades. Far fewer are contending with what Susan had to face. It began with severe pain, stiffness, and inflammation in her feet so severe it was hard to walk. Puzzled, she and her parents waited to see if this would disappear as suddenly as it came. It didn't, so they visited their doctor. At this point, Susan had only this very disruptive symptom, and the doctor had no idea what was underlying it. Shortly thereafter, she developed severe arthritis throughout her body's joints. The doctors were now sure . . . "clearly this is a case of juvenile rheumatoid arthritis."

For another year, this is how Susan and her family explained her pain, increasing fatigue, and new symptoms. Meanwhile, Susan, a sports fanatic, tried to keep up with her active lifestyle, especially in playing her beloved softball. This was one of the many times Susan used positive coping techniques, which have helped her mind-body health throughout. Finally, she developed a foot lesion, and her doctors performed a biopsy and a diagnostic test that offered some accuracy in diagnosing SLE. Susan's test came back positive. This young girl and her parents had no idea what SLE was, so they used a second positive coping technique: They did a great deal of research to learn as much about SLE as they could.

Year two ended, and with it appeared a new symptom to further test Susan's limits. She developed pleurisy, or inflammation of the lining of her lungs. She still hadn't caught on to the patterns of her illness; all she knew as she tried to keep up with the rest of the marching band in high school was that she could barely breathe and had chest pains. She then told her parents of the new symptom. Her doctor immediately hospitalized her to remove the fluid from her lungs. Susan recalls laughing at the doctors' shock about how much fluid was removed. That's the third positive coping technique: humor. Her ability to retain her humor throughout her pain and loss have allowed her to make the gains and develop the control she has over her health. Until this time, she'd largely ignored new symptoms, a frequent response to chronic illness. After this though, she became more aware of her body and its changes and now takes immediate action so her illness doesn't escalate in severity. This is her fourth mode of healthy and proactive coping.

A fifth mode is knowing what works for her and doing it: "sleep and reducing my stress level." I asked her about the latter, and she described a technique she calls her "mental attitude check," one of her best tools. She reminds herself of the larger universe around her and that she and her particular life are much smaller in comparison. She uses moderate, balanced self-talk, such as "of course, I'd like to do well at work, but it isn't worth my getting sick over."

These are words we would all do well to repeat in our minds when we're hell-bent on proving we're perfect at work, at home, and everywhere. Susan's sixth positive coping tool includes a very well-thought-out stress coping plan. Rather than just reacting and trying to reduce stress each time her symptoms intensified, she introduced the continuous stress reduction and mind-body unifying practice of yoga. She says, "This keeps me balanced and in touch with myself." Again, Susan's health-building humor is evident as she laughed about how easy it is to forget about our proactive, preventive measures when symptoms, pain, and fatigue lessen: "How soon we forget!"

Susan now values herself enough so that she no longer strives for perfection and takes time off from work if necessary. How many of us value ourselves enough, and aren't overly reliant on external praise and validation to feel good about ourselves? Susan is clear and positive about her gains from this experience: "Most people only find out what is important about life when they're much older, if ever. I figured it out when I was only twenty-three! I learned I can take something from this illness. I have a choice: I can focus on all the negatives and losses and be miserable, or I can enjoy the life I now lead, push myself to see how much I can do while respecting my health, and be happy. When things are bad, I tell myself things could be worse, and they really could be. I try to do things I want and like to do. Sure, it's hard when I see my friends in great jobs accomplishing important things." I asked, "Who do you think is happier and more satisfied overall?," and she laughed brightly, knowing what I meant. "Yes, I've learned the important lessons. I don't need a fantastic job or the adulation of others. This is important if I need to go back down to part-time or even leave work for a while for my health. If I push too much, I pay. It's a simple but hard lesson for us real achievers to learn. This is similar to my use of anti-inflammatory drugs. Even if I'm feeling great, I still need to take some because if I don't, I'm going to feel lousy tomorrow." Balance, I asked? "Yes," she laughed knowingly. "For me, healing now is just having a normal day, not too much pain, going to work, having a good eight hours in a day, and being active any way I can. My healing also includes what I've been fortunate to learn so early: to value the present and live each moment as fully, positively, and completely as possible. I know I can be sick again merely by becoming overly stressed."

You might be interested to hear what medications and tools help Susan deal with the illness. She has been on Plaquenil since the first year. Her dosage increased over the years, but now she is back to just slightly above the initial level. She attributes this to an increased sense of control over her life and the new mental and physical techniques she uses to reduce her distress, symptoms, and pain. What else helps? "Water therapy and swimming, or even baths. I also learned biofeedback, which helps so much with pain. Massage is great, but my most powerful medicine has been sleep! The steroids I finally had to take at my worst worked instantly, but they also were terrible for me in terms of side effects and I'll try all the alternative techniques I can if I get that sick again." What would you tell someone diagnosed with SLE? "Be happy with what you can do. Don't focus on all the losses or what you can't do. If you choose to focus on the negative, you're going to live an awful life. There is no need for that!"

CHAPTER 9

Sjogren's Syndrome

The healing system is the way the body mobilizes all its resources to combat disease. The belief system is often the activator of the healing system.

—Norman Cousins

If asked about Sjogren's syndrome (SS), most people would reply that they had never heard of it. This underscores again how scant and erratic is the knowledge of autoimmune conditions. It's unusual for a disorder to be so unfamiliar when more than four million people have what Sue Dauphin (1987) terms the "sneaky arthritis." In fact, she puts it second to RA in terms of frequency. The word syndrome is used instead of disease when no clear-cut etiology or cure exist, and when the illness is a collection of often diverse symptoms. These reasons and the fact that research started fairly recently helps partially explain the lack of knowledge of this illness.

Another reason, common to all of the autoimmune conditions, is the intense segmentation of today's health care system. The partitioning of medical services makes accurate diagnoses difficult. Dauphin describes her own travels as she went "... to an opthamologist for an explanation of blurred vision, a dermatologist about dry and irritated skin, a urologist about recurring infections, and an internist about the aching and swollen joints.... Dentists ... constantly admonish[ed] her about the build-up of plaque and excessive cavities ... in spite of ardent brushing and flossing." Med schools are the starting point of such ignorance, and Dauphin estimates that doctors forty years old and up have heard minimally about SS and were probably taught the chances were slim they would need to treat such a "rare" condition. This fact plus the wide array of SS symptoms increases the risk of incorrect diagnosis. The delay between symptom onset and getting the correct diagnosis is often twenty years or more. Women who experience these differing symptoms out of the blue at different times, after being dismissed as fakers or hysterics, or being pushed through the system incorrectly diagnosed, may give up trying to get an answer or trying to heal.

What Causes SS?

Many causes have been proposed and studied. Blood sample studies suggest that the sex hormones involved in SLE are also involved in SS (Manthorpe 1981, 1986). People with SS also tend to share certain genetic factors in their blood: anti-Ro (SS-A) and anti-La (SS-B) antibodies, and HLA-DR3, DR2, DR4, DRw52, and other histocompatibility antigens (Dauphin 1987). What we know now is that for some reason, the immune system produces lymphocytes that generate self-reactive proteins, or autoantibodies, which attack the salivary, tear, and other moisture-producing glands. This destroys the glands and their ability to produce vital substances. Someone genetically predisposed probably needs a trigger, whether it's bacterial, viral, a physical or emotional stressor, a chemical exposure, or even a food allergy.

SS can be confused with SLE due to an overlap in symptoms. Both involve the extreme fatigue seen in so many autoimmune disorders. For at least some conditions, the same dynamics underlying the fatigue may exist. According to Dr. Robert Schwartz (1989), the inflammation of ARCs causes white blood cells, the lymphocytes, to emit certain signals. A lymphokine or peptide, interleukin-1 (IL-1), causes certain brain cells to emit another peptide, which causes sleep. In healthy people, this is a protective, healthy response as it induces those with a cold or other illness to get the sleep they need to heal. However, if you have one of certain autoimmune-related illnesses, your immune system is overactive and the inflammatory response occurs all over your body. The last thing you need is less energy and more fatigue.

Symptoms and Signs

The AARDA states that hallmark symptoms of SS are severe dryness of the eyes, mouth, vagina, and other mucous membrane tissue. Joint pain and inflammation are also typical. Mouth dryness can lead to chronic dry coughing, drinking inordinate amounts of fluid, difficulty chewing and swallowing, and resulting heartburn and chest pain. Eyes may feel extremely dry, burning, itchy, or gritty, and nasal dryness and ulcers may result. These symptoms are the result of lymphocytes attacking and damaging the glands responsible for lubricating the eyes, mouth, and joints. However, people with SS may also experience a wide array of ever-changing symptoms. These include multiple bladder infections, skin problems, and a mouthful of bad teeth and gums! SS patients can also cause various digestive and nervous system problems. Those with SS can experience any of a number of other symptoms given the vagaries of the condition and the propensity to have other arthritic conditions or autoimmune syndromes or illnesses.

Related Conditions and Look-alikes

Besides the similarity in the dynamics of autoimmune conditions, another similarity is diagnostic difficulty. People with autoimmune conditions often have more than one type. If you have SS, your most likely autoimmune-related companion is RA, as 30 to 50 percent of SS patients also have RA. You may also have one or more of the connective tissue diseases or another autoimmune disorder, such as scleroderma, SLE, polymyositis, or dermatomyositis. Because SS causes severe fatigue, SLE may be wrongly diagnosed (though they can occur together).

When a person has at least two out of the three typical SS symptoms, including dry eyes, dry mouth, and painful joints, without an accompanying connective tissue or rheumatic disorder, she is said to have primary Sjogren's syndrome (sicca complex). In Latin, "sicca" means dry, and the link between this name and the syndrome is obvious. If a woman has these symptoms with one of the aforementioned connective tissue diseases, she has secondary Sjogren's syndrome. People with SS do tend to have an array of changing symptoms, making it difficult to properly diagnose the condition. While not frequent, other problems that can occur with SS and increase diagnostic confusion are hepatitis (liver inflammation), cirrhosis, pancreatic inflammation, and inflammatory bowel disease. Many SS patients do report the annoying presence of a variety of allergies, with the symptoms of stuffed-up noses and rashes, but they must be cautious because their post-nasal drip, stuffy head, and swollen glands may be due to SS and not allergies. Correct diagnosis is essential, as antihistamines for allergies can cause trouble if the symptoms are due to SS.

Rheumatoid Arthritis

SS is often misdiagnosed as RA because they share symptoms such as dryness of the eyes and mouth, joint pain, and damage to muscles, lungs, skin, blood vessels, and nerves. In fact, 30 to 50 percent of RA patients are also diagnosed with SS. For more on RA refer to chapter 7. Recent improvements in differential diagnosis have improved the ability to distinguish between the two.

Lupus

As many as 30 percent of SLE patients may also have SS, and certain underlying causes, such as sex hormone activity, may be similar (Manthorpe 1981). Those with both conditions may share similar genetic disruptions with respect to their immune systems. Some of the shared symptoms include swollen glands, skin problems, joint pain, and extreme fatigue. It's harder to distinguish between

SS and SLE than between SS and RA. What is most difficult is distinguishing between primary SS with shared symptoms of SLE and Sjogren's syndrome secondary to SLE.

Scleroderma

About 4 to 5 percent of people with SS also have scleroderma, a systemic, chronic connective tissue disease. An early sign that you're developing scleroderma is the onset of Raynaud's phenomenon, in which fingers are extremely sensitive to cold and may turn from red to white to blue while feeling numb or tingly. The Arthritis Foundation (1983) states that scleroderma also involves inflammation of the fingers and toes and thickening of the skin and sometimes internal organs. The confusion between SS and scleroderma arises from scleroderma's similar effects on skin, joints, blood vessels, kidneys, and the respiratory, muscular, and digestive systems.

Polymyositis, Dermatomyositis, and Fibromyalgia Syndrome

Polymyositis and dermatomyositis are rare, occurring in approximately five people out of one million, and are characterized by the immune system's attack on the muscles (Dauphin 1995). This leads to pain, loss of muscular function, heat sensations, and inflammation. See chapter 12 for more on Fibromyalgia.

The Courses of Sjogren's Syndrome

This is a chronic autoimmune illness in which the immune system, as in other autoimmune conditions, turns against itself. In this case, lymphocytes damage exocrine (mucus-secreting) glands, such as tear glands and salivary glands, misperceived as foreign invaders. Once injured, the glands no longer produce enough lubrication of the eyes, joints, mouth, and other body parts. Some early symptoms include: severe mouth and eye dryness; eye secretions that interfere with vision; eye grittiness, burning, or itching; and changes in taste and smell. You may see halos or light flashes and have light sensitivity.

The typical SS dry mouth results from lymphocytes attacking the salivary glands on each side of the face and the resulting disruption in saliva production. Results range from the least harmful (though embarassing)—having food particles stick to your teeth and difficulty swallowing dry foods—to the most harmful—having severe tooth decay because there is insufficient saliva to remove food deposits and bacteria. You may get frequent cold sores in your mouth and at the corners of your lips, and the extreme dryness and irritation can increase candidiasis yeast infections (Hernandez and Daniels 1989). You may find that your increased thirst results in frequent urination. If this happens often at night, it may be difficult to get adequate sleep. One of the most disheartening symptoms comes from inflammation in the glands around the mouth, causing swelling beneath the ears and noticeably enlarged jaws. This often appears in conjunction with redness and fever. Don't ignore this swelling. If you detect a hard lump in these areas, report it to your health caretaker to rule out a tumor. Also, because your saliva may be deficient in epidermal growth factor, which regulates stomach wall growth, your stomach wall may be thin and prone to infections or ulcers.

As regards the third typical symptom of SS, joint pain, there is some good news for people with primary SS, as this symptom is typically less severe than in RA. Also, if you've been diagnosed with primary SS and haven't experienced joint pain, it's unlikely you'll develop RA after this. Confusion between SS and RA is common as they even share a pattern of joint pain and swelling (i.e., simultaneous affliction of the same joints on both sides of the body).

About 25 percent of people with SS also experience symptoms involving the blood vessels, kidneys, pancreas, muscles, and thyroid. One might wonder where the effects of SS stop, as the central and peripheral nervous systems and digestive system may also be affected. For example, lymphocytes may cause kidneys to malfunction and excrete water in the form of urine even when there is no excess water; fortunately, this symptom is rare. Other problems may arise based on your dietary habits. High-fiber foods often recommended to keep your digestive system functioning smoothly may backfire in SS because they act by absorbing moisture in the digestive system to create bulk. You probably understand why high-fiber foods can be trouble for people with SS, who already have insufficient amounts of liquids, including digestive substances, throughout their systems. In your case, high fiber may cause constipation, indigestion, abdominal pain, nausea, and ulcers. Often, SS patients have stomachaches arising partly from a *lack* of sufficient acid in the digestive system. The resulting irritation of the stomach lining leads to the burning, pain, and nausea experienced by many people with SS. Problems arise when a doctor attributes it to excess acid that frequently underlies stomach upset in the general public and prescribes medicines which are the opposite of what you need.

Though it's a controversial idea, there may be a link between the central nervous system and SS. Some studies show interference with higher cognitive functions, like memory and concentration, and mild mood swings. This area requires further study.

If you've been diagnosed with SS, it's essential to remember that the progression described here is only a generalization. Your case can differ greatly from the norms. However, you must educate yourself as this is the start of the most effective coping you can do. Learn what to expect in general, what your options are, who the specialists in your area are, and what the most effective healing methods are.

Testing for Sjogren's Syndrome

As with other ARCs, there is no single, definitive test to unerringly diagnose SS. As research continues and more is learned, this may become possible. At present, your doctor should rely on a variety of information: your reports of current and past symptoms; factors you believe are related to symptom changes; any previous health-related concerns, illnesses, operations or allergies; medications; physical or emotional stressors (past or ongoing); lifestyle habits (diet, exercise, smoking, drinking, drugs, toxin exposure); your social history and childhood experiences related to your current physical health; your family's physical health history; the doctor's own physical exam; data from other doctors you've seen; and various tests. Be prepared with as much information as possible when you visit your health caretaker.

Here is a brief discussion of some specific tests used to identify SS and rule out other diagnostic possibilities. These descriptions can help you decipher a doctor's medi-speak (should it sound like a foreign tongue) and will help you use this jargon a bit if necessary. Being an assertive partner in your healing increases your control and chances of improvement.

Given the relatively poor accuracy in diagnosing SS, it's essential you find an expert who is well-educated and experienced with the condition. Your health professional should be thinking about SS if you present with complaints of continuous dryness of the eyes, mouth, vagina, and nasal passages. She should conduct a thorough physical exam, which often detects enlarged lymph nodes in the neck, swollen salivary glands, irritated eyes, and a sore tongue. Your physician may take an X-ray called a sialogram after dye has been injected into your parotid gland to determine how well your salivary gland is working.

If the doctor doesn't refer you to an ophthalmologist, ask for a referral or locate your own. The resources in appendix I will help you locate a referral. An eye doctor will examine your eyes by putting a drop of dye into the eye and examining the cornea with a slit lamp. This allows her to detect whether the cornea is injured or dry. In addition, she can place a particular type of thin paper under your lower eyelid to measure the amount of tears secreted by your tear glands (Schirmer test).

Biopsies are another frequently used method of testing for ARCs, and of all tests for SS, the most common may be a lip biopsy. This is performed by removing a bit of tissue from a salivary gland and studying it under a microscope. The researcher is looking for the infiltration of lymphocytes. If found, the diagnosis of SS is typically considered confirmed. Certain blood tests for autoantibodies should also be used to accurately define the diagnosis. As you know by now, these tests don't pinpoint SS as the cause, but they're useful in ruling out other causes. In this case, diagnostic difficulties can arise because SS shares certain blood factors with both RA and SLE. A medical professional not too familiar with the overlap among ARCs or the particular patterns of shared diagnostic indicators and symptoms might note the lupus indicator or the rheumatoid arthritis indicator and diagnose one of these two disorders rather than SS. A physician looking at the abnormal results of an antinuclear antibody blood test may conclude, as is frequently the case, that this indicates RA. Unfortunately, blood tests of SS patients indicate that up to 50 percent of SS patients have rheumatoid factor and as many as 90 percent have antinuclear antibodies. Therefore, distinguishing between RA and SS isn't a simple procedure. Similar abnormal results on these blood tests can also suggest SLE, scleroderma, and connective tissue disease.

Lupus erythematosus cell preparation was initially used to diagnose SLE, as the LE cell is present in those with active SLE about 90 percent of the time. However, the same cell is found in other autoimmune disorders, such as SS, RA, and scleroderma. Another problem in SS occurs when lymphocyte multiplication is so excessive that clusters are formed. These may appear to be tumors when diagnostic tests are used; while they're not inevitably malignant, they must be watched as they can eventually develop into true lymphoma. If you have these clusters, your doctor must monitor your blood serum components. Should the level of immunoglobulin drop from a high level and a decrease in RA factor be noted, a lymphoma state may be developing. Don't panic unnecessarily, as fewer than 5 percent of people with SS develop lymphoma (Pavlidis et al. 1982). Just keep this information as part of your SS database and have regular check-ups.

What You Can Do

Remember, your body is unique. The last thing in the world you should do is ignore symptoms simply because they don't fit descriptions you've read or heard about. You must be in touch with your body and its changes. If you suspect something is amiss, even though it doesn't follow any rigid description, see a professional. The sooner you determine whether something is wrong and what it is, the sooner you can form your plan of attack, research the illness and good health professionals, work on your attitudes, and thus reduce the speed of progression or degree of damage. This all fits into your toolbag for beating the odds. Also, your unique mind-body state means you may need different types of healers and alternative methods. After all, there is no such thing as 100 percent certainty in any doctor's diagnosis or prognosis. You'll have to develop a cohesive mind-body integrity so that as you travel your unique path, you connect with your SHOC team in a timely way if medications aren't working, if side effects crop up, or if things take an unexpected turn. Recall the role your mind and thus your emotions and behavior have in improving or worsening your health.

Because there are few if any magic pills to "cure" your condition, the aim of your treatment will be to discover ways to provide relief, improve your quality of life, enhance your energy, increase your satisfaction, and even derive mind-body growth. Just as your individual experience of SS will differ, so too will the treatment and healing. The key lies in integrating appropriate types of conventional and alternative measures. This is just another example of the healing inherent in balance, which will work in all areas of your life. Make this a key component of your SHOC, because extremes can trigger relapses or intensify symptoms. Moderation and balance take hard work but greatly increase your odds of living life to the fullest. Learning to maintain balance in your life is one of the paths toward growth promised to those who decide to take the challenge.

Some treatments people with SS end up using, including prescribed medications, can actually increase certain symptoms. Again we see the damage that arises from misdiagnosis of autoimmune conditions. For example, NSAIDs are often used to relieve distress in people with arthritis and related conditions.

Because SS is often confused with RA, many people with SS end up being pre-scribed medicines for RA. In particular, NSAIDs are trouble, because they decrease production of prostaglandins (chemicals that increase stomach mucosal secretions, thereby increasing stomach lining protection). With a further reduction in already low levels of mucus, the already thinner walls and susceptible tissues are made even more vulnerable to infections or damage by chemicals.

Corticosteroid drugs like prednisone are often used to reduce severe inflamm-ation, but another effect is that prednisone reduces your body's supplies of vita-mins C and B6, zinc, and potassium. Furthermore, corticosteroids cause trouble by actually suppressing the immune system over time, thereby increasing the possibility of infections, which your body will have difficulty fighting off. When infections arise, people may end up too frequently being prescribed antibiotics. If this happens often and long enough, antibiotics suppress the immune system's proper functioning and destroy the good bacteria in charge of warding off infec-tions. Your doctor may unintentionally cause a worse scenario than that with which you began.

Medications and Remedies

To prevent problems, make sure to have regular check-ups with your eye doctor and dentist. Lubricating ointments and artificial tears can help reduce eye irritation and damage. Use of moisturizers and vitamin E will greatly benefit your dry skin. Your environment directly impacts your symptoms, so maximizing the humidity where you live and work will reduce your symptoms. Vaginal dryness can cause pain during intercourse and increased susceptibility to infections, but there are many helpful vaginal lubricants you can use. You may wish to confer with your health professional to see whether she recommends a particular brand.

In fact, it's essential you remain in frequent contact with your physician, rheumatologist, and other treatment professionals, given the frequent changes of SS and the infrequent though serious problems (i.e., lymphoma) that may arise. Below you'll find a description of how you can be directly involved in scouting out this possibility, slight as it is. Early diagnosis is key in lessening illness sever-ity and may even be life-saving.

Buyer Beware

Many seeking alternative treatments believe that because they're "natural," they can cause no harm. While these tools can be incredibly effective, you do need to treat them with caution. Just as with conventional medicine, you must assume an active, responsible role and ensure you're working with trained professionals with appropriate certification or license (if applicable), training, and experience. Do your best to find one who has worked extensively in and possi-bly even researched or written about your particular disorder. This should be a basic element in the design and practice of your SHOC. You simply owe it to yourself.

Self-Monitoring

Lymphoma from SS is rare, and your commitment to regular check-ups, together with technological advances in finding and diagnosing lymphomas, greatly increase your chances if lymphoma is detected. You can also take steps at home toward the same goal. Pay attention to body changes, like weight loss or lumps or swelling in the groin and armpits. Frequent checks for breast cancer are invaluable, as is examining your head and neck behind the ears, working downwards along the neck and underneath the armpits. If you have an enlarged lymph node, you'll be able to see it, feel it, or both. If so, report this to your health caretaker right away. Many people, when they discover something may be amiss with their body, do their best to avoid their doctors. While denial is often a natural reaction to poor health, it may also be very dangerous. Ignoring symptoms, changes in health, or pains won't make them disappear and often opens the door to mind-body illness.

Nutritional Enhancement

While this book discusses nutrition, illness, and health, it isn't meant to be a sole source of information on this subject, so check with your health professional before making any changes to your diet. This is an area in which you can benefit by being open and not limiting yourself to conventional remedies.

Depending on the orientation of the healer you're consulting, you'll hear different stories about diet modification in treating autoimmune disorders, such as SS. Many conventional doctors don't believe that what you eat greatly impacts the course of the disease, beyond the need to maintain a balanced, nutritious diet. Healers from alternative schools often disagree with such views and believe that dietary changes greatly impact the nature of the illness. One thing is certain with respect to SS, and that is that while most people benefit from high-fiber foods to keep the digestive system working smoothly, these can be harmful for people with SS. You already have insufficient amounts of liquids, including digestive substances, throughout your system and thus if fiber absorbs the minimal amount of liquid you do have, you can develop severe constipation, indigestion, abdominal pain, nausea, and ulcers. It's definitely worth your while to consult with your physician, health care professional, and/or nutritionist to construct an optimal eating plan.

Overall, there is support for a diet low in fat, animal protein, and salt. For one, this combination is an easy one for kidneys to tolerate. Secondly, all fats are not equal and must be treated differently: Use olive oil or canola oil, but avoid other types of oils. If you have more than one autoimmune disease, be sure to take note of the nutritional guidelines in the other chapters as well. Discuss the following with your health professionals to determine what to incorporate into your SHOC:

- The essential fatty acids provided by oily fish, such as sardines, are helpful for individuals with various autoimmune-related conditions, such as lupus.

- For dual diagnosis patients, dietary sulfur is central in repairing and rebuilding connective tissue, cartilage, and bone, and in absorbing calcium. Sulfur is found in foods such as garlic, onions, eggs, and asparagus. Avoiding nightshade vegetables (eggplants, peppers, tomatoes, and white potatoes) is important because they contain solanine, which increases pain and swelling. Steering clear of red meat, dairy products, caffeine, acidic fruits, tobacco, salt, and sugar is beneficial.

- Fresh pineapple contains bromelain, an enzyme central in reducing inflammation.

- Under certain conditions, iron supplements can help if your diet is lacking sufficient amounts of this nutrient. (However, if you have SLE as well, taking iron in supplementary form may backfire by increasing pain, inflammation, and the destruction of joints.)

- Some regard consuming significant amounts of alfalfa as risky becuase it may trigger some genetically predisposed people (see SLE and RA chapters). The issue is controversial; if you choose to use alfalfa, do so only after discussing it thoroughly with health professionals experienced in nutrition, autoimmune conditions, and SLE in particular.

Vitamins, Minerals and Supplements

Given that SS is an autoimmune disorder, any substances that boost immune system functioning are critical. Garlic has been touted for hundreds of years as a health aid; for your purposes, it improves immune system functioning and protects important enzyme system functioning. It's best to disperse consumption throughout the day. Vitamin C (3,000 to 8,000 mg per day) and zinc (maximum of 100 mg per day) also help our immune systems and assist in healing. Speak with your health care professional about raw thymus and raw spleen glandulars, as they can improve the immune processes of the spleen and thymus.

It's also wise to take a comprehensive multivitamin/mineral complex. You may more easily tolerate and better absorb nutrients from the liquid forms of such multivitamin/minerals.

Three factors that deplete vitamin C and call for increased consumption are cigarette smoking, frequent aspirin use, and use of birth control pills. Vitamin C can be derived from various herbs and foods including citrus fruits, berries, tomatoes, potatoes, peppers, cayenne, garlic, kelp, plantain, papaya, raspberry, rose hips, and watercress.

Anti-Inflammatory Nutrients

Given that many SS patients have joint pain and inflammation, arthritic conditions, or other ARCs, the following may be particularly helpful. Nutrients with anti-inflammatory properties can reduce symptoms like pain, swelling, and stiffness.

- Vitamin B complex daily with primrose oil, an omega-6 EFA; also seeds, nuts, beans

- Omega-3 fatty acids by supplement or eating at least two servings per week of tuna, salmon, shark, herring, and mackerel. Deep sea fish also helps reduce fatigue and painful joints due to anti-inflammatory properties. Other omega-3 EFAs are canola and flaxseed oils, which should be consumed in supplement or natural forms while avoiding heat exposure.

- Grape seed extract and shark cartilage

- Vitamin C: 3,000 to 10,000 mg per day in several doses with bioflavonoids, 500 mg per day, which increase vitamin C's potency (Balch and Balch 1997)

- Fresh pineapple, which contains the anti-inflammatory enzyme bromelain.

- Anti-TGF-B injections reduce joint inflammation 75 percent (Balch and Balch 1997).

- Bee venom (may also boost immune system functioning)

Sweet and Gooey: What a Pain

It's convenient and tasty to start the day off with some donuts and coffee. A few hours later, when you're feeling lethargic and low, it's time for that candy bar and cola. When lunch hour rolls around and you're off to do some errands, you may have just enough time to hit the drive-thru, pick up a greaseburger, fries, and shake, and gobble it down while rushing back to the office or home. When the inevitable four o'clock slump arrives, you pray that the vending machine selling candy or chips down the hall is working or that you have some sugary or fatty snacks if you're at home. Dinner . . . well, you get the picture.

Maybe it's a different scenario for you. Exhausted, stiff, and in pain, you barely manage to get out of bed or off the couch at times. You certainly don't feel up to making a fresh, healthy meal or cutting up crisp fruit and veggies for a snack. Maybe you can toss some frozen food into the microwave and get the fatty, bland stuff down. Or maybe that's still too hard and you're feeling depressed, so a nice bag of cookies or chips sounds like the perfect prescription.

Whatever the cause, it's so easy to fall into unhealthy eating habits these days. Sugar, fat, and caffeine are real trouble, particularly if your SS causes severe pain and stiffness. These substances may give you a rush or surge in energy. As you probably know, this peak is temporary and soon you crash. What is harmful about these elements? In effect, they trigger your body's fight-or-flight stress response. Most of us have too much unnecessary stress in our bodies and don't need any more from our food! The results of prolonged distress, like decreased cortisol, blood vessel constriction, and tightened muscles and tendons, increase the inflammation, pain, and stiffness of SS.

Refined, fatty carbohydrates (cookies, pastries, chocolate, etc.) and other fats (lunch meats, whole-milk dairy foods, red meat, palm and coconut oils, etc.)

worsen SS pain by adding weight. Additional weight, unless you're underweight, further stresses your body by putting your joints under more pressure and making your muscles work overtime! Each gram of fat contains twice as many calories as a gram of protein or complex carbs. What you want to strive for with food, as in all areas of your life, is balance. Include fresh fruits and vegetables (primarily nonacidic fruits), certain carbs, fish, and other low-fat proteins in your diet. Minimize sugary foods, unhealthy fats, white bread, caffeine, alcohol, red meat, and dairy products. Remember that people with SS often need to watch the amount of fiber they consume. It's a good idea to work with a nutritionist in order to maximize the benefits from your diet.

Antioxidants

Antioxidants, one of today's health buzzwords, include natural substances in our bodies, as well as vitamins, minerals, and enzymes. They protect you against free radicals that damage your cells and immune system and are linked with infection, disease, and aging. Some free radicals arise as a result of exposure to chemicals, cigarette smoke, radiation, excessive sun exposure, and natural body processes. However, in the body's wisdom, we also have free-radical scavengers whose job is to neutralize the free radicals threatening your body's internal integrity. These enzymes are assisted by vitamins, herbs, minerals, and hormones with antioxidant properties.

Elements with antioxidant properties are important in combating SS. That multi-talented nutrient, garlic (Kyolic), interferes with free radicals that cause joint damage. The suggested dosage is two caps three times daily with meals (Balch and Balch 1997). Grape seed extract, germanium, vitamin C, vitamin A (beta carotene), and selenium are potent free-radical scavengers that reduce the inflammation and pain of SS.

Candidiasis

Persistent mouth dryness and other SS characteristics can contribute to oral candidiasis infection. Fortunately, there are many remedies to deal with this parasitic, yeastlike fungus. In general, we all have this fungus, which operates in concert with other bacteria and yeasts. But in certain instances, such as SS, this fungus can multiply rapidly, weaken the immune system further, and lead to the candidiasis infection. People with candidiasis may go on to develop sensitivities to elements like tobacco, exhaust fumes, and chemical odors. This same sensitivity appears in autoimmune-related conditions, like CFIDS and FMS.

Various nutrients can help you beat candidiasis: EFAs like black currant seed oil and flaxseed oil; caprylic acid, an antifungal substance that destroys candida; acidophilus (nondairy type); garlic; and vitamin C which, besides its immune system enhancement and antioxidant properties, also protects the body from the candida toxins. Candida thrives in sugars so avoid fruits, sugar, and yeast products. To prevent reinfection, replace your toothbrush each month. Also try eating plain yogurt with live yogurt cultures. There are antifungal medications to treat this condition; however, over time they lead to the development of stronger candida strains requiring ever-increasing dosages. These amounts weaken the immune system and damage organs. So, for SS, medications are not the primary choice of intervention. See the Herbal Remedies section below for treatment.

Dental Dilemmas

After going from dentist to periodontist to root canal specialist, always losing teeth and money, Kelly finally found a dentist who gave her a simple answer for questions she'd had for years: The cause for her teeth and gum problems was a deficiency in saliva production. Unfortunately, neither this doctor nor the many others she'd seen gave her helpful information about what she could do. Even when she asked about SS, they'd vaguely say that there was little hope. One even flatly told Kelly that "they" (people with SS) just lose all of their teeth. Just like that . . . no crystal ball, no stack of empirical studies, and certainly no belief in fostering a positive stance to enhance self-healing. Through her own research and by finding a well-trained, empathic dentist, she got the information she needed to beat the odds. She learned about things she could do to increase salivary production, like using Biotene mouthwash, toothpaste, and gum; using fluoride rinses, like ACT; using the new electric toothbrushes for two to three minutes; flossing and drinking water throughout the day; and having teeth cleanings three to four times a year. SS patients must find dental professionals knowledgeable about SS who are willing to communicate and give guidance.

Herbal Remedies

The cold sores inside and outside the mouth are painful, disturbing reminders of SS. To deal with the external cold sores, take a medical-type gauze and saturate it with nonalcoholic goldenseal extract. Put this on the sores overnight while you sleep or during the day if you'll be resting for a few hours. This reduces irritation and helps speed up the healing process. To prevent the development of these sores, try taking the amino acid L-lysine. Another benefit of this nutrient is that it helps the immune system defend against viral infections.

With respect to candida, certain herbs are said to be effective against this fungus. Pau d'arco is a remarkable herb because it has myriad benefits for many illnesses and physical problems. It is naturally antibacterial, cleans the blood, assists in healing, and is helpful for all types of infections, including candidiasis. It also helps in treating symptoms of many autoimmune-related conditions, like irritable bowel syndrome, cardiovascular disorders, and rheumatism. If you've tried it but it hasn't seemed to work, or if you're looking for a change, try new avenues. Both clove tea and maitake tea can help rejuvenate your body's efforts to fight infections such as candida.

You may also want to try the herb myrrh, which has antiseptic effects. It's helpful in treating mouth problems as it helps prevent the development of unhealthy bacteria in this area. It also helps in treating ulcers, an unfortunate consequence for some people with SS. Milk thistle is helpful for SS because it has antioxidant properties, helps protect the kidneys, soothes bowel problems, and is thought to be good for weakened immune systems.

As balance is central to your healing, you shouldn't rely only on herbal remedies to deal with your autoimmune condition. In this case, you're most likely to obtain maximum benefits by integrating guidance from conventional doctors and alternative professionals, such as holistic nutritionists, herbalists, and the like. Remember to do your part in finding the most knowledgeable, helpful experts to be on your SHOC team. Later chapters and appendix II offer more information on relaxation techniques, acupuncture/acupressure, massage, chiropractic, breathing, coping skills, and cognitive techniques (that is, using your mind to modify mind-body interaction and boost overall health).

C H A P T E R   1 0

Graves' Disease and Hashimoto's Thyroiditis

Statistics are the triumph of the quantitative method and the quantitative method is the victory of sterility and death.

—Hilaire Belloc

These self-destructive thyroid diseases represent two sides of the same ARC coin. When the result of autoimmunity is excess production of thyroxine (thyroid hormone), the condition is hyperthyroidism. The most common type of this disorder is Graves' disease (GD). When autoantibodies attack the thyroid gland, causing insufficient thyroxine production, the condition is hypothyroidism. Hashimoto's thyroiditis (HT) is the most common cause of this type. HT affects 5 percent of American adults, while GD affects an estimated 2.5 million Americans. About 37,000 Americans receive a diagnosis of thyroid disease for the first time each year, and most are from twenty to forty years old. The prevalence of GD is significantly higher in women than in men with an estimated ratio of seven to one.

When it was first discovered that thyrotropin (TSH) regulated thyroid functioning, many scientists concluded that hyperthyroidism in GD simply arose from the pituitary gland's error in secreting too much TSH. Several decades ago this theory was rejected when sophisticated instruments revealed that people with GD didn't have elevated TSH levels. Different theories arose when it was found that GD patients serum contained a thyroid-stimulating antibody, TSAb. This was the start of today's theory that GD is an autoimmune disease. Apparently, the TSH receptor antibodies' constant stimulation of the TSH receptors causes the thyroid cells to produce excessive thyroid hormones.

The hypothyroidism of HT (also known as Hashimoto's thyroiditis, chronic lymphocytic thyroiditis, or myxoedema) stems from the immune system's erroneous attack on the thyroid gland. HT is characterized by antibodies to several thyroid elements, a chronically inflamed thyroid, and lower than normal thyroxine. The antibodies damage the thyroid gland, causing insufficient thyroid hormone production. Both body metabolism and heat generation decrease, leading to typical symptoms. As in GD, female prevalence is greater (5:1) and age is generally in the late thirties to forties.

What Causes Graves' Disease and Hashimoto's Thyroiditis?

If you have GD, your autoantibodies target your own body's TSH receptor protein. The thyroid cell can't determine whether the TSH receptor protein is responding with the normal stimulator, TSH, or with the abnormal protein, the thyroid-stimulating antibody called TSAb. As it can't distinguish, your thyroid is stimulated to continuously produce excessive thyroid hormones. What could cause this mutiny of your immune system?

As with many autoimmune conditions, there is evidence for a genetic component. If one identical twin has GD, the other has a 50 percent chance of developing it. As is typical in ARCs, the genetic contribution may be necessary but not sufficient. Other factors must be present to trigger the disease. While bacteria and viruses trigger some autoimmune conditions, no bacterial or viral involvement has been found in GD, and the illness can't be transmitted directly from one person to another. Some studies have examined the role of cigarette smoking as a trigger. Patients with protruding eyes (Graves' orbitopathy) are significantly more likely to be smokers. Smoking may increase the chances of immune system dysfunction, leading to GD and orbitopathy. Further studies of this possibility are needed. Also true to form for ARCs, GD and HT may appear in the same family. There is even greater overlap between these two disorders: If you've had GD for a while and haven't been treated, your condition can change to HT. This also works in the reverse.

As mentioned, one element of developing these disorders is the existence of antibodies targeting your own thyroid gland. In GD, antibodies attach to and stimulate hormone receptors on the thyroid gland, causing increased production of thyroxine. The pituitary gland produces thyroid-stimulating hormone (TSH), which normally then stimulates the thyroid gland to produce thyroxine. The autoantibodies take over thyroid receptors that usually receive TSH from the pituitary gland and trick the thyroid to believe it's getting the go-ahead from the pituitary gland to make more thyroxine. Another possible trigger for GD, typically a factor in developed countries, is excess iodide. Iodide was often used in medicines in the past; some cold and sinus medicines still contain significant amounts. If you have thyroid disease, steer clear of these, including Iophen, Organidin, Par Glycerol, and R-Gen (Surks 1993). Also watch for the iodide present in the material injected during certain CT scans and X-rays. Table salt also contains iodide, so it may be wise to avoid consuming a lot of salt.

If you have HT, your body's white blood cells (lymphocytes), which are central to the immune response, flood the thyroid and finally crowd out your normal thyroid tissue. As a result, your thyroid grows in size and various symptoms appear. As the thyroid gland grows, it may first release too much thyroid hormone, as in GD. But eventually the thyroid gland produces too little thyroid hormone. After the thyroid is overwhelmed by lymphocytes, scar tissue forms, the lymphocytes depart, and the thyroid shrinks. The next step of the autoimmune process remains a mystery. In HT, the self-attacking antibodies target several components of the thyroid, causing inflammation and insufficient thyroxine production. The autoantibodies go after two central elements of the thyroid gland: thyroglobulin and thyroid microsomes. This interference disrupts the thyroid's duties. One model suggests that the antibodies themselves or as part of an immune complex attach to cells inside the thyroid gland, which are then mistakenly destroyed by the body's own killer lymphocyte cells. The presence of these antibodies in the blood is used to diagnose HT. With this condition, you have an 80 percent likelihood of both antibodies appearing in your blood (Surks 1993). As in GD, iodide can also be a factor in thyroid dysfunction. Insufficient iodide may be a trigger of hypothyroidism, though this is rare in developed countries because salt and food products contain iodide.

Graves' Disease Symptoms

GD may creep up with little notice. Often, a woman feels something is "wrong" but does nothing. If she's lucky, her health system allows regular physical checkups and she may be diagnosed. If she's even more fortunate, she'll have a doctor familiar with thyroid disorders who will find it early. If you think you may have a thyroid disturbance, visit an internist who will conduct a thorough physical examination and take certain blood tests. If something is awry, she'll refer you to an endocrinologist (a doctor specializing in the endocrine or hormonal system). Due to the endocrine system's complexities and the harmful consequences if your hormonal system isn't working well, it's essential you be assessed and treated by an endocrinologist.

The immune system targets the body's thyroid gland and causes an increase in thyroid hormones, thus impacting almost all bodily organs and disrupting metabolism. Physical changes affect the hair, skin, nails, and muscles (causing muscle weakness.) The less severe symptoms of GD include insomnia, sweating, weight loss, increased appetite, hand and body tremors, anxiety, diarrhea, frequent bowel movements, and elevated body temperature. These symptoms make sense if you think of the body as perpetually revved up, using all its available energy, producing excess heat, and needing more energy to keep it running fast.

Because thyroid glands affect the heart, GD patients may have a faster heart rate and stronger heart contractions than normal; these can feel like heart palpitations.

In severe GD cases, there may be abnormal changes in the heartbeat (arrhythmias). If atrial fibrillation occurs (when the heart beats so quickly it can't effectively fill with blood to pump it out to the body), it can cause blood clot formation in the heart, which may spread through the bloodstream. Even stroke is possible if a clot moves to block an artery leading to the brain. Other severe symptoms include light sensitivity, finger clubbing (extreme swelling), and swelling of the legs and eyes. The eye swelling (orbitopathy) is one of the most widely recognized signs of GD. In extreme cases, shock, coma, or cardiovascular collapse can occur. The brain is also affected by the thyroid glands. If you have GD, you may feel nervous, moody, irritable, and have difficulty paying attention for any length of time.

Hashimoto's Disease Symptoms

In HT, chronic thyroid gland inflammation results from autoantibodies that target several thyroid components and decrease thyroxine production. Hypothyroidism and insufficient thyroid hormones lead to opposite effects on the metabolic system compared to hyperthyroidism. Without sufficient thyroid hormones, you'll have decreased metabolism and heat generation. If you have HT, you'll feel cold even in warm surroundings—though this won't necessarily register on a thermometer. As the heat your body generates decreases, your body tries to keep warm by moving blood away from your skin, which causes the pale skin characteristic of hypothyroidism.

Other symptoms are very dry, flaking skin; thin, brittle nails with lines across them; dry, brittle hair; and hair loss from the head and other body areas. This often develops later in HT, and if you're treated early enough you may not lose much hair. Many of these symptoms are quite difficult for women due to the great value we are taught to place on our appearance. Another such symptom is weight gain resulting from slowed metabolism. Weight gain also occurs from the buildup of bodily fluid characteristic of HT. The fluid accumulation leads to swelling, most noticeable around the eyes but occurring elsewhere, including internal bodily tissues. Just like metabolic rate, the rate at which food passes through your digestive tract slows, and constipation may be so severe as to require enema use.

One process that *won't* slow is your menstrual cycle. You may actually have increased flow and frequency as a result of the failure to produce eggs, resulting in the infertility that is common in hypothyroidism. Since your body isn't producing eggs, your estrogen continues stimulating your uterus lining because it isn't getting the signal to stop. For some, this is the most disturbing result of hypothyroidism. Some women with HT become pregnant, but pregnancies are usually high risk due to the elevated occurrences of miscarriages, stillbirths, and premature births. Once hypothyroidism is treated, successful pregnancies are much more likely.

Other symptoms include muscular and neurological problems. HT interferes with motor movements, making it hard for you to perform everyday activities in a smooth, flowing manner and requiring you to really focus on movements to avoid accidents (or what you or others might see as clumsiness). Muscular functioning is worsened by accompanying muscle pain, which is similar to that of other ARCs, ranging from a general aching to focused and severe. A slower heartbeat and decreased blood flow to muscles and organs further impair muscle movements, making you feel more fatigued than warranted by the level of exertion.

As you know, physical changes mean mental changes. You may have a decreased ability to concentrate, increased difficulty with problem solving, and decreased interest in activities and relationships. Take another look at these symptoms. Do they remind you of any other disorder? In fact, these are some of the defining criteria for the diagnosis of depression. When my clients come in for depression, I always ensure they have a medical check-up to rule out hypothyroidism or other physical causes.

Related Conditions and Look-alikes

GD is often equated with swollen, bulging eyes, but the thyroid-stimulating antibodies that cause harmful overproduction of thyroid hormones may not be at the root of the eye disorders sometimes seen in GD. People with extreme hyperthyroidism may have no eye disease, while some with mild hyperthyroidism may have a serious eye disorder. We don't know if the eye disease is an element of GD or a separate ARC (Surks 1993). Other GD symptoms are mood swings, irritability, anxiety, and constant tension. Recall the overlap in symptoms between HT and depression. The same pattern occurs with GD: a woman with these symptoms may have a doctor briskly conduct a superficial assessment and conclude she has an anxiety or mood disorder. Such situations explain some of the gender discrepancies in mood and anxiety disorders. I'm not denying there may exist a difference, one arising from many causes (Ravicz 1998), but physicians do relate women's physical problems to emotional disturbances much more often than they do with men (Smith 1992).

The protruding eyes and stare of orbitopathy occur in about 50 percent of GD patients, but if a woman has orbitopathy it doesn't mean she has GD. Other causes are severe nearsightedness, losing or gaining a lot of weight, having certain liver disturbances, and having received a lot of drugs containing cortisone. Other conditions that increase thyroxine levels also cause diagnostic confusion with GD: the pill, pregnancy, postmenopausal estrogen treatments, and hepatitis. Fortunately, certain tests can be done to determine if GD is involved.

HT symptoms may be confused with conditions like depression, and if you're female, you're more likely to get referred to one of us "shrinks." I'm not diminishing the benefits psychologists can have whether depression is primary or secondary, but your overall well-being requires proper medical treatment as well.

Please find a well-trained, experienced, and caring medical doctor who will perform a thorough mind-body assessment.

The enlarged thyroid gland characteristic of HT may raise your doctor's concern about thyroid cancer. However, people with HT don't seem to be at significantly increased risk of thyroid cancer. According to Surks (1993), complex scans or biopsies should only be done if a very hard area is detected in the thyroid gland, the typical TPO antibodies aren't seen in the blood, or there seems to be no clear cause for thyroid inflammation. The type of enlarged thyroid gland tells much to experienced professionals. People with HT have a symmetrical, swollen thyroid gland devoid of small lumps and with a firm, flexible texture. If the cause of the swelling is other than HT, the gland is usually softer.

Other causes of TSH deficits that lead to hypothyroidism must be ruled out to diagnose HT. While rare (occurring in less than 5 percent of hypothyroid clients), underlying hypothalamic or pituitary problems must be treated differently. If the true cause is pituitary gland failure, as from tumors, then other glands controlled by the hypothalamus and pituitary, like the adrenal cortex and ovaries, will also function suboptimally. How would this be detected? If tumors cause pituitary or hypothalamus damage, you'd also experience headaches and visual problems. Adrenal gland problems would lead to low blood sugar, hunger and anxiety after eating, dizziness, and fatigue. Ovarian disruption would appear as a loss of pubic hair, sexual disinterest, and few or no periods. For all of these, typical thyroid hormone treatment could cause severe side effects, which makes testing for the cause of hypothyroidism critical. HT is thought to cause hypothyroidism when serum T_4 is less than 5 micrograms/dl. serum TSH is more than 5 microunits/ml and TPO antibody levels are elevated. If serum T_4 is less than 5 micrograms/dl but serum TSH is normal or not more than 5 microunits/ml, your doctor should consider whether pituitary or hypothalamus problems are underlying the hypothyroid condition.

Type I diabetics are at increased risk for both GD and HT. Thyroid hormone affects how fast hormones, including insulin, are cleared from the blood; if thyroid hormone is low, insulin stays in the blood too long. If you're diabetic, discuss this connection with your doctor.

Graves' Disease and Hashimoto's Thyroiditis

The thyroid gland is critical in infancy and childhood because it influences brain and bone development, but it's also essential for adults because it controls functioning of muscles, mental activity, and bone development. The first symptom people with GD may notice is a swollen thyroid gland, which isn't always painful. It may be found if you're touching the area or see swelling in front of your neck in a mirror. Sometimes someone else will inform you. The gland may be three to four times its original size, causing you to feel pressure at the area with head movement or when swallowing. Other early symptoms are feeling very hot, day/night perspiration, rapid heartbeat/palpitations, nail and skin changes, and hair texture changes or loss. For many people with GD, mood swings, irritability, and feeling "revved up" occur early in the course.

You may start losing weight despite eating the same or even more, and bowel movements may increase. Relaxation and concentration may be difficult and you may feel driven to "do" even when exhausted. Your eyesight can change; if you're one of the 50 percent of GD patients with orbitopathy, you may get double vision, dryness, sensitivity to light and wind, infections, pain, and color reduction. Most people have stable or worsening severity, though 20 to 40 percent have periodic symptoms. Surks (1993) suggests there are characteristics that give clues about the future severity of your illness. Remission is more likely if hyperthyroid symptoms are mild, thyroid gland is less than twice normal size, treatment is received only several months after onset, and onset was linked with a serious crisis. If so, confer with your doctor, as it may be best to use antithyroid drugs rather than having parts of your thyroid destroyed through radioactive iodide.

Hypothyroidism develops slowly at first, with few apparent symptoms, so many women attribute the changes to "just getting older" or to being over-stressed, overwhelmed, or just plain exhausted. As with other ARCs, symptoms come and go and come again. Symptoms of hypothyroidism aren't specific to the disease, so diagnosis can take a very long time. Again, we run smack into the problem of gender bias and the generality of the symptoms. A woman may present to her doctor with symptoms of fatigue, weight gain, temperature fluctuations, or in more severe cases, a loss of interest in personal relationships, apathy, and increased sleepiness. Many conventional doctors would conclude she's having hormonal problems or that her physical symptoms are just emotional, perhaps caused by depression.

As time passes without an accurate diagnosis, symptoms continue to worsen. If you have access to preventive health care, today's medical equipment makes it possible to detect hypothyroidism even before the detrimental symptoms develop. This makes delay not only a great shame but also unnecessary. If untreated, HT can lead to fluid accumulation (often in the legs), high cholesterol, weight gain, difficulty thinking, slowed heart rate, lowered fertility, heart disease, and coma.

Ava's Story

The setting of this case and part of the treatment approach I used differed somewhat from the norm because I was working with a group of employees of a large corporation. The firm offered a weekly group meeting for employees to attend on a voluntary basis. A number of people came regularly and had developed solid, trusting relationships.

Ava was a thirty-six-year-old wife, mother, and employee in the bank. Her peers described her as a kind, dependable woman dedicated to her children, husband, and friends. She always managed to be on top of her job, in control of her household, and involved in community groups. When these same friends were questioned carefully about the pervious six to seven months, they paused and modified their previous descriptions. Yes, there had been times recently when she'd forgotten to do some things for her friends or co-workers. She'd been given a warning at work for making more and more simple errors. Come to think of it she was more distracted and had less spunk than before. They didn't like to admit this, but they felt Ava was upset about her new figure, since she was now much heavier and clumsier than before. Her hair and nails looked unkempt sometimes, but they thought maybe she was working too hard or something. Her close friend recalled Ava begging off their early morning walks complaining of extreme cold, a surprising change.

Her co-workers were concerned, but only her best friend knew Ava had been seeing doctors for her weakness, fatigue, heavy periods, and now self-hatred for her appearance. Ava opened up willingly now and described seeing an endocrinologist and telling him she couldn't concentrate, had gained weight, and was always cold and clumsy now. He noted her skin was cool and dry and her pulse quite slow at fifty-five beats per minute. He felt around her neck and spent a long time feeling one place. When she asked, he explained that in palpating her thyroid gland, he'd noticed it was larger and more firm than usual. He thought her thyroid gland might be involved, and she responded that her cousin was treated for some thyroid problem that had caused her to lose a great deal of weight.

Ava was surprised when the doctor asked if she'd felt pricking in her hands and whether it worsened at night; she responded in the affirmative. When he tapped the inner part of her wrist gently, she sucked in her breath in pain; it felt as if an electric current were running down her hands into her fingers. He explained that this pain probably stemmed from carpal tunnel syndrome, in which the median nerve passing from the forearm into the hand through a narrow portion called the carpal tunnel was being subjected to too much pressure. The kind doctor told her that many people with hypothyroidism also have carpal tunnel syndrome. He explained this to her as well as the concept of ARCs. She felt comfortable since he seemed to know so much about her symptoms and pain. He encouraged her to research the disorder, ask her cousin about her thyroid disorder, and seek a second opinion. He said he'd be happy to take her on if she pursued treatment as he was experienced with thyroid disorders.

Ava educated herself about the disorder, helped greatly by her co-workers' research. She also sought a second opinion, which confirmed the first. She returned to the first endocrinologist because he made her feel comfortable, encouraged her active role in her treatment, and was always open to her questions. When she chose to use herbs, he checked for negative interactions with her meds and when he found none, was secure and open-minded enough to support her, stating that conventional medicine didn't hold a monopoly on healing.

Testing for Graves' Disease and Hashimoto's Thyroiditis

When compared with some other ARCs, recent testing advances have made it easier and cheaper to better diagnose these disorders. However, the blood tests don't always reveal the presence of telltale antibodies, and your doctor still needs to conduct careful and thorough assessment screenings. Your doctor should rely on a variety of information sources: your reports of current and past symptoms; factors you believe are related to changes in these symptoms; previous health-related concerns, illnesses, operations, allergies; medications; physical and emotional stressors (past, ongoing); lifestyle habits (diet, exercise, smoking, drinking, drugs, exposure to toxins); your social and childhood experiences possibly related to your current physical health; your family's health history; the doctor's own physical examination; data from your other doctors; observations of your illness; and tests. In fact, examining the levels of serum T_4 and serum thyroid stimulating hormone (TSH), as discussed below, may be today's most effective, efficient way to diagnose both hyper- and hypothyroidism. Be prepared with all your information when you visit your health caretaker.

Let's look at some specific tests used to identify GD and HT and to rule out other possible diagnoses. These descriptions can help you decipher your doctor's medi-speak (should it sound like a foreign tongue) and help you use his jargon if necessary. Being an active, assertive partner in your treatment increases your control and chances of improvement.

The physical exam is an essential part of assessing for GD or other thyroid disorders. What follows is a fairly typical scenario performed by your doctor while examining you prior to diagnosis and at other points in time. The major structure in your neck is called the thyroid cartilage; it's the highest bonelike form found in the center of the front of your neck. Find it by searching for the region that vibrates when you say "Aahh . . . aahh . . ." Directly below this is the cricoid cartilage, a wide band of cartilage. Below this you'll feel a vertical series of thin, round bands that make up your trachea, through which your breath passes. Your thyroid gland, composed of two sections with one on each side of your neck, is located at the same level in your throat as the cricoid cartilage. Since each portion of your thyroid gland is just a bit over one inch in length and the texture is soft, this gland is difficult to feel when in a normal state.

Your doctor will probably want to examine your thyroid gland while you are seated and have your chin raised. Take a moment now to sit this way, putting your fingertips on your trachea and swallowing several times. As you swallow, your trachea goes up and then down. Since your thyroid gland is attached to your trachea, it follows the same motions as you swallow. When your thyroid is normal, there is nothing notable about it when you swallow. However, if your thyroid develops lumpy nodules or if it's swollen, a visual and tactile inspection may reveal this. Your doctor will feel areas of your neck, focusing on your trachea and asking you to swallow. He must include this swallowing portion in your exam, for if it isn't done, he may not detect any thyroid abnormalities.

When It's Hyperthyroidism

If you have developed orbitopathy or eye disorders seen in 50 percent of GD patients, your doctor will probably first order the blood tests described below for hyperthyroidism. If the blood tests come back negative, he'll want to assess the size of your eye muscles using one of the following techniques (in order of decreasing costliness): magnetic resonance imaging (MRI); computerized tomography (CT scans); or ultrasonography. If any of these indicates enlargement of eye muscles in both eyes, the GD diagnosis may be given at that time. Recent tests for these disorders are less costly and difficult compared with the earlier tests relying on radioactive iodide. If your symptom presentation and the doctor's own discoveries during the physical suggest a thyroid disorder, he'll look for confirming information in the form of abnormal concentrations of thyroid hormone in your blood. In particular, a so-called serum T_4 measurement test will be run. (This test is also used to diagnose HT.)

When T_4, one of the hormones secreted by your thyroid gland, is elevated, a hyperthyroid condition is suggested. Another test that is somewhat more expensive but also more sophisticated is a free T_4 test. If this is used, the former serum test need not be used. In addition, a test measuring the quantity of serum thyroid stimulating hormone (TSH) is a good way to determine thyroid abnormalities. Other very sophisticated testing techniques aren't necessary if the goal is just to determine the presence of thyroid disturbances. However, they are essential if you or your doctor detects lumps (nodules) in the thyroid that may be either benign or malignant. These imaging methods include a thyroid sonogram or ultrasound, magnetic resonance imaging (MRI), and computerized axial tomography (CT scan). For further information on MRIs and CT scans, refer to chapters 5, 6, and 7.

The best method for diagnosing hyperthyroidism is for your doctor to measure your serum T_4, together with your serum thyroid stimulating hormone (TSH). If your thyroid gland is excessively active, the tests will reveal levels of serum T_4 above the normal levels (more than 12 micrograms per deciliter) and TSH serum levels lower than normal (less than .1 micro International Unit per milliliter). However, other factors may also increase serum levels, such as pregnancy, the birth control pill, postmenopausal estrogen treatment, and hepatitis. In this case, the best combination is a free T_4 measurement combined with the serum TSH measurement. If hyperthyroidism is present, the same pattern discussed above will be observed. Martin Surks (1993) advises that if your doctor orders a radioactive iodide uptake or thyroid ultrasound test before blood tests have been taken, you should ask why this is so. Blood tests only take a few days and upon their return, if warranted, the other, costlier exams can be ordered.

When It's Hypothyroidism

When T_4, one of the hormones secreted by the thyroid gland, is lower than normal, the same blood measurement tests discussed above are used for diagnosing hypothyroidism is suggested. A more sophisticated, expensive alternative is a free T_4 test. In addition, a test measuring TSH helps determine the proper dose of thyroid hormone. Patients with hypothyroidism show declines in serum T_4 to less than 5 micrograms per deciliter and increases in serum TSH to greater than 5 micro International Units per milliliter. The assessment of antithyroid microsomal (TPO) antibodies is critical. When elevated levels are present, HT is believed to be the cause of hypothyroidism. In addition, the physical exam is central in diagnosing HT; it usually reveals a swollen thyroid symmetrical in form, devoid of lumps, and quite firm to the touch.

Just as in hyperthyroidism, recent advances in testing have made some earlier methods unnecessary. For example, neither the thyroid ultrasound nor the thyroid radioactive iodide uptake test are required. Even if a decline in radioactive iodide uptake is noted, this doesn't necessarily indicate hypothyroidism, as a number of conditions may cause this (Surks 1993).

What You Can Do

One critical issue to remember in treating thyroid disease is that the significant increase or decrease in one's metabolic rate can have undesirable consequences when it comes to prescription medication. Namely, this metabolic factor can directly affect the metabolization of medications. In hyperthyroidism, your body eliminates certain drugs much more quickly than usual; in hypothyroidism, the opposite occurs. Your doctor should obviously be aware of these dynamics when prescribing your medications.

You need to ask yourself whether you truly require treatment at all. As with all ARCs, any particular case can range from very mild to extremely severe. If you have few if any symptoms of hyperthyroidism, it's in your best interest to discuss honestly with your doctor whether any treatment is truly necessary. (Although even some mild cases of hyperthyroidism have certain assessment findings that do indicate conventional treatment.) This is a time when it's essential you have an open, trusting relationship with an experienced, knowledgeable professional willing to work with you on your SHOC.

Conventional Medical Treatments for GD

As is too often the case with ARCs, we do not yet know how to attack, modify, or remove the specific cause and must be content with treatment offering control, symptom relief, and sometimes some restoration to normal thyroid functioning. This, of course, represents the view held by the Western school of scientific thought. To treat GD, the focus is on decreasing thyroid gland activity. In the past this was done fairly crudely by removing most of the thyroid gland. In cases that don't respond to other available treatments, surgery and radiation may be required. Unfortunately, the techniques and medications now available don't target the main problem, which is the immune system's production of the TSAb autoantibody that causes the thyroid gland disturbances of GD.

Most GD patients are initially treated with antithyroid medications that suppress thyroid function, such as methimazole or propylthiouracil (PTU). These are the two medications currently approved to treat hyperthyroidism in the U.S. They have different effects and rates of onset, so discuss them with your doctor. These drugs are typically effective, with about 20 to 30 percent of patients going into long-term remission. However, there are potentially serious side effects.

While it's rare (one out of 200 to 300 cases), some GD patients develop agranulo-cytosis, which is the loss of many of the white blood cells necessary for your body to fight infections. You'll need to take your medicine as prescribed, because it can take up to several months before you notice symptom decrease and improved mind-body well-being: Your constant feeling of being overheated decreases and disappears, your fast heartbeat slows, palpitations decrease, strength returns, and anxiety and appetite decrease.

Another effect that's often distressing to women in particular is the possibil-ity of weight gain. Your previously elevated metabolic rate allowed you to eat large amounts of food without gaining weight, but if you continue this way, whether out of habit or reliance on food to meet needs other than hunger, in all likelihood you will gain weight. Please be patient with yourself as you learn to readjust your eating habits to your body's new requirements. You'll have to tune in to what your body is telling you and eat only when your body signals hunger. This can be a difficult change, particularly if you were using food in these ways: to satisfy dependency, nurturing, or control needs; in an attemp to appear perfect, at least superficially; or to stuff your feelings of loneliness, inadequacy, shame, fear, and the like. If this is the case, you must strive to get in touch with how and why you are using food this way. Only with such insight can you develop a workable thought and behavioral program to modify your eating habits. You may benefit from working with a psychologist, attending a support group, or par-ticipating in a program like Overeaters Anonymous.

You should think carefully about one treatment approach used by some doc-tors. This involves prescribing very large short-term and long-term doses of anti-thyroid medications. Because such high doses would cause hypothyroidism if given in isolation, thyroid hormones are also added. There are at least two prob-lems with this intervention that could affect you adversely. Firstly, it's certainly more expensive to pay for two medications, but secondly and more importantly, by taking such large dosages of antithyroid medications, you're greatly increasing your risk of developing negative side effects. Make certain your doctor has suffi-cient justification for using this approach so that it's consistent with your SHOC.

It may be best to have lower levels of medication, since the longer you are on appropriate antithyroid medication, the greater your chances of remission. Obviously, remission is the goal of those who use medication. Medicine can't yet cure the disease, but it helps control the symptoms while you hope for remission. If and when this occurs, you still need to have regular exams by your health pro-fessional. If tests show TSAb lingering in your blood and your exam reveals decreased TSH levels and increased serum thyroid hormones, it's likely you'll have symptom recurrence shortly thereafter. The regular check-ups help prepare you for possible return of symptoms even before they begin. Regular health care visits are also important so that if you're one of those who develops hypothyroid-ism after a long-term remission of GD, you will be ready to take appropriate action.

Physicians often want clients to continue their designated medications for up to two years to give them a chance for remission. This lengthy period is used because remission may occur within a broad time frame—from several weeks to two to four years. Some health professionals say that if you haven't experienced remission by two to four years of treatment, you probably never will. At this point, you need to make an informed choice, together with your health care support team, whether to continue with medication or pursue radioactive iodide treatment, as well as adding or modifying alternative techniques in your SHOC.

Radioactive iodide is used to decrease the number of thyroid cells and their ability to produce the excessive thyroid hormones that typify hyperthyroidism and GD. If you receive this treatment, you must take some precautions for yourself and your loved ones (Surks 1993). After taking the liquid or capsule of radioactive iodide, avoid exposing others to radioactivity. For the first few days, stay five to ten feet from others and limit your presence around pregnant women, children, and babies for a week. Also, as some of the radioactive iodide remains in your saliva, avoid intimate contact and kissing, and use separate silverware, dishes, and glasses. You also need to take care of your own body. While most of the radioactive iodide heads to your thyroid gland, some is excreted in your urine. Drink plenty of water so you increase the transit time and amount of urine and thus decrease the amount of time the iodide is in your body. Within one to two days, most of the iodide is in your thyroid gland, and every week or so thereafter, the radioactivity decreases by another 50 percent.

The effects of this treatment are not immediate and vary greatly among people. You may experience decreased symptoms in several weeks, though it takes from three to six months before the dosage has its full effects. Frequent visits to your health care professional are essential, because up to 50 percent of GD patients treated with radioactive iodide develop hypothyroidism within ten years and require thyroid hormone treatment, often for the rest of their lives.

Other medicines can be used as primary treatments or as adjuncts. For those for whom medications don't work, surgery and radiation may be used. These methods are used for thyroid ablative treatment, which destroys part of the thyroid to reduce thyroid tissue and the effects of its overactivity. Treatment with antithyroid drugs during pregnancy, if used very carefully, may lead to a safe birth and healthy baby, but obviously it's preferred that the client isn't pregnant.

Conventional Medical Treatments for HD

The treatment of HD depends on the factors contributing to its development and the stage and severity of the disease. The chances are less than 10 percent that HT will disappear without treatment. Your physician is likely to prescribe treatment with thyroid hormones, which generally help your thyroid gland return completely or almost (if significant scarring is present) to its normal size and reduce other disease-related symptoms. On a positive note, this is one ARC for which proper treatment generally leads to a return of your previous asymptomatic lifestyle. As is the case with GD, the amount of iodide in your body can underlie the onset of HT. In our country the risk of insufficient iodide as a trigger is low, but in the world population as a whole, iodide deficiency is the primary cause of hypothyroidism. Iodide can be associated with hypothyroidism through other means as well. As discussed, the diagnostic testing and treatment of this condition may require the injection of large amounts of iodide into the body. If testing of T_4 and TSH suggest hypothyroidism and you haven't been treated with radioactive iodide or thyroid surgery, the chances are great that you have HT. This fact can be confirmed by examining the blood for the presence of the TPO antibodies discussed above.

Under certain circumstances such as in thyroid cancer, a total thyroidectomy (in which the thyroid gland is totally removed) may be performed. When this causes hypothyroidism, continuous treatment with thyroid hormones is required. Another cause of hypothyroidism (15 to 50 percent chance) is previous surgical treatment for GD (often subtotal thyroidectomy). After such a surgery, your health caretakers continue to play important roles in your SHOC, as the risk of hpothyroidism remains elevated. Radiation therapy for GD may also trigger hypothyroidism (10 to 30 percent chance). The chances remain elevated throughout the years, and at the ten-year mark about 50 percent of treated individuals will have hypothyroidism and require thyroid medications for the rest of their lives (Surks 1993). Another treatment causing hypothyroidism, with a likelihood of 25 to 50 percent (though this is not widely known), is external radiation to treat Hodgkin's disease or neck and head tumors.

When HT has been discovered early in the disease process, the signs typically include the presence of the TPO antibodies and a thyroid gland that is larger than normal. At this point, the course is uncertain and variable, so different physicians treat the condition differently. In this early stage, some doctors suggest no medications be used and that intermittent check-ups be given to watch for HT. Other doctors may immediately prescribe thyroid hormones. The best treatment course is debatable, for at such an early stage the chances of experiencing the characteristic symptoms of hypothyroidism at some point range from 12 to 30 percent. All avenues are open: some women experience a remission in the form of shrinkage of their thyroid gland, some women remain in an asymptomatic phase for years, and others will develop hypothyroidism plus greater thyroid size. If HT signs and symptoms are clear and thyroid enlargement with a firm texture is present, it's in your best interest to begin treatment with thyroid hormones. The likelihood of HT spontaneously remitting is less than 10 percent, and thyroid hormone treatment is very effective.

Treating hypothyroidism and HT has come a long way, starting with the transplantation of pigs' or cows' thyroid glands into people, followed by patients consuming animal thyroid glands, moving on to providing pill forms of animal thyroid glands, and most recently to administering manufactured thyroid hormones. Many forms of hormones are available today, but the most frequently used is synthetic L-thyroxine, because when it's ingested it triggers the normal body's response of generating its own T_3. In addition, while all of the many synthetic thyroid treatments lead to development of normal serum TSH levels and normal thyroid functioning, only L-thyroxine results in the development of the most normal serum thyroid hormone levels.

There are certain issues that you need to discuss with your doctor regarding the use of this medication. One such issue involves the initial dosage, which will be based on considerations such as your weight, age, and the presence of other illnesses, particularly heart disease. If you are older and heart disease may be a consideration, initial levels will be lower. The higher the initial level, the faster your body's return to normal functioning and health. In three to six weeks, you'll notice greater energy, decreased muscle cramping, aches, and body weight, and a return to balanced body temperature. Another issue that is important to discuss with your physician is the use of generic versus name-brand medications. Generics are generally much cheaper and often just as good as name-brand medications, but there have been cases of generic preparations without sufficient amounts of the synthetic thyroid hormone, causing a return of hypothyroidism. Your physician may prefer you stay with name-brand medications, such as Levothroid, Synthroid, Levo-T, and others.

Buyer Beware

Many who seek alternative treatments believe that because they're "natural," they're also harmless. While these tools can be incredibly effective, you do need to treat them with caution. As with conventional medicine, you must assume an active, responsible role and ensure that you're working with trained professionals with appropriate certification or license (if applicable) and experience. Your SHOC requires that you find healers with extensive experience and understanding of your condition. You owe it to yourself. The key lies in integrating appropriate conventional and alternative methods. This synthesis is akin to the general notion of keeping balance in all areas of your life, a key component of your SHOC. Extremes trigger relapses or a worsening of symptoms. Moderation and balance take work, but they greatly increase your odds of living your life to the fullest, obtaining the most satisfaction, and growing and thriving. Learning to keep balance in your life is one of the gifts of growth promised to those with ARCs who decide to take the challenge.

Nutritional Enhancement

While this book discusses nutrition and its role in illness and health, it isn't meant to be a sole source of information on this subject. The suggestions presented here can't replace direct consultation with your doctor, nutritionist, or other trained health professional. Check with your SHOC team before changing your current diet, exercising, or adding supplements. At the same time, you need not limit yourself to conventional remedies and can gain much from consulting herbalists, holistic nutritional counselors, and the like. Depending on your healers' orientations, you may hear quite different stories about the efficacy of diet modification in treating ARCs like GD and HT. Many conventional professionals don't seem to believe that what you eat affects the course of the disease, beyond the need to maintain a balanced, nutritious diet. Alternative healers often disagree and believe dietary changes greatly impact your healing.

In keeping with the revved-up body functions of GD, digestion is also much more rapid than usual. As a result, not as many nutrients, vitamins, and minerals are extracted and absorbed from foods before they pass through the digestive tract. This means that what you eat is more important than ever. Nutritional supplements, vitamins, and minerals available in liquid or sublingual form may be more effective for people with GD. Another consequence of having a faster metabolism is that you should definitely avoid taking in caffeine, refined sugar, and nicotine. These foods are helpful in treating GD as they help suppress thyroid functioning:

- Vegetables: brussels sprouts, cauliflower, broccoli, cabbage, spinach

- Fruits: pears, peaches

- Fatty acids: omega-3, omega-6

Overall, there is support for a diet low in fat, animal protein, refined sugar, and salt. As discussed previously, all fats are not equal and must be treated differently. You may use olive oil or canola oil; avoid other oils. The suggestions presented here are helpful in treating GD; however, you must contact your physician and other health professionals to determine what is right for you to incorporate into your SHOC.

For HT, various nutritional recommendations can help. As with many ARCs, it's best to include organic, natural foods and avoid refined, processed foods, such as white flour and refined sugar, whenever possible. It's also important that you watch what you drink; because fluoride and chlorine are both present in tap water, you should try to drink steam-distilled water instead. Yes, you also need to avoid using fluoride toothpaste because fluoride is rapidly absorbed into mouth tissues. The reason for avoidance is that both fluoride and chlorine block the thyroid's iodine receptors, leading to decreased production of hormone containing iodine. This can be associated with hypothyroidism, and if you're already dealing with this condition, you want to avoid factors that can worsen the situation.

James and Phyllis Balch (1997) suggest that the following foods are helpful for individuals with HT: proteins including chicken, cheese, fish, and raw milk, as well as fruits such as dates, apricots, and prunes. They also indicate that the following foods should be eaten in moderation because they can interfere with iodine uptake into the thyroid gland: fruits like peaches and pears and vegetables like brussels sprouts, spinach, broccoli, cabbage, turnips, and kale. If you have severe symptoms, completely avoid these foods, as they can suppress thyroid functioning even further.

Vitamins, Minerals, Herbs, and Other Supplements

Given that GD is an ARC, any substances thought to boost immune system functioning are critical. Garlic has been touted for hundreds of years as a health aid, and for your purposes it improves immune system and enzyme system functioning. You can follow the label directions, but be sure to disperse ingestion to several times throughout the day. Vitamin C (3,000 to 5,000+ mg per day) helps our immune systems, improves stress tolerance which is essential with this disorder, and assists in healing. Taking a vitamin B complex (50 mg three times per day) assists thyroid functioning, improves immune system functioning, increases energy, and helps in the proper functioning of cells and organs. Because GD causes rapid digestion and difficulty in absorbing sufficient nutrients, it's important you take potent forms of these vitamins. In addition to the vitamin B complex, you can take: vitamins B1, B2, and B6 (each 50 mg twice per day).

The essential fatty acids (EFAs), both omega-3, found in fish oil and vegetable oils, such as flaxseed and canola (consumed as supplements or pure liquid; not heated as this can create harmful free radicals) and omega-6, found in seeds, beans, and grape seed and primrose oils, are helpful for people with ARC. They're particularly important for GD patients as they help regulate glandular functions. You can consume foods high in EFAs or take supplements.

Two other essential additions to your regimen are a multivitamin/mineral complex and vitamin E. The former is very important again as a result of the revved-up speed at which your body is operating. Find a comprehensive, high potency multivitamin/multimineral complex and take it faithfully. Vitamin E is a useful vitamin and powerful antioxidant but you should not take more than 400 International Units each day, as greater amounts can stimulate your thyroid gland further (Balch and Balch 1997).

For HT, try vitamins A, B, C, and E and zinc, which help immune system functioning but also have other positive effects. Some of these have antioxidant properties, the benefits of which are discussed in the following section. Vitamin A is an important antioxidant and a requisite for good immune system functioning (15,000 IU per day; if pregnant restrict to 10,000 IU per day) (Balch and Balch 1997). Vitamin A also strengthens the skin and mucous-containing regions, which are the body's first line of defense against invading bacteria, viruses and the like. Vitamin A is optimized when you also consume the same quantity of natural beta-carotene. Beta-carotene is a precursor to vitamin A and is another strong free radical scavenger; however, those with diabetes can't process it and should steer clear of it.

Vitamin C, an antioxidant that stimulates certain key autoimmune-related components, is essential. It aids in stress tolerance and helps detoxify the body. Vitamin C is also important in protecting vitamin E, another important antioxidant that improves immune system functioning. Zinc, which also has antioxidant properties, maintains stable vitamin C levels and helps with vitamin A absorption. For people with HT, both zinc and EFAs (see above) maintain healthy glandular and immune system functioning. Taking a vitamin B complex daily is essential as it improves digestion, thyroid functioning, immune system functioning, and energy.

As discussed in the medical techniques section above, your doctor will likely prescribe a type of synthetic thyroid hormone or natural thyroid extracts to help you regain normal serum thyroid hormone levels. Talk to your SHOC members about consuming saltwater fish, seafood, and kelp. These foods have good quantities of iodine necessary for healthy thyroid gland activity.

Sweet and Gooey: What a Pain

It sure is convenient and tasty to start the day off with one or two donuts and some hot coffee. A few hours later, when you're feeling lethargic and low, it's time for that candy bar and cola. When the lunch hour rolls around and you're off to get some errands done, you have just enough time to stop at the drive-thru, pick up a greaseburger, fries, and a shake, and gobble it down while rushing back to the office or home. You grab a late afternoon junk-food snack and for dinner, well, you're too tired to fix a fresh, healthy dinner.... It's incredibly easy to fall into unhealthy eating habits these days. Sugar, fat, and caffeine are a troublesome trio since they give you a rush and then let you crash. These elements are harmful because they trigger the fight-or-flight stress reaction, and most people with ARCs already have excessive, unnecessary negative stress and certainly don't need any additional "help" from our food! Results of prolonged, frequent negative stress, like decreased cortisol (in long-term stress), blood vessel constriction, and tightened muscles and tendons, are physically and mentally unhealthy. Refined, fatty carbohydrates (cookies, cakes, pastries, chocolate, etc.) and fats (lunch meats, whole-milk dairy foods, red meat, oils including palm, coconut, and palm kernel, etc.) also reduce our energy and cause muscle pain as they make us gain weight. This is already a problem for many women with HT. Unless you're underweight, gaining weight puts further pressure on your joints and makes your muscles work overtime. A gram of fat contains twice as many calories as a gram of protein or carbohydrates. You want to strive for balance in your foods just as throughout all areas of your life.

Antioxidants

Antioxidants are a current health buzzword ... but what are they and why do they matter? Antioxidants include naturally occurring substances in our bodies, as well as vitamins, minerals, and enzymes. They're essential in protecting against free radicals that damage our cells and immune systems and are linked with infections, diseases, and aging. Some free radicals occur in the body from exposure to chemicals, cigarette smoke, radiation, excessive sun, and natural body processes. In the body's wisdom, we also have free-radical scavengers whose job is to neutralize the free radicals. These enzymes are helped by vitamins, herbs, minerals, and hormones with antioxidant properties.

For GD, Vitamins C and E are suggested—but don't exceed 400 IU daily, as greater amounts may stimulate the thyroid gland further (Balch and Balch 1997). The antioxidants important for HT were described above under the vitamin section (vitamin A, C, and E and zinc).

Three factors that deplete your levels of vitamin C and call for increased consumption are cigarette smoking, frequent aspirin use, and use of birth control pills. Remember that vitamin C can also be derived from a variety of herbs and foods including alfalfa, catnip, cayenne, dandelion, garlic, horseradish, kelp, plantain, papaya, raspberry, rose hips, strawberry, and watercress. However, you should know that it's been suggested that excessive use of alfalfa may be associated with the development of autoimmune symptoms in vulnerable individuals.

Other Techniques

Since women with GD often experience nervousness, irritability, insomnia, tremors, and fatigue and women with HT may feel depression, distress, and fatigue, additional techniques discussed in the third segment of this book can be helpful. Refer to later chapters on breathing, relaxation, massage, biofeedback, meditation, and cognitive tools.

C H A P T E R 1 1

Type I Diabetes

For a long time I felt like damaged goods. I was obsessed with the
question "What is wrong with me?" But I just kept doing the work.
A part of me knew that I was not locked into anything. My cells replace
themselves completely every seven years ... Of course I could change.

—Saphyre, quoted in *The Courage to Heal*

It's fitting that the chapter on type I diabetes follows the discussion of Graves'
disease and Hashimoto's thyroiditis, for if you're diagnosed with TID, you're at
greater risk for certain ARCs, including GD and HT. (People with TID are five
times as likely to have thyroid disease as people who don't have TID.) You'll read
about this tendency and associated ARCs in the diagnosis section below. If you
know Latin and Greek, you'll know much about this condition through its technical name, diabetes mellitus. "Diabetes" is the Greek word for excess urination,
while "mellitus" is the Latin word for honey. Centuries ago it was recognized
that urine from diabetics was replete with sugar and smelled and tasted sweet.

Current estimates indicate that sixteen million people in the U.S. have the
disease (Campbell 1998). This overall figure includes type I, type II, and gesta-
tional diabetes (which develops in pregnant women with no previous history of
diabetes). It's assumed that 5 to 10 percent of these individuals, about 1.6 million,
have TID. Each disorder differs somewhat, but all share the central problem of
difficulty moving glucose out of the blood and into the body's cells where it

provides energy for the body. TID is of interest here because it is an ARC. Formerly known as juvenile-onset diabetes (50 percent of people with TID are less than 20 years old when they are diagnosed), it's now called type I diabetes, or insulin dependent diabetes mellitus, as it also affects a number of young adults. Besides age, other TID factors are being Caucasian and having a family history of diabetes.

Let's take a quick look at the digestive process so you can see where the TID problem arises. When you digest food, your body breaks down much of it into sugar (glucose). Your blood carries glucose into your cells to provide energy for your body. Insulin, a hormone produced by the pancreas, is essential here as it assists the sugar in entering your cells and also controls your blood sugar level. Without enough insulin, the cells of your body can't absorb enough sugar from your bloodstream.

If you have TID, your autoantibodies attack the insulin-producing cells of your pancreas, thereby destroying the ability to generate insulin. Accordingly, people with TID require regular injections of insulin to maintain normal levels of blood glucose. In type II diabetes (TIID), the pancreas can generate insulin, but the insulin doesn't work properly in concert with the glucose. The result is that too much sugar stays in the blood and hyperglycemia (hyper = too much, glycemia = glucose in the blood) develops. This condition leads to frequent urination, great thirst, fatigue, and other symptoms. If the condition is left untreated, severe medical problems can arise. While many of these problems can be life-threatening, you can control your blood sugar level with various treatments available today.

What Causes Type I Diabetes

As with other ARCs, TID doesn't have a single etiology but results from the complex interplay of various factors. Some researchers suggest that TID can sometimes result from a viral infection or some type of pancreatic injury. However, there is substantial evidence that it also may result from an immune system disorder, and the former two causes may be triggers for the disease in an already genetically predisposed individual. Overall, the etiology of TID mimics that of ARC in general. That is, one necessary factor is genetic endowment, as most TID patients have inherited a genetic vulnerability from both parents. The probability of a child inheriting the disorder from a father who has TID is one in seventeen. If the child's mother had TID and she had the child prior to age twenty-five years old, the child's risk is one in twenty-five, whereas if she had the child after twenty-five years of age, the risk is substantially lowered, to one in one hundred. If a child's mother experienced TID onset before the age of eleven, the child's risk of developing the disease is twice as great. Finally, if both parents have TID, the risk of their child having the disease is between one in four and one in ten (Culverwell 1995). Of course, most children born to two such parents never develop the disease. Obviously then, other factors are necessary.

In TIID, obesity, lack of exercise, negative stress, hypertension, high blood cholesterol, and unhealthy diets are triggers, but these elements seem to have little to do with the onset of TID (Fromer 1993). However, they must be considered in treatment once the disease has developed. Looking again at genetics, there is substantial support for its role in TID. Comparable to other ARCs discussed so far, evidence suggests several genes—rather than a single gene—increase the chance of developing TID. Recall the discussion of the HLA genetic region and its role in ARCs. This region on chromosome 6 and 11 may partially explain why and how one develops the disease.

In terms of environmental factors precipitating TID, viruses may be associated. On a number of occasions a sudden increase in diagnoses of TID has occurred after a viral epidemic. Records also show that TID can appear just after a person has a viral infection. We can't assume that any viral infection causes TID, but viruses may trigger the disease in genetically vulnerable individuals. These include viruses causing German measles, mumps, and a virus closely related to the one that causes polio. These particular viruses include proteins highly similar to the proteins in pancreatic cells that produce insulin. The immune system may be confused by this similarity, so the body's defense system may mistakenly target and destroy these pancreatic cells and the body's ability to generate insulin.

Another environmental factor that can trigger TID is chemical exposure. So far, three such substances have been found, two of which are prescription drugs: L-asparaginase, used to treat cancer, and pentamidine, used to treat pneumonia. The third chemical known to cause TID in humans is pyriminil, a hazardous substance used to kill rats. Other chemicals are known to trigger diabetes in animals, but it's unknown whether they produce the same reaction in humans. Note that the three substances described above produce TID through the same mechanism as other TID triggers, namely, by destroying the beta cells or insulin-producing cells in the pancreas. Another trigger being explored is prolonged exposure to cold weather (Fromer 1993). A final potential—though controversial—trigger is cow's milk. Infants who consume cow's milk rather than breast milk may have a greater chance of developing TID. The process through which this could occur is the same as that for viruses. Cow's milk is thought to contain protein similar to the protein in the pancreas' beta cells. If the baby develops antibodies to the protein in the cow's milk, these antibodies may then go after the body's own pancreas protein cells.

Symptoms and Signs

As with the other ARCs discussed thus far, there is incredible variety with respect to symptoms, signs, and disease pattern. The hallmark symptoms of TID are perpetual thirst and excessive urination. The central symptoms are interrelated: The excessive thirst and dry mouth lead to consumption of great quantities of fluids, increased urination, and thus discernible weight loss from significant losses of body fluids. Along with increased thirst, you may have an increase in appetite, though some people experience decreased appetite. Other symptoms include body fat loss, muscle tissue reduction, and severe fatigue. There is often an increased risk of infection, usually manifest in skin or vaginal infections, as well as blurred vision and strange sensations on the hands or feet, such as itching or burning.

Related Conditions and Look-alikes

TID places you at greater risk for developing four other ARCs. Two of these involve the thyroid gland, another involves the gastric parietal cells lining the stomach, and the other involves the adrenal glands. The first of these ARCs is Hashimoto's thyroiditis (HT), covered in the previous chapter. HT develops when your immune system attacks your thyroid gland, causing it to release insufficient thyroid hormone. On the other hand, the ARC known as Graves' disease (GD) represents the other side of the thyroid coin. In GD, excessive amounts of thyroid hormone are produced. How is this disorder related to insulin and diabetes? Excessive thyroid hormone can lead to insulin resistance, which can easily disrupt efforts to control diabetes. Because of the associations between TID and GD and HT, some experts believe people with TID should be screened to see whether the thyroid self-antibodies are present. This idea is supported by the fact that if these antibodies are going to be present, they'll already be detectable around the time TID can be diagnosed. Even if your diagnosis of TID was confirmed years ago, it's still a good idea to be tested for thyroid disease, because thyroid disease may show up years later. If you're positive for thyroid autoantibodies, you need to be cautious even if you don't have any hypothyroid symptoms yet. This is because the risk of developing this disorder increases with every year of your life. The same goes for detecting the status and development of GD.

Another of the four ARCs TID patients are at risk of developing is pernicious anemia, in which the autoantibodies target the gastric parietal cells. Half of people who test positive for gastric parietal cell autoantibodies (PCA) have very low functioning of their gastric parietal cells. The autoimmune reaction that destroys the parietal cells causes low intrinsic factor levels, thereby interfering with the absorption of vitamin B12. As you may know, vitamin B12 is central to red blood cell generation and nervous system functioning. Long-term low levels of intrinsic factor and corresponding long-term deficit in vitamin B12 absorption bring on pernicious anemia, which is destructive to the spinal cord and brain. As with GD and HT, many experts think all TID patients should be tested for PCA, especially if thyroid autoantibodies are found.

The final ARC associated with TID is Addison's disease. This disorder arises when adrenal glands damaged by autoimmunity yield insufficient cortisol and aldosterone. Cortisol is essential to healthy blood pressure, stress reactions, and hypoglycemia prevention, while aldosterone prevents low blood pressure and dehydration. If both of these hormones fall to very low levels, a dangerous "Addisonian crisis" may be triggered. Early testing is essential.

As TID is often associated with other ARCs, the following list will help your understanding of your particular case and will make you an informed member of your very own SHOC team so you can comprehend and question your health care experts. *Hashimoto's thyroiditis and Graves' disease*: People with TID are five times as likely as nondiabetics to develop thyroid disease. The ratio of female diabetics affected with thyroid autoimmune disorders compared to men is two to one. Ten percent of new mothers with TID develop thyroid disease postpartum, while only 5 percent of new mothers without TID develop thyroid disease postpartum. *Pernicious anemia*: People who test positive for thyroid autoantibodies have a 20 percent chance of testing positive.

The Courses of TID

Remember that the symptoms and patterns described above are only generalizations and your individual case can differ greatly. There is just no single typical progression of the disease. Symptoms can come up slowly over days, weeks, or months or may appear suddenly. You must educate yourself as much as possible, as this is the start of the most effective coping technique. You'll learn what to expect in general, what your options are, who the specialists in your area are, and what the most effective treatments are. TID can be very serious, and treatment should be sought as early in the disease process as possible.

If you have TID, your symptoms will likely begin with a perpetually dry mouth and a great thirst. You'll need to urinate frequently and will notice weight loss resulting from the excretion of so much body fluid. You may be one of those who experiences an increased appetite along with the increased thirst, or you may find yourself with a decreased appetite. You might have feelings of burning or itching on your hands or feet and may have visual changes, often blurry vision. Over time, you may develop infections, most likely of the skin or vagina.

If TID is left untreated, serious medical complications can arise. For example, a woman might develop heart or cardiovascular disease and experience strokes. While cardiovascular disease is the primary cause of death in our country, and for women the rates are growing ever higher, TID patients are at much greater risk of developing this disorder. Kidney disease, nervous system disorders causing leg and foot infections, and even blindness are consequences of untreated TID. While diabetes is one of today's leading killers, this need not be the case. By following certain practices to keep your blood glucose level within normal limits, you can live a happy and healthy life. You'll need to learn to frequently monitor your body's functioning and learn how your body reacts to different factors known to raise and lower blood glucose levels.

Testing for TID

As typical of ARCs, TID symptoms are variable and can be evasive. Unfortunately, up to 20 percent of people with TID have already sustained some damage, such as to the eyes or kidneys, by the time they're diagnosed (Fromer 1998). Fortunately, testing for TID is more straightforward than for other ARCs. In fact, the diagnosis comes directly from the testing.

Blood tests are the primary testing method. Tests report glucose levels and factor into the final treatment plan. Blood glucose can be measured in two ways.

One way is a test called random or casual blood glucose, in which your blood sample is taken and analyzed at a random point in time during the day. For this test, a result of 200 milligrams/deciliter indicates diabetes. The second method of testing examines your blood after ten to twelve hours of fasting. With this measure, levels of 140 mg per dl or more at two different sessions until recently indicated diabetes. The new requirement is 126 mg/dl.

Besides your glucose measurement numbers, your doctor should rely on a variety of information: your reports of current and past symptoms; factors you believe are related to symptom changes; previous health-related concerns, illnesses, operations, or allergies; medications; physical or emotional stressors (past or ongoing); your lifestyle habits (diet, exercise, smoking, drinking, drugs, toxin exposure); your social and childhood history related to your current physical health; your family's health history; the doctor's physical exam; data from your other doctors; and blood and urine tests. This represents the ideal of what a medical doctor or health professional would pursue prior to diagnosing and treating any illness. If you feel shortchanged, you can always seek a second opinion to maximize your SHOC. Prepare for your appointments by having as much relevant data as possible. Being an active, assertive partner in your treatment increases your control and chances of healing.

While you can do some home glucose testing, your doctor must perform the glycosylated hemoglobin test (HbA1c or A1c test). Your own testing tells you daily how close you're sticking to your goals, but this other test tells you how well you're doing over time. The figure provides your average blood glucose levels over three to four months. Nondiabetics' figures are about 5 percent and people with TID should try for a figure less than 7 percent.

What You Can Do

Remember, your body is unique. The last thing in the world you should do is ignore symptoms simply because they don't fit descriptions you've read or heard about. You must be in touch with your body and its changes. If you suspect something is amiss, don't just wait for it to go away. See a professional; the sooner you determine whether something is wrong and what it is, the sooner you can form your plan of attack, research the illness and good health professionals, work on your attitudes, and reduce the progression or degree of damage. This all fits into your toolbag for beating the odds. Also, your mind-body uniqueness means you may benefit from integrating alternative healing methods with conventional methods. Remember, there is no such thing as 100 percent certainty in any doctor's diagnosis or prognosis. You'll have to develop a cohesive mind-body integrity so that as you travel your unique path, you connect with your SHOC team in a timely way if medications aren't working, if side effects crop up, or if things take an unexpected turn. Recall the role your mind and thus your emotions and behavior have in improving or worsening your health. Accepting that complete control over this disease is highly unlikely (I don't like to say "impossible") will reduce the self-blame and guilt that exists when you're not doing as well as your internal critic tells you you "should" be. Focus instead on what you can control, such as glucose monitoring, taking your insulin, eating a healthy diet, getting exercise, and so on.

Because TID arises from insulin deficiency, increasing available insulin is key. The central factor in avoiding long-term health damage is your glucose control: your goal after fasting is 80 to 140 mg/dl and after a meal it's 100 to 180 mg/dl. While some TIID patients can maintain normal blood sugar through diet and exercise, in all likelihood you'll need insulin to regulate your levels. The three-pronged approach that's most effective includes nutrients, exercise, and medication. If your glucose levels aren't where you'd like, several factors may be interfering. Your SHOC team will look at: disease or sickness; your overall negative stress from home, work, kids, being ill, etc.; your actual diet and exercise vs. the plan; your work habits; errors in insulin treatment; and interactions between your insulin and other medications, herbs, or homeopathic remedies. Other factors can also raise blood glucose and sabotage your treatment, including menstruation, contraceptives, pregnancy, and the dawn phenomenon. TID patients who get sick need to watch for increased glucose that may accompany illness, as well as some cold medications, which also increase glucose.

Exercise and Your Glucose Level

Some exercise is critical, but more isn't necessarily better. People with TID must take care when it comes to exercise. Balance and moderation are key, but some exercise is essential in improving your mind-body health. Check with your SHOC members before beginning any exercise program. TID patients need to be cautious because after glucose stored in muscles is used up in exercise, the liver releases glucose stored in the liver. Insulin helps the body use glucose for continued energy but since people with TID lack insulin, ketoacidosis (a life-threatening condition) may arise when this glucose is released and isn't matched with sufficient insulin. Test your blood glucose pre- and post-exercise; if it's above 240, you need to test your ketone level before and after as well. Ketones appear in the blood when your body is burning fatty acids and serve as a warning signal. If they're present, don't exercise until you modify your glucose level. If your blood glucose is 240 to 300 but ketones aren't present, go ahead and hit the track (after checking with your health care professionals of course). No matter the ketone level, if your blood glucose is over 300, you're not going anywhere but to work on getting your glucose back under control (Fromer 1993).

Periods, Pregnancy, and Your Glucose Level

About once a month, female TID patients have a more difficult time keeping a desirable glucose level. In some women, progesterone and estrogen changes linked with monthly periods increase blood glucose, while in others it's the opposite. Depending upon how you're affected, you can take the measures discussed in this section to shift your level back to normal. Pregnancy also affects women differently: Some pregnant women with TID don't have insulin requirement changes, while others must increase their insulin dosage. This increased requirement often peaks in the last trimester, when hormonal changes trigger insulin resistance. All three elements of the three-pronged approach should be involved (medications, exercise, and diet), though pregnant women must increase their communication with their SHOC team.

Negative Stress

Suffice it to say here that part of the negative stress response is the release of certain hormones that trigger a big jump in glucose. You will learn techniques to handle stress later in the book.

Food: What, When, and How

What you put into your mouth determines the amount glucose in your system. Besides giving enjoyment, your diet must also help you keep a normal blood sugar level. You'll maximize your SHOC by working with a dietitian experienced in TID. Check with your doctor for referrals, but also get guidelines directly from your doctor about what to eat, what not to eat, and how may calories to consume. Purchase an inexpensive food scale to help you stay on track. (See appendix I for contact info for the American Diabetes Association.)

Most importantly, choose carefully what you put in your mouth. By focusing on foods high in complex carbohydrates and fiber and reducing saturated fats, you'll make big strides in healing. Also, spread your food intake throughout the day, as the three-meal-a-day habit may result in you going too long without food. Avoid sabotaging your meal plan by not buying foods you shouldn't be eating. However, you don't have to completely restrict yourself from certain foods, just eat small portions. Banning foods often leads to cravings for those very foods and thus bingeing. Sure, this planning takes time compared to your previous lifestyle, when you rushed about grabbing coffee, donuts, fast food, and sugar-laden snacks. But your downtime will be much less now, and so you'll gain productivity overall. Prepack your breakfast, lunch, and other meals and carry a protein snack, such as cheese and crackers, or fat-free lunch meat and crackers, in case you don't have access or time for a meal when your body calls. Carry some glucose tablets, raisins, or a few hard candies in case your blood sugar drops precipitously. The condition of hypoglycemia and what to do about it is discussed in greater detail below. With these dietary changes and some forethought, your body will thank you in other ways than keeping a stable blood sugar level. Your wallet will often thank you too.

Besides keeping a healthy blood sugar level, your eating plan helps reduce cholesterol. Watch for trans fatty acids and saturated fats; there are plenty of products to replace them. Because cholesterol and triglyceride levels are linked with heart disease and other disorders, your doctor should check your cholesterol and triglycerides every three to six months.

Dawn Phenomenon

Your body operates on a schedule and rhythm regulated by internal and external factors. While each person's clock is different, certain commonalities allow for conclusions about timing and body functioning. During early morning hours, your body starts to release hormones preparing it to wake and the liver to release glucose to give you energy. (I'm sure many of us would like some caffeine with that glucose, but think of the coffee houses that would be out of business!) These inner mechanisms underlie the dawn phenomenon, the rise in glucose level from four to eight A.M., which partly explains higher morning glucose levels. If this is your case, consult your SHOC team as possible remedies, like increasing you're morning insulin dose, modifying eating habits, or taking morning insulin earlier can help.

Self-Management

Self-managing TID these days is much easier because of the home tools that are available, including glucose meters and test strips, supplies for urine testing, and glucose tablets. The American Diabetes Association Buyers' Guide, updated annually and presented in the *Diabetes Forecast* magazine, describes many such tools (800-232-6733).

One essential tool is the blood glucose meter, which measures glucose in your blood at any given time. This is vital information because it allows you to make swift changes if your glucose level is off. It's also useful over the long term so you can track your treatment's efficacy and make changes in your diet, medications, insulin levels, exercise program, and other relevant lifestyle factors. Ask your doctor about different brands and measurement types (for example, readings may be given through color changes or through numerical changes). Check whether your insurance company covers these expenses. Some new meters can even read your glucose levels aloud if you're visually impaired.

You may want to buy a urine testing kit, for while they're no longer used to assess glucose levels (they've been replaced by accurate blood glucose meters), they still provide essential data on ketone quantities in the blood. When your insulin level is really low, glucose can't enter cells to give energy, and cellular starvation may result. To forestall this, the body starts burning fat for energy and ketones appear in the blood as a result. They're warning signals that insulin levels are off and that you're in a bad state. People with TID must measure ketones when they're sick, particularly if a fever is present.

Hypoglycemia

When glucose levels fall too low (from too much insulin or exercise or from missing a meal), which occurs even in the most diligent, symptoms of a hypoglycemic reaction arise. Hypoglycemic reactions can be triggered if blood glucose is below 70 mg/dl. Symptoms are fatigue, jitters, weakness, hunger, concentration difficulties, and in extreme cases, loss of consciousness. Rapidity of response is essential, so glucose tablets can be critical. If they're not available, try other fast-acting sugars like sugar cubes, fruit juice, hard candy, raisins, or grapes. While these are cheaper than glucose tablets, the tablets work faster, don't taste as yummy as candy (reducing snacking temptation), and the packages clearly indicate dosages needed to obtain specific glucose changes. You need this ease when you're having a hypoglycemic attack as it's often hard to think clearly.

Dangerous Secrets

One of my TID clients, Kay, tries to hide her illness from most everybody. Unfortunately, this has caused dangerous incidents, including serious car accidents. Recently, at a dinner party, she tried to hide the fact she was taking her insulin and, distracted, took too much. Fortunately, her husband was there and noticed the now too-familiar signs of her hypoglycemia. She began speaking unintelligibly and swaying as if drunk. Back in the hotel room, he had one minute to shove chocolate into her mouth before she lost consciousness. He was terrified and feeling helpless. Kay carried no glucose tablets because it reminded her too much that she was "sick." Her eyes were wide open, blank, and he thought he'd lost her. He kept trying to get sugar down her and monitored her glucose. Finally, she regained consciousness and typically recalled nothing about her erratic behavior or her husband's terror. This time though, he had tape-recorded the episode. She finally "heard" the severity of her illness and for the first time in her life bought a medical ID tag. You certainly have the right to privacy, but be careful not to carry this to the extreme.

Helping Yourself Get Help

It's vital for insulin-dependent TID patients to wear a medical identity tag. If you prefer, you can carry a medical card, though you're less likely to get separated from a medical tag. This information gives emergency personnel the essential information they need to make the right decision in caring for you. Deadly mistakes have occurred when people, under the assumption that someone whose mental functioning is impaired is merely drunk, don't help diabetics get treatment. There are myriad medical tags in the marketplace. Some women I've worked with have somehow personalized their tags and feel proud to wear them. See appendix I for more information.

The Ties That Free: The Facts about Insulin

People with TID must take insulin as a central part of their treatment plan. One of the first steps to take on your SHOC is to educate yourself about the insulin type your doctor prescribes (i.e., its time of use, peak action, and duration). Your doctor or pharmacist can tell you how best to store, use, and inject your insulin, as well as how to best dispose of the residuals or kit.

While both animal and synthetic human insulin are available, it's suggested that people with TID use the human form (Campbell 1998). The miracle of genetic engineering underlies this synthetic human insulin—its molecular structure is identical to that of our natural insulin. Another result of scientific advances is that three types of insulin now exist: short-acting (SA), intermediate-acting (IA), and long-acting (LA). This variety gives you greater flexibility to fit into your schedule and also more closely mimics Mother Nature's intricate designs. While the science of medicine is phenomenal in these developments, the art of medicine is just as significant. If you've just been diagnosed with TID or any ARC, you'll probably have to go through a trial-and-error period with your medication. Given each person's uniqueness, we're as yet unable to prescribe the amount that is (as in Goldilocks' search) "just right." You'll have to be patient (or challenge yourself to be as part of your SHOC) with yourself and your health helpers as they use their teamwork and knowledge to find what type and duration works for you. Also ask them about causes of low blood sugar and how you can respond to these. After this, the ball is in your court, and you must do the mind-body work described in this book to incorporate treatment into your daily schedule and see insulin as the lifesaver it is. Then you avoid wasting your valuable energy on resentment and self-pity and instead use it to grow, create, love, and focus on important things in life.

As I describe each type of insulin, you can refer to the table below for a visual summary. Short-acting insulin takes only thirty to sixty mintues to take effect, peaks in several hours, and is out of your system in six to eight hours. Your doctor may prescribe you short-acting insulin like Novolin, Velosulin, or Humulin. Intermediate-acting insulin starts to work in three hours, peaks anywhere from six to twelve hours, and terminates action in twenty-six hours. Long-acting insulin takes four to six hours to take effect, peaks in twelve to eighteen hours, and is gone by thirty hours. IA and LA differ from SA because they include substances like zinc to slow their absorption and increase their duration of action. A new form of short-acting insulin analog, Insulin Lispro or Humalog, which I call very short-acting insulin, (VSA) offers very fine control in insulin timing. As it takes effect in five to fifteen minutes, you can really synchronize it well with meals, both planned and unplanned. When used right before you eat, Humalog helps prevent blood sugar from rising too high after a meal. More than typical short-acting insulins, Humalog's very brief duration reduces the chances of hypoglycemia. Since Humalog only works for about two hours, it can't cover your whole day and you must supplement it with other forms of insulin (either intermediate- or long-acting types).

Type	Onset	Peak	Termination
VSA	5 to 15 minutes		2 hours
SA	30 to 60 minutes	2 to 4 hours	6 hours
IA	1 to 3 hours	6 to 12 hours	18 to 24 hours
LA	4 to 8 hours	12 to 18 hours	approx. 30 hours

Usually when a woman with TID first appears at her doctor's office, she has no idea she has TID, most or all of her insulin-generating pancreas cells are destroyed, and she has one or more symptoms. Since her body is literally starving for insulin, she needs a fair amount to set it back on track. The actual amount depends on her unique body as well as her weight, diet, and activity level. Her doctor may then reduce her insulin and tinker with it until her glucose normalizes. If she goes into remission, glucose levels stay fairly stable and no major symptoms occur. But she can't let down her guard. This can actually be a danger point because some women are lulled into a false sense of security and think they can be free of insulin. This is usually misleading and some who go off it, only to have to resume it, find they've developed an allergy to it. By now the last pancreatic insulin-producing cells have been destroyed by the autoimmune response, and the body can no longer generate insulin. Typically, insulin requirements again climb but then even out when an appropriate plan is found.

Insulin injections remain central to TID treatment. Other techniques are being developed or tested, like a surgically implanted "pump" to deliver insulin, an insulin patch, and insulin nasal sprays. Further research is being conducted and hopefully new methods will be available.

Doctor Visits and Regular Testing

In addition to your home monitoring, your healing routine must also include tests performed by experts. TID patients need to have examination by an opthamologist at least once a year. You also need to have your thyroid function, cholesterol, and triglycerides checked every three to six months. Your doctor may want to perform urinalysis depending on your glucose level and to monitor your progress. Check with your doctor about how often you need HbA1c tests.

Alternative, Complementary Techniques

Your key to optimizing your healing and health lies in accurately combining appropriate conventional treatments with appropriate alternative measures. This is akin to the general notion of keeping balance in all areas of your life, a key component of your SHOC. Extremes trigger relapses or the worsening of symptoms. Moderation and balance take work, but they greatly increase your odds of living life to the fullest, obtaining the most satisfaction, and growing and thriving, whether in spite of or because of your illness. Maintaining balance in your life is one type of growth promised to those with ARCs who take the challenge.

Buyer Beware

Many seeking alternative treatments believe that because they are "natural," they can cause no harm. While these tools can be incredibly effective, you do need to treat them with caution. Just as with conventional medicine, you must assume an active, responsible role and ensure you're working with trained professionals with appropriate certification or license (if applicable), training, and experience. Do your best to find one who has worked extensively in and possibly even researched or written about your particular disorder. This should be a basic element in the design and practice of your SHOC. You simply owe it to yourself.

Later chapters on coping and optimizing and the appendices on certain alternative methods will prove invaluable. This chapter focuses on symptom management and healing specific to TID.

Nutritional Remedies

By following a plan low in fat and high in fiber and complex carbohydrates, you're doing much to heal yourself. Aim for whole grains, beans, root vegetables, fruits, soybeans, fish, low-fat cheeses, other dairy products, rice cakes, and unsweetened oat cookies. Try to avoid salt, fatty foods, and refined products like white flour and refined sugars that rapidly increase blood sugar (unless you're using them to avoid an insulin reaction). To read more about the negative effects of eating fats and sugars, refer to the section Sweet and Gooey: What a Pain in previous chapters about the individual ARCs. The foods recommended above help decrease the amount of insulin required, help normalize blood sugar, and reduce undesirable fat. Never change your insulin amounts without first consulting with your physician and SHOC team members.

Eat Me, Drink Me, and Read This!: Alice's Commandments

You don't have to cut out all of these substances completely and immediately. You may become resentful after doing this and resume eating the "forbidden" foods, a cycle perpetuated by self-criticism, anger, and the feeling of being out of control. Reframe this situation: It isn't a punishment, just as having the illness is not a punishment for your being a bad person. First, remember you do have a choice, even here. You don't have to change your diet, and this is under your control. When you think through the consequences, and you have in all likelihood already experienced them painfully enough, you'll probably *choose* to modify your diet to make yourself feel better. Remind yourself this is something you want to do for yourself and see it as a challenge, difficult perhaps, but offering great rewards. Secondly, tell yourself these changes are not just another thing that you have to do as a person with TID. Most of these changes are recommended to everyone to improve their mind-body health. Thirdly, to help see this as a challenge and maintain your motivation, create some goals and rewards for yourself. Be creative! There are so many fat-free, sugar-free, and preservative-free foods these days that your palate won't be able to discern many of these changes. Build a sense of mastery by learning about new fruits, vegetables, seasonings, and low-fat cheeses and other protein sources. You have enough loss and restriction in your life, so don't make eating, a great pleasure, another of these. By using your self-talk, reframing and setting up the chance for prostress, you'll be happier and healthier.

Vitamins, Minerals and Supplements

People with diabetes should proceed with caution and a doctor's advice or steer clear of certain supplements. Given the nature of TID, this section starts by listing supplements you should avoid. If you have diabetes, stay away from *beta-carotene*, a precursor to vitamin A, as your body can't convert it into vitamin A. Another popular type to steer clear of is *fish oil supplements and products with significant para-aminobenzoic acid (also listed as PABA)*. While amino acids are also popular, you need to stay away from *cysteine*, which can inactivate insulin. *Chromium picolinate* is also popular these days and is touted as good for diabetes; however, most research and effective findings come from TIID rather than TID. TID patients need to take care with this supplement, for if it's taken without direction from a doctor, it can shift insulin requirements and possibly cause a harmful insulin reaction. Speak with your doctor and SHOC members about these nutrients.

Antioxidants

Antioxidants are a current health buzzword . . . but what are they and why do they matter? They include naturally occurring substances in our bodies, as well as vitamins, minerals, and enzymes. They protect against free radicals that damage our cells and immune systems and are linked with infections, diseases, and aging. Some free radicals occur in the body from chemicals, cigarette smoke, radiation, excessive sun, and natural body processes. In the body's wisdom, we also have free-radical scavengers that give protection by neutralizing these free radicals. These enzymes are helped by vitamins, herbs, minerals, and hormones with antioxidant properties. The antioxidants recommended for TID include vitamins A, C, and E, grape seed extract, and zinc.

Let's look at vitamins, minerals, and supplements from which you can benefit. Vitamin B complex aids fat metabolism, circulation, stress tolerance, immune system functioning, and energy, and when taken with biotin, helps metabolize glucose. Take B vitamins together to maximize benefits. Coenzyme Q10 stabilizes blood sugar and enhances circulation. TID patients often have insufficient manganese, which is central to glucose metabolization and pancreatic health. Garlic boosts immune system functioning and stabilizes blood sugar. Vitamin A, an antioxidant that aids immune system functioning, helps the body use proteins, protects against infections, and protects the eyes. Given the eye disorders associated with TID, this is critical. Maximum dosage is 15,000 IU per day (if pregnant, 10,000 IU per day). Vitamins E and C are helpful antioxidants that improve circulation, autoimmune-related activities, stress tolerance, and detoxification. However, people with TID must stick to normal daily requirements, or insulin efficacy can be compromised. Zinc, another antioxidant, maintains vitamin C levels and improves vitamin A absorption. Importantly for TID patients, it helps healthy glandular and immune system functioning. Watch for smoking and frequent aspirin use, which deplete vitamin C and require increased dosages.

Herbal Remedies

Integrating herbs into conventional treatment can be very effective. Herbs are natural, but not always safe. Pay attention to the following warnings as well as suggestions. Goldenseal can be helpful, but it shouldn't be taken for longer than a week at a stretch and must be completely avoided if you're pregnant. People with TID and people with glaucoma or cardiovascular disease (which often accompany TID) should not take this herb without working closely with a physician and other SHOC members. The herb known as huckleberry can assist insulin production, as can dandelion root, bilberry, and buchu.

Smoking

If you have TID and smoke cigarettes, you're greatly increasing your risk of developing the worst potential consequences. TID patients who smoke have much greater chances of developing diseases of the cardiovascular and central nervous systems and kidneys. Quitting will be one of the hardest things you'll ever attempt. However, if you care about your future and that of your loved ones, you must take this step. Fortunately, there are now tools like nicotine gum and patches that can make the process a bit less difficult. While these help with the physical addiction, you also need to address the psychological addiction. Many find it useful to attend structured programs which educate and support you after you've stopped smoking. Others find informal support groups like Nicotine Anonymous helpful. For some people, therapy with a mental health professional helps them address the emotional needs underlying their smoking habit. Whatever you need to do to quit smoking, do it.

CHAPTER 12

Fibromyalgia Syndrome

*What I've had to tell myself again and again is "Trust yourself."
When my body tells me to stop, I stop. When my body tells me to go,
I go. I used to push myself beyond my limits, and I'd always get sick.
Now I've learned to listen so I don't have to go to that point. I trust
myself because I'm my own greatest healer. Even the best therapist
can't help me heal unless I listen to my body."*

—from *The Courage to Heal*, by Ellen Bass
and Laura Davis

Fibromyalgia syndrome is the most recent name for a disorder first called "fibrositis" and then described as and written about scientifically as "muscular rheumatism" in the 1800s. Despite its long history, FMS is regarded by a large portion of the medical profession as controversial. But to people with FMS, there is no doubt as to its reality. FMS is a typical example of disorders appearing primarily in women, relegated to "it's all in your head" land, with very little serious attention or research until recently.

The current name conveys at least one symptom accurately: "fibro" (fiber), "my" (muscle), and "algia" (pain). The word "syndrome" is used, rather than "disease," because at present there isn't consensus in the medical community as to any particular cause or specific diagnostic test. The American College of Rheumatology set forth the diagnostic criteria for FMS as follows: chronic pain with a duration greater than three months; pain in the four body quadrants, including the spine; painful tenderness in at least eleven of eighteen specified locations. Diagram 12-1 below shows the tender point locations both front and back. Estimates of FMS vary greatly, from three to ten million people. FMS is second to osteoarthritis as the most widespread arthritis-associated disorder. As is typical with ARCs, women far outnumber men, by nine or ten to one (Goldenberg 1998).

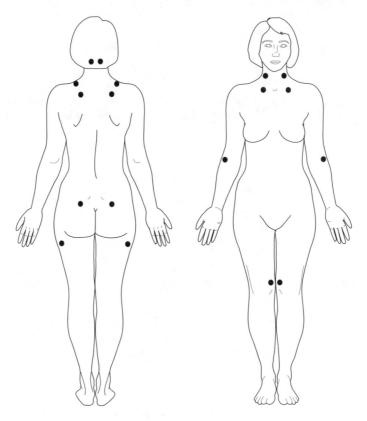

If There Ain't No Such Thing, Why Do I Feel So Sick?

If you consider prevalence statistics over the last several years, you might think FMS is spreading at a rapid clip. More likely, this increase is due to belated, often grudging decisions by doctors to apply this diagnosis. Of course, they're not entirely to blame, as little has been known about FMS, and even less attention has been paid to it in medical educational systems. When it comes to misdiagnosis, the doctor shuffle, and the "it's all in your head" routine, FMS and chronic fatigue immune dysfunction syndrome (CFIDS) are certainly among the top contenders. Of all of the ARCs in this book, these two are probably the most difficult to cope with in terms of facing continuous disbelief on the part of doctors, insurance companies, employers, friends, and family. Over and over, we hear, "You look fine. How can you be sick?" We begin to wish our external appearances, so carefully maintained, would show the true ravages of what we're experiencing internally. You're also likely to hear the dismissive, "Sounds like you have a lot of stress in your life. Maybe you just need to talk to someone." For reasons you'll read about, these conditions have met with great resistance and been considered psychological problems.

Long before I wrote this book, I was fascinated by what I'd noticed repeatedly about women with FMS. Over and over, I encountered women who had been very high-achieving, driven, busy individuals. More recently, I've come across this observation in other articles and texts. But it's hard to believe the theory that FMS is created by the very women for whom these symptoms would be anathema. It's also hard to believe that so many women, each supposedly trying to shirk their responsibilities, would make up conditions with the very same symptoms. So, while there may be personality characteristics shared among *some* with FMS and CFIDS, this by no means indicated that this is the cause of these conditions or that they are shared by all.

While all ARCs illustrate the necessity of including the mind-body factor in healing as it was involved in the onset of illness, it's essential to use this fact as the basic framework for FMS. Consider one example: FMS involves suppression of the hypothalamus gland (the so-called "master" gland, as it controls many bodily glands). Part of the FMS fatigue arises from this suppression, with one of many results being immune system disruption and decreased ability to prevent infections, such as bowel infections. This is critical as it interferes with absorption of nutrients necessary for mind-body health (Teitelbaum 1996). Not only are we unable to absorb sufficient nutrients from food, but we also don't absorb enough from some types of vitamins, minerals, and supplements we take to improve our health. The real backlash is that while we're unable to fully utilize nutrients we consume, FMS also increases our needs for certain nutrients. Our bodies can't meet increased demands while losing necessary energy; the result is fatigue and other FMS symptoms. Let's look at a behavioral part of the cycle: When we're so fatigued, in such pain, or feeling depressed, we may not eat healthfully, perpetuating the cycle of fatigue and pain. This is but one example of how all mind-body parts—the glands, immune and digestive systems, thoughts, emotions, and behaviors—interact with external factors, like viruses, bacteria, and accidents, to generate and perpetuate the cycle of damage.

What Causes FMS?

Many theories have been proposed to explain the onset and long-term, possibly chronic, presence of FMS. Very little is known about the possible causes, and great controversy reigns regarding their relative merits. Because there is as yet no identified cause, there is no cure, although progress is being made.

Genetic Theory

Genetic theories suggest a genetic predisposition to FMS that can affect many of the body's processes. About 40 percent of people with FMS have a close family member with comparable symptoms, supporting this notion. An article entitled "FMS Gene Found" discussed the possibility that the discovery of a new antibody in the blood of 50 percent of FMS patients (with higher percentages in people with severe FMS and those who meet the listed diagnostic criteria) may implicate a particular gene in causing FMS (Sumner 1999). This is exciting, and it's hoped this can be used as an FMS diagnostic marker in the near future. At present, little is known about the genetic components of FMS. As is the case with other ARCs, the extreme prevalence in women as compared to men may relate to a male Y chromosome's protective influence in those with a genetic predisposition. Interestingly, some FMS characteristics look like premature aging of the musculoskeletal system, and perhaps one gene waiting to be discovered as contributing to FMS will be associated with aging (Fransen and Russell 1996).

Jay Goldstein (1996) suggests that disturbances in prefrontal cortex functioning are due to a combination of primarily genetic and secondarily developmental and environmental factors. This is a good example of a model in which genetics serves as a foundation, but not the only factor, involved in FMS (and CFIDS) development. You'll read abut CFIDS in the next chapter, but briefly, Goldstein acknowledges the role of genetics but adds that exposure to infectious agents, a person's developmental history and the resulting particular neurochemical patterns, and limitations in brain adaptability are also involved in the development of CFIDS. The prefrontal cortex has the essential function of determining whether sensory input is relevant to your other experiences and attitudes. If it's not working properly, it allows unimportant information to enter or assigns excessive importance to it. FMS patients can relate to this: the "blasting" music others say isn't loud; the slight impact feeling like a strong jolt each of the many times we bump our hands, arms, or legs; and our extreme sensitivities to smells, lights, and chemicals. Support for the role of genes in FMS arises from the fact that it often runs in families, either by itself or with CFIDS or other ARCs.

As Dr. Goldstein's contributions to the study of FMS and CFIDS are invaluable, I've included significant information on his theories. Other theories and models are also included because they may add pieces to the puzzle. Goldstein's theory differs in essential ways from others. He sees FMS and CFIDS as neurosomatic disorders caused by defects in how information received through our senses is processed and handled by our brains. The primary problems lie in the prefrontal cortex, with resulting disruptions in the primitive limbic system. Simply put, we may be overly sensitive to unimportant (mild) external input, have problems learning and seeing newness in stimuli, and have problems effectively processing and so performing familiar activities.

Sleep Theory

FMS sleep theories arose from studies that prevented subjects from getting deep sleep; the subjects then developed symptoms and tender points like those of FMS. There are many theories for the disturbed sleep and FMS symptomatology. For example, studies show that when people with FMS enter delta wave deep sleep, alpha waves (generally present while awake) interfere, causing awakening or a retreat to a lighter, easily disturbed sleep level. This is called the alpha-delta sleep anomaly, and research suggests that up to 90 percent of FMS patients have it. Delta sleep is a critical stage, for this is when the pituitary gland produces the most somatotropin, or growth hormone (GH). If FMS patients are deficient in delta sleep, logic says they'd have low levels of GH, which is exactly what tests show. Why is GH critical? Even in adults it plays a central role in repairing muscle tissue, which develops tiny tears and damage as we do our daily activities. Further, it's possible that people with FMS have a genetic predisposition for greater microtrauma to the muscles. GH insufficiency interferes with essential repair for daily muscle functioning and health, with one potential result being many minute muscle tears throughout our body that aren't being repaired. The result? You got it . . . typical FMS muscle aches and pain.

Today's investigations focus on the role of neural hormones in causing FMS symptoms. Neural hormones are messengers that are as essential as the cytokines discussed earlier. The former are involved in central functions, like emotions, sleep, pain, and immunity. In a 1992 issue of the *Journal of Arthritis and Rheumatism*, Dr. Bennett and associates described the results of a study of hormones and their interactions. Two groups of women participated: fifty-five "normies" and seventy FMS patients. When the blood was compared between the groups, it was found that women with FMS had less somatomedin C (a hormone related to the pituitary gland). As this hormone's production is based on GH's activity, we see similar results of a deficiency. Somatomedin C is also involved in muscle repair/upkeep, and deficiencies contribute to the muscle pain and fatigue that FMS patients experience. Our GH deficiency also adds to our aches and pains, as it's central in removing lactic acid and substances produced when muscles are used. Insufficiencies of GH allow these substances to build up and cause more pain and interference with normal muscular functioning.

Dr. Goldstein maintains that not only is the alpha-delta anomaly a culprit in disturbed and insufficient sleep, but there are also other reasons for disruptions in slow wave sleep (SWS). For one, there may be damage to areas in the brain like the caudate nucleus (seen in neurosomatic disorders) that also reduces GH amounts. The greater than normal level of pain neurotransmitter, substance P, in people with FMS and CFIDS may be acting as a stimulating neuromodulator, causing symptoms of tooth grinding, night sweats, awakening in a panic, or nightmares. One result of this type of arousal is that it overwhelms the influence of adenosine, an inhibitory neurotransmitter that increases the likelihood of uninterrupted sleep. Another mechanism offered by Goldstein involves depletion of certain neurotransmitters associated with arousal, decreasing fatigue, and triggering behavior, including glutamate, norepinephrine, dopamine, and the neuropeptide, corticotropic releasing hormone. Obviously this can interfere with arousal and energy and increase fatigue. Further, low levels of dopamine and serotonin, which regulate mood, are linked with negative mood states that themselves interfere with good sleep. Serotonin also decreases movement and input processed through the senses, both of which are central in healthy sleep.

Another reason for some FMS patients' disturbed sleep is sleep apnea, in which excessive closure of the air passage during sleep can lead to complete closure and blockage of airflow into the lungs. Results of sleep apnea are snoring or, in the case of complete closure, shallow sleep, which opens up airway passages. Snoring partners and pain also disrupt sleep. People with FMS must be cautious of pain medications, as many react in extreme or unique ways to chemicals. Drugs that make others drowsy might energize you. Even common drugs like aspirin and ibuprofen can interfere with your sleep. Another substance you may think of as a relaxant, but which can greatly interfere with sleep, is alcohol. Also avoid caffeine and refined sugar, which trigger the fight-or-flight stress response, something you don't need when trying to settle down for the night. Finally, I've spoken with many FMS patients with higher than normal rates of teeth grinding while asleep (bruxism), jerkiness and leg spasms while trying to fall asleep (restless leg syndrome), and sudden movements while asleep that interfere with deep sleep or even cause awakening (nocturnal myoclonus). If you have any of these conditions, speak with your doctor. If bruxism is the problem, you'll also need to see your dentist. A device to prevent grinding can be worn while you sleep; it's essential because grinding can also cause severe dental damage. If limb jerking and muscular spasms are problems, take 400 to 800 IU of Vitamin E and/or calcium and magnesium, preferably together in a supplement (Williamson 1996).

If you have FMS, you may feel drawn to sleep theory, as it helps explain the awful sleep experiences many of us have. It also helps explain what I used to think was only my own sleep experience, namely that though I hadn't yet found corroborating evidence, I was certain a huge truck rushed through my house nightly to trample me. How this could happen to me while leaving my cat and husband unscathed was a mystery. By now though, I've heard the same truck analogy from many women with FMS. Is there a team of large semis doing nightly damage to FMS patients? While I'm making light of the situation here, I want to convey the seriousness of this problem, as poor sleep contributes to fatigue, concentration, and memory problems and other symptoms. It's also a primary treatment area. While sleep theories have merit, they're not the sole etiology, as "normies" can also show the same alpha-delta anomaly.

Immune System Theories

Sleep theories are relevant to a discussion of the immune system's role in developing and perpetuating FMS, in that insufficient healthy sleep is associated with decreased immune system functioning. This is discussed in greater detail below. Due to the widespread attention given to AIDS over the past years, when most people think of immune system problems, they think of underactivity or inability of the system to ward off outside infectious agents. By now you know that the immune system can be overly activated and can malfunction by destroying its own body's tissues and organs. As of yet, it's not known exactly how or to what extent the immune system is linked with the onset of FMS, though there is recent growing evidence of linkages. It's posited that GH may be involved in this relationship. GH deficits are associated with the immune system by affecting the activity of cytokines, the proteins that control certain immune system cells, protect against viral infections, and increase the growth of cells, such as blood cells (Williamson 1996). Many immune system chemicals get their "instructions" on how to function from cytokines. GH by-products may slow cytokine generation with deficits in such GH by-products allowing excess production of cytokines. In fact, some symptoms of flu and other contagious illnesses, like fatigue and general achiness, may stem from excess cytokines. If excess cytokines are present in FMS, as appears to be the case, this could underlie the fatigue, aches, and pains.

Cytokines play a much greater role in immune system functioning than was initially believed. Macrophages, part of the body's first line of defense, release cytokines that act as messengers to warn and further stimulate the immune system to respond to an antigen threat. For example, cytokines prod helper T cells to release substances and affect B cell activity. Negative stress may harm the immune system by interfering with cytokine production. Cortisol, released by adrenal glands as part of the distress response, especially in situations of helplessness and lack of control, inhibits cytokine release and macrophage activity (Kemeny 1998). While some ARC patients have lower than normal amounts of cytokines, it isn't clear that quantity is the sole determinant of health. Studies show that in ARCs, parts of the immune system are overactive while others are underactive. In particular, those with FMS and CFIDS may have elevated cytokine levels (Kemeny 1998). The FMS serotonin deficiency also disrupts cytokines and thus immune system functioning and decreases endorphin (natural painkiller) activity. Deep sleep deficiencies increase cytokine activity and mean that antibody production, the immune system's defense against external antigens, isn't proceeding healthfully. People with FMS may have hyperactive immune systems, which explains frequent allergies, excessive or odd responses to medicines or chemicals, and rapid adjustment to drugs (making them ineffective).

A second model focuses on cortisol, a hormone regulating the immune system, blood pressure, and other important elements. Many people with FMS have cortisol deficits that lead to overactive immune systems. People who don't have FMS have daily cortisol fluctuations: a burst of morning production followed by a smaller burst at night. FMS patients have a smaller than normal morning cortisol burst followed by a greater than normal evening burst. This fits with the severe morning fatigue and inability to sleep at night (Fransen and Russell 1996). FMS is also linked with abnormal natural killer cell activity, further suggesting immune system malfunctioning.

Brain Structures and Functioning

Many FMS patients have memory and concentration difficulties, speech disruptions, and mental fogginess, and it isn't surprising that researchers have found differences in brain functioning. The limbic system, a collection of structures around the brain stem that controls primitive functions and affects memory, emotional regulation, and motivated activities, such as anxiety, aggression, sexuality, eating, and drinking, may be involved. Another camp suggests the cause is in the hypothalamus, a structure with widespread connections to the limbic system and other structures, involved in motivated behaviors like eating, drinking, sex, fighting, body temperature regulation, and overall activity. Of importance in FMS is the fact that the hypothalamus regulates hormonal secretions through its relationship with the pituitary (or master) gland. Researchers supporting the role of these brain structures in FMS suggest that either a virus or long-term excessive stress disrupts and causes structural changes in these systems.

Recent technological developments let us see causes of cognitive dysfunction and FMS in a new way. PET scans, BEAMs, and SPECTs show not only brain structures but also how the brain is functioning, areas involved in different activities, and deviations from the norm. One study using SPECT technology to explore regional cerebral blood flow in FMS patients found decreased blood flow in the brain regions of the caudate nuclei, central in memory, pain control, and concentration (Mountz and Bradley 1993, 1994). Another study highlighted brain functioning differences among FMS patients and CFIDS patients by using SPECT technology to examine the brains of thirty-three CFIDS patients, fifteen of whom also had FMS. Again, blood flow deficits to areas in the brain were found in all subjects, but blood flow restrictions were greatest in CFIDS patients with FMS (Goldstein 1993, 1994). It's unknown if the restricted blood flow and resulting oxygen deficit to various parts of the brain is a cause or symptom of FMS.

Some have explored the particular brain area most deprived of oxygen flow, the limbic system, to determine its potential in causing or maintaining FMS. This system is composed of the amygdala, hippocampus, and hypothalamus. The limbic system is self-regulating and maintains body homeostasis. Problems in this system cause disruptions throughout the body. Dr. Ronald Dubner at the University of Maryland maintains that pain for days or hours at a time causes changes in the central nervous system (CNS) and peripheral nervous system (PNS), made up of nerves allowing communication between the CNS and the rest of the body. If these changes disrupt the balance between the CFS and PNS, pain spreads and intensifies. This view mirrors the philosophy of Chinese medicine, which emphasizes the need for balance between opposing elements. Also akin to the Chinese notion, when the limbic, nervous, and endocrine systems are out of balance, mind-body problems arise. It's been posited that all three are out of balance in FMS and CFIDS. Goldstein maintains that the primary problem occurs in the prefrontal cortex, with dysfunctions cascading down to disrupt the limbic system. What happens if there are limbic system problems? The results could come directly from a list of FMS complaints: sensitivity to chemicals, odors, and foods; depression; difficulty with balance and dizziness; confusion; and memory and concentration problems. As mentioned, Goldstein sees FMS and CFIDS as information-processing problems in which the limbic system is overly sensitive to certain stimuli and doesn't screen out adequately. Processing is accurate, but problems lie in the "gating," or control of data input and output from processing centers.

Controversy exists as to whether a viral infection could cause FMS, but efforts to find a "FMS-causing virus" haven't yet been successful. Many FMS patients have had viral infections at the same time, but this doesn't necessarily indicate the latter causes the former. They may both somehow be related to a malfunctioning immune system.

Hypoxia and Muscle Tone Changes

FMS may result in part from insufficient oxygen reaching muscle tissue (hypoxia). Studies of FMS patients' muscles reveal reduced muscle-tissue oxygen pressure in affected areas and to a lesser degree in other areas. A problem in the sympathetic nervous system may underlie oxygen deficits to the muscles, or people with FMS may have imbalances of certain substances in the muscles, such as excess calcium, which leads to inordinate muscle contraction and the inability of oxygen to enter the tissues. They may also have deficits in the high-energy phosphates ATP, ADP, and phosphocreatine. Decreased ATP synthesis may lead to the muscle tissue breakdown and mitochondrial damage seen in FMS biopsies, which could explain widespread aching and specific muscle pain (Abraham and Flechas 1992). If so, this might explain the energy boost and pain reducing effect of malic acid, which may remedy decreased energy production and glycolysis, especially in conditions of hypoxia. Subjects given malic acid have reported decreased pain that returns to higher levels when malic acid is discontinued.

Muscle pain and damage may also stem from our increased muscle tone, which has many causes. The tension of increased muscle tone requires greater oxygen availability, meaning there must be increased blood flow to the muscle to carry this oxygen. Increased blood flow is hampered because tight muscles put too much pressure on blood vessels and prevent them from expanding to carry more blood. This pressure and the resulting oxygen deficits add to aches and pain and interfere with cleanup of muscle waste, furthering pain. Since hypoxia and poor waste removal both cause increased muscle tone, our muscular system is caught in a vicious cycle with ever-increasing pain. All of this is worsened by negative stressors. The imbalance continues as our stronger, toned muscles compensate for weaker muscles and muscle tension increases in response to pain. The excess muscle tone is deeply ingrained and brings about physical changes. Highly toned, tight muscles start to pull on their tendons and the structures connecting tendons to the bones, causing hypoxia and pain in these areas. Tendons become fibrous and problems with joints begin. The compensation by stronger muscles for weaker ones becomes exaggerated and established, making previously coordinated movements jerky and poorly coordinated. By this point, specific muscle changes well established in chronic pain appear (Chaitow 1995). Dr. Paul St. Amand uses guaifenesin, an over-the-counter expectorant, to draw unhealthy phosphates and chemicals from muscles; while many have benefited, no empirical support yet exists (Starlanyl 1998). Guaifenesin increases serotonin, which could also explain improvements. You can learn more about this treatment option by reading Devin Starlanyl's *Fibromyalgia Advocate* or by calling Dr. St. Amand (see appendix I).

Neurotransmitter and Hormone Imbalance

Even though the predominance of FMS in women is glaring, shockingly little attention has been paid to the possible role of sex hormones in FMS. Many FMS symptoms like fatigue, muscular achiness, mental confusion or memory loss, and poor sleep also occur in menopause. In fact, sleep disruptions, which suppress the immune system and cause great fatigue, can start as early as eight to ten years before menstruation ceases (Vliet 1995). Early effects of hormonal changes seem to underlie some FMS cases. In fact, Dr. Elizabeth Vliet notes that the most likely times for the onset of FMS are when estrogen is low (i.e., postpartum, perimenopause, postmenopause, several years after tubal ligation or hysterectomy, and during disruption of a woman's menstrual cycle). In fact, Vliet has teased out a vicious cycle in FMS: declines in estrogen level interfere with sleep and intensify the susceptibility of nerve endings to pain; FMS pain interferes with sleep; and prolonged interference with deep sleep further intensifies pain and causes further decreases in estrogen.

People with FMS have low levels of serotonin, (which regulates sleep and mood) and dopamine, (which stimulates thought/behavior, reduces fatigue, and manages mood). Low dopamine goes with high stress vulnerability. Our serotonin deficit increases pain in two ways: 1) less serotonin results in reduced efficacy of endorphins (body's natural painkillers) and fewer serotonin-derived neurotransmitters (epinephrine and dopamine) to reduce pain; and 2) less serotonin results in increased amounts of pain neurotransmitter (substance P). Cerebrospinal levels of substance P are three or more times higher in FMS patients, one very clear sign about which you can educate disbelieving physicians. Our low norepinephrine makes sense, as it's inversely related to substance P and explains heightened sensitivity to external stimuli and concentration/attention problems. These imbalances help us understand FMS symptoms, but we don't know why or how they occur.

Another significant aspect involving serotonin again highlights gender differences in relation to ARCs. As mentioned above, Vliet (1995) notes that the most likely time for FMS to appear is when estrogen levels are low. Low estrogen levels cause lower pain thresholds and decreased serotonin. Further, the stress of chronic pain leads to decreases in ovarian hormones, resulting in a vicious cycle. Such findings may explain the prevalence of FMS in women, as serotonin is central in sleep and pain. We may be more vulnerable to this and related pain disorders due to biology. It isn't yet clear whether hormonal disruptions cause or result from FMS, though we know there are low levels of serotonin, GH, and endorphins and increased substance P, among other imbalances. Studies have looked at deeper causes for these and other FMS dynamics. One school explores possible dysfunction along the hypothalamic-pituitary-adrenal axis (HPA). If there are HPA disruptions, imbalances like these could occur. One cause of HPA axis disruption is the body's response to distress. The hypothalamus, which some see as part of the limbic system, regulates temperature, hunger, thirst, weight, hormone activity, the immune system, and the stress response. When you experience distress, your hypothalamus' neurons release corticotropin releasing hormone (CRH), targeting pituitary cells that respond by releasing ACTH hormone into the blood. ACTH causes the release of a third hormone, cortisol. People in distress usually have high cortisol levels. High levels of cortisol usually feed back to the hypothalamus and pituitary glands, causing them to stop generating CRH and ACTH, but distress disrupts this feedback loop, causing all three hormones to continue being released. This inevitably leads to mind-body damage. Many studies show distress disrupts the immune system; one way may be through continued production of these arousal hormones, placing excess wear on the immune system.

Physical and Emotional Trauma

Physical trauma and FMS . . . another chicken and egg question. People with FMS have often had some major physical trauma, such as a car or sports accident or illness, weeks to months before symptom intensification. There isn't yet enough data for conclusions to be drawn. What I can say with certainty, and as many FMS patients know, is that minor and possibly major accidents can increase greatly *after* FMS onset. This may arise from muscle weakness or cognitive problems called "fibrofog." I know I've become much more "clumsy." Perhaps some of this is due to inattention and muscular weakness, but in my experience it seems there have been real changes in my visual-spatial skills. I pay attention and scan the typical obstacle path, but rarely fail to make contact with the bed corner, desk legs, or doors! This makes for great slapstick and often I easily join others in laughter, but at times I become frustrated and sad about my "clumsiness." I know I'm comparing present abilities with past, one of the popular "enemy thoughts" that cause us to feel depressed and regretful about losses: "I've had years of gymnastics and used to move quickly, powerfully, and gracefully. Maybe I've just gotten clumsy and uncoordinated . . . " At this point, I yank my thoughts back to focus on the present, valuing what I do have and working toward what I want in the future. While the issue of whether physical trauma causes FMS is unclear, many FMS patients don't doubt FMS is associated with more accidents!

In my interviews and work with FMS patients, one subject emerges over and over. Like a bad record stuck on a sad refrain, I hear from women who experienced great emotional stress or long-term stress before the arrival of FMS. It seems we often create much of our distress by pushing ourselves so hard and so fast, trying to be perfect in all areas, and taking care of others rather than ourselves. Is this worry and hurry sickness a trigger in those who are genetically predisposed, or does stress increase as a result of FMS? Probably both, but research in this area is sorely needed. Studies have explored possible linkages between FMS and childhood emotional trauma from physical or sexual abuse. While a few studies support the link, most (including those performed with good scientific guidelines) don't support emotional trauma as causing FMS.

Multiplicity

Some researchers believe the fungus *Candida albicans* or some parasitic invasion causes FMS. Other suggestions are vitamin deficiencies, mercury poisoning from amalgam fillings, hypoglycemia, allergies, hypothyroidism, and anemia. The challenge is that FMS may come from many of these causes, together with those discussed above. As one problem arises, it has a domino effect and causes other mind-body problems. Researchers usually follow up on all of the trails caused by the domino in order to get back to a single original "domino." The biggest challenge may be for those with Western perspectives to strive to accept multicausal, multidirectional influences and the impact of each unique person's mind-body state at different points along the domino trail. If you've read FMS theories, you may have settled on one that matches your beliefs and experiences, or like many, you may be confused because most or all of them seem plausible. As you'll see in the following story, this reflects the true variability of FMS.

Symptoms and Signs

One problem with diagnosing FMS is that it presents with a bewildering array of symptoms that wax and wane. Your symptoms may lead your doctor to think of a completely different disorder. The following list includes the percentage of people experiencing particular symptoms in a sample of those with FMS and/or CFIDS (Chaitow 1995): chronic fatigue, cold extremities, and impaired memory: 100 percent; frequent urination: 95 percent; depression (secondary or part of FMS/CFS) and sleep disturbances: 94 percent; balance problems: 89 percent; muscle twitching: 80 percent; dry mouth, muscle aches, and headaches: 68 percent. Other symptoms are pain and sensitivity when touched, fatigue upon awakening, diarrhea and/or constipation, concentration and communication problems, and painful or absent menstruation. Armed with this list of FMS signs and symptoms, you may be able to make your doctor take FMS and your pain more seriously. To understand these symptoms, you must read the earlier section, What Causes FMS?

Heather's Story

If you saw this friendly, attractive, and hard-working woman, you'd have difficulty believing she is forty-one. When we met for this interview at a popular coffee house, she came inside energetically, dressed in a flattering business suit, and explained she'd come directly from a business meeting. Had I not known her story, I would never have known she had any illness or serious physical problems. Heather was diagnosed with FMS when she was thirty-nine and in her last semester of graduate school. Right away I recognized the classic pattern of a woman trying to do too much, too fast, and too perfectly, while caring for others but not herself. She'd been finishing a difficult graduate program while continuing to work full-time (fifty hours a week) at a daunting job and teaching exercise classes three days a week at 6:00 A.M! She also crammed other activities into her schedule. "I was doing all of these things and all of a sudden I was just exhausted. I couldn't get out of bed anymore. It was such a struggle to get up at 4:30 A.M. to teach that exercise class. I don't know how I did it." Heather didn't want to let her class members, who'd become like family, down by not showing up. She didn't want to give this part of her "normal life" up, because on some level feeling like she'd "failed" would be an admission that something was truly wrong.

Her exhaustion worsened and she had several viral infections. Physical illness and pain weren't new, as she'd already had a disorder that ate away at the muscles in her colon. Finally, she went to see the internist who'd helped her through the colon disorder. She listened to Heather, and, suspecting FMS, referred her to a rheumatologist. Both her internist and rheumatologist knew of FMS, and Heather attributes their caring and knowledge to their being women. The rheumatologist did a thorough health history, learned of her childhood asthma, the many allergies her parents told her were in her head, and her sleep problems, and did tests like the manual trigger point test. Both doctors felt certain about the diagnosis, and while her rheumatologist suggested sleep medication, Heather chose not to pursue this in favor of exploring alternative techniques. Her nutritionist tailored a plan of protein and vegetables with A.M. carbs. Heather found this helpful, but as happens to many people with FMS, an infection, in her case hepatitis B, appeared "out of the blue" and landed her in bed for five weeks. She was both physically traumatized and ". . . emotionally destroyed. Maybe it was a problem with the nutritional supplements, it could be anything. I'm still convinced nutrition is the key and is about 80 percent of the answer. A long year passed and I felt better, but recently I've begun feeling tired again."

You can see typical characteristics: cyclical symptoms, chronic sleep problems, allergies and asthma, major physical trauma (colon disease), and a high achieving, perfectionistic personality. I listed some FMS-related problems and she, surprised, confirmed her migraine headaches, her chronic tendonitis, which requires steroid treatment (itself a stressor on the body); her Reynaud's; and her doubts about her immune system's health given her lifelong susceptibility to colds and infections. Perhaps all of these infections overtaxed her immune system and brought on the FMS. Perhaps it was the poor sleep or the physical trauma of the colon disease. Maybe the allergy theory was "right" and all of those childhood allergies had led to FMS. Perhaps she'd just worn herself down with type A behaviors and perfectionistic self-expectations.

Heather has been athletic and taken care of herself physically throughout her adult years. Should we conclude exercise, diet, and lifestyle don't prevent FMS and become junk-food eating couch potatoes? Probably not. Recall that she exhibited childhood FMS-type symptoms. Recent research has explored FMS in children; Heather may have been genetically predisposed, which when combined with distress from overwork and overload or some type of infection or other trigger, might have led to FMS. Had she not been leading a healthy lifestyle, FMS might have appeared full blown years earlier or might be more severe at present. As it is, she can still exercise, socialize, and work.

When asked what she had learned from FMS, she spoke of her anger and depression, and said that the refrain, "This is not the way I want to live my life," often ran through her mind. While she admitted that she hasn't totally accepted FMS as part of her life, she has reduced her negative self-talk, because she realizes it worsens her mind-body health. As she spoke, she could see herself more objectively as a woman who'd grown from berating and judging herself to a woman who was learning to stop her negative, hopeless self-talk and impossible strivings to be perfect, and was instead able to be tolerant and accepting of herself. She has recognized that by always pushing herself, she'd lost touch with her mind-body state; she sees her greatest lesson as learning to listen to what it says to her. "I've learned to say 'no' to people and situations that use up my time and energy and I don't feel guilty about these decisions because I'm not getting into that negative head dialogue." She now has the knowledge and self-esteem to act on a new, empowering belief; namely, that she is the best person to make decisions about herself. When asked what she would recommend to other FMS patients, she answered: "You have to make your health a priority. You have to find good people to work with, people who you respect and with whom you feel comfortable. Remember, you're the best one to make decisions about your health and healing. You listen to experts, ask questions and do your own research . . . and then you decide. For me, my health comes first or I pay a severe price. I've chosen to take an alternative approach using herbs, vitamins, and minerals, biofeedback, nutrition, exercise, and bodywork, and I haven't delved into medications much. I may need to later, and am willing to do so. You just need to think rationally and in a balanced, open way even when you're exhausted, stressed, and in pain."

Related Conditions and Look-alikes

Because so many symptoms and disorders are associated with FMS, the following will help you understand your particular case and what your doctor's medi-speak means. Here are some diagnoses confused with FMS due to shared symptoms and patterns that can also exist in conjunction with FMS: CFIDS, myofascial pain syndrome, mitral valve prolapse, SLE, SS, Lyme disease, MS, hypothyroidism, and RA. The following often accompany or are FMS symptoms (percentages indicate how many people with FMS have these conditions): generalized pain: 97.6 percent; fatigue: 81.4 percent; morning stiffness: 77 percent (Wolfe 1990); migraines/headaches: 53 percent (Williamson 1996); irritable bowel syndrome (IBS): 40 to 70 percent (FMS network); paresthesias (a burning or tingling sensation): 62.8 percent; anxiety: 47.8 percent (Wolfe 1990); PMS: 40 percent (Chaitow 1995); amenorrhea: 40 percent; Raynaud's phenomenon: 30 to 50 percent (Chaitow 1995); facial pain (including temperomandibular): 25 percent (Wolfe 1990).

CFIDS

CFIDS is covered in the next chapter. Suffice it to say that there is great overlap between FMS and CFIDS symptoms, and it's estimated that 50 percent of those with FMS also have CFIDS and vice versa. One theory proposes that they're one and the same, based on results like those from Don Goldenberg's 1993 study of fifty FMS and fifty CFIDS patients, looking at symptoms like chronic cough, sore throat, rashes, and low grade fevers, in which percentages were almost equal in both FMS and CFIDS patients. However, a symposium stemming from Dr. Moldofsky's 1988 work differentiated CFIDS and FMS, stating that CFIDS more often develops after an infection. Others distinguish CFIDS and FMS by saying that severe generalized and specific pain are FMS typical, while extreme fatigue is

CFIDS typical. Both assumptions are questionable, as Moldofsky compared a group of CFIDS patients with FMS patients, all of whom developed the condition after a bout of infection. He also included FMS patients who hadn't developed it as a result of an infection. He used an objective measure, EEG brain anomalies (electrical brain waves), of the three groups and found them the same. More support for CFIDS and FMS similarities came from comparisons of fatigue, pain, and tender points that indicated equivalent responses between groups.

Myofascial Pain Syndrome (MPS)

MPS is similarly confused with FMS. Some believe one triggers the other, others believe they are one and the same, and others believe they are distinct. Certainly one can have both. The pain of MPS is derived from connective tissue and muscle fiber. Similarities include: tension headaches; symptoms intensified by cold; ineffectiveness of anti-inflammatory meds; numbness and tingling and Raynaud's phenomenon; excessive sympathetic nervous system activity; and some of the same trigger points (Baldry 1993). Differences include: FMS has generalized achiness while MPS has local specific areas of pain; FMS has tender points on the body causing pain directly and specifically in the area pressed while MPS diagnosis requires trigger points on regions of tight muscles causing pain in distant locations when pressed (however, this isn't a good diagnostic indicator, as FMS patients often have trigger and tender points); FMS points don't disappear, whereas MPS points do; FMS' cause is unknown while MPS is caused by injury; FMS strikes women while MPS strikes both sexes equally; FMS is systemic while MPS is neuromuscular; tricyclic antidepressants can improve FMS but not MPS; FMS is long-term with difficult recovery; FMS has dysmenorrhea, IBS, and joint swelling while MPS doesn't.

Mitral Valve Prolapse (MVP)

MVP involves problems with one of four valves moving blood through the heart. MVP allows blood to move backward into the adjacent chamber. There is no pain with MVP, and it's generally discovered when a heart murmur is found through a stethoscope. Similarities between FMS and MVP are: fatigue, headaches, and diarrhea and/or constipation. MVP isn't truly serious but can be if other heart problems exist. People with MVP may need to take antibiotics prior to dental work to protect against bacteria entering the heart and causing infections.

Lupus

SLE generally requires testing and review to rule it out as it's prevalent in women and involves fatigue, fibrositis, muscular pain, cold extremities, and painful joints, all of which can appear in FMS. Up to 50 percent of people with SLE may have FMS. One way to differentiate is by which treatments work (for example, anti-inflammatories help SLE but not FMS). Tests for antinuclear anti-bodies in SLE can help but often aren't effective during early SLE.

Sjogren's Syndrome

SS is another ARC that shares symptoms with FMS, including intense fatigue and dry eyes and mouth. Like most ARCs, it's more common in women. Blood tests for specific SS autoantibodies help in differential diagnosis. Joints are primary targets of SS while muscles are targeted in FMS.

Lyme Disease (LD)

Lyme disease may be tested first to rule it out as some believe FMS indicates LD and isn't a disease itself. Of 100 Lyme center patients, 25 percent had FMS, not chronic LD; however, in 70 percent of these, FMS was thought to have occurred after LD. This would seem to support LD as a cause of FMS but as you know there are many causes of FMS and LD may be one potential cause. FMS and LD involve muscle weakness, poor sleep, extreme fatigue, flulike symptoms, neck/back pain, general or migrating aches, and headaches. LD is discussed in Chapter 8.

Mupliple Sclerosis

Early symptoms include clumsiness, imbalance, numbness, tingling, cold sensitivity in extremities, fatigue, and muscle weakness, just as in FMS. Neuro-logical exams are essential in diagnosing MS.

Hypothyroidism

Insufficient thyroid activity shares symptoms with FMS like fatigue, muscle tension, and depression; some FMS patients benefit from thyroid treatment. Test-ing reduces confusion as test results generally indicate hypothyroidism when it is present.

RA

Characterized by muscle and joint pain, RA is often confused with FMS. Up to 20 percent of RA patients may have FMS. Make sure your doctor is certain in diagnosing RA or connective tissue disease.

Other Symptoms

Other symptoms that may lead to diangostic confusion include:

- cognitive problems (memory, concentration, attention, organizational abilities, problem solving)

- circulatory problems (causing cold extremities or possibly Raynaud's)

- bladder problems (frequent, burning, painful urination; must rule out bladder infections)

- IBS (painful diarrhea, constipation; rule out colitis and Crohn's)

- low blood sugar (tremors, shakes, light-headedness, dizziness, perspiration; rule out true hypoglycemia)

- PMS (painful periods, headaches, emotional symptoms, back/abdominal pain)

- underactive thyroid (fatigue, depression, muscle weakness and pain, constipation, cognitive problems; rule out hypothyroidism)

The Courses of Fibromyalgia Syndrome

After the doctor-go-round and being told time and again you look fine and it's all in your head, you may actually feel relief when you're correctly diagnosed at last. FMS patients I've interviewed said they finally no longer worried they were losing their minds or making up symptoms, as so many other doctors had led them to believe. If your health expert isn't experienced in FMS, hopefully she'll refer you to a rheumatologist or neurologist. At any rate, it's important you remember that the symptoms and patterns described here are only generalizations, as each individual case differs greatly. There is no single typical description of the progression of FMS. While it used to be termed a self-limiting (i.e., not chronic) condition, recent evidence doesn't support this. I declined steadily for years, and was finally dubious as people with FMS told me it would go away or disappear for long periods. I haven't truly seen this in myself or in my clients or subjects, but I've had and seen cycles of good improvement. Recall that FMS is hard to diagnose because it mimics many diseases or illnesses; however, we now know many of the characteristic symptoms and signs. Educate yourself thoroughly, as this is the start of your effective coping.

One variable element of FMS is its severity and degree of impairment. There are cases so severe that lives are greatly restricted. The findings of a survey of 394 FMS patients showed 25 percent of women and 27 percent of men were so impaired they could no longer work. Almost one-third of the sample was affected this severely, and most of the remaining two-thirds said their job performance was significantly impaired (Goldenberg 1993). Those who stopped work didn't have significant declines in symptoms or pain, which showed that removing one potential stressor isn't enough to "cure" FMS, a finding confirming this book's call for a holistic, active approach offering a sense of control and addressing mind-body needs in healing.

While many have waxing and waning symptoms, it's easy to not acknowledge these lighter periods. Often I've heard my clients focusing only on the worst times and their endless pain and fatigue. I need to point out that last week they were pleased that they'd awakened with little or no pain and had accomplished quite a bit that day. I'm not downplaying FMS' severity and its great toll, but I've seen that when people pay attention to and recall positive times, even if journaling is needed to recall it, they experience a decrease in hopelessness and depression.

Trigger Points

The trigger points of FMS lead to diagnostic confusion with MPS. It's helpful to learn about how trigger points develop and "work" in case you develop these along your FMS course. Trigger points are areas on the body that are painful when touched and also refer pain to other areas in the body. New trigger points tend to develop over time. (Note that 80 percent of trigger points are in the same areas as Chinese acupuncture points [Chaitow 1995].) Trigger points are areas where oxygen deficits arise due to poor circulation plus an increased need for energy. These situations conflict and underlie much FMS pain. Trigger point muscles are taut and shorter than normal so treatment must remedy this. Until the situation is modified, pain will continue even if it's temporarily decreased by treatment.

Testing for Fibromyalgia Syndrome

There is no single definitive test to unerringly diagnose FMS, which is one of the reasons the medical community has been reluctant to accept the disorder. For now, your doctor should rely on a variety of information: your reports of current and past symptoms; factors you see as related to symptom changes; previous health-related concerns, illnesses, operations, or allergies; medications; physical and emotional stressors (past or ongoing); your lifestyle habits (diet, exercise, smoking, drinking, drugs, toxin exposure); your social history and childhood experiences as they relate to your physical health today; your family's health history; the doctor's physical exam; data from your other doctors; and various tests. Be armed with as much information as possible, and don't forget that your medical records are all accessible to you. I'm including a discussion of some of the tests that are used to identify FMS and rule out other diagnostic possibilities. This will help you decipher your doctors' medi-speak (should it sound like a foreign tongue) and allow you to use it if necessary to ask questions or state preferences. Being an active, assertive partner in healing increases your control and chances of improvement.

Blood tests detect the presence or absence or levels of certain chemicals, nutrients, neurotransmitters, and the like. While general blood tests may appear "normal" for people with FMS, specific tests are more revealing. Some FMS patients have problems with the synthesis of collagen in their body. Collagen is used by the body to make connective tissue, which binds the body together. Blood tests can reveal a shortage of collagen in people with FMS. Another important blood test determines if your GH is low, which is typical of FMS. Other special blood tests determine whether you have other FMS characteristics like low levels of serotonin and its offshoots, dopamine and epinephrine, elevated substance P, and low cortisol levels. You may also have low levels of thyroid hormones, but doctors performing thyroid panels may read results as "normal" even when they're not. For important specifics, refer to the Testing section in chapter 12 on CFIDS. Underactive thyroid glands cause fatigue, muscle stiffness and pain, and depression, all of which may be familiar to you. This is another reason you must ensure your SHOC doctor is FMS-knowledgeable as she'll have to do a thorough thyroid panel and read it appropriately. Sex hormone imbalances and changes must also be examined. If your doctor laughs it off, "forgets," or tells you it has nothing to do with FMS, it's time for a new, more open and educated doctor.

The manual trigger and tender points test should be done. Recall that the diagnostic criteria is that at least eleven of the eighteen points are painful when touched with moderate pressure. Make sure your doctor knows the location of these points and how to perform the exam.

Cutting-edge brain-imaging techniques add valuable information. Doctors haven't been successful with typical testing techniques to rule out or rule in FMS (one reason many are hesitant to "believe in" FMS). This arises in part because FMS is a neural network disorder involving problems with circuitry throughout the brain. Doctors look for structural changes or evident brain tissue damage to confirm a true "physical" disorder, but due to the nature of neurosomatic disorders like FMS, the best way to discover disruptions and brain differences is using relatively new brain imaging (functional) techniques. For example, SPECT, quantitative EEGs, evoked response mapping, and positron emission tomography (PET) find real differences in regional cerebral blood flow and brain activation of FMS patients (Goldstein 1996). In this era of managed care it's often hard to have much choice in doctor selection, but if at all possible, find yourself an FMS expert or at least one who believes in FMS.

What You Can Do

Remember, your body is unique. The last thing in the world you should do is ignore symptoms simply because they don't fit descriptions you've read or heard about. You must be in touch with your body and its changes; if you suspect something is amiss, don't just wait for it to go away. See a professional soon so you can quickly form your plan of attack, research the illness and good health professionals, work on your attitudes, and reduce the progression or degree of damage. This all fits in your toolbag for beating the odds. Also, your unique mind-body means you may benefit from integrating alternative healing methods with conventional ones. Remember, there is no such thing as 100 percent certainty in any doctor's diagnosis or prognosis. You'll develop a cohesive mind-body integrity so that as you travel your unique path, you'll connect with your SHOC team in a timely way if medications aren't working, side effects appear, or if things take an unexpected turn.

Recall the role your mind and thus your emotions and behavior have in boosting or worsening your health. Accepting that *complete* control over this disease is highly unlikely (I don't like to say "impossible") reduces self-blame and guilt when you feel you're not doing as well as your critical inner voice tells you you should be. Instead focus on what you can control, which you'll read about below.

Given the many systems affected by FMS, you may have an array of SHOC members from a family doctor, to a neurologist, ophthalmologist, psychologist, dermatologist, rheumatologist, massage therapist, nutritional counselor, spiritual helper, and the like. Whatever the composition of your SHOC team, you must feel comfortable with them and their FMS knowledge and expertise in their fields. Deep, empathic relations may not develop, but you should have their respect and sense their desire to help. If you feel they don't and your reaction isn't misplaced anger or hostility at yourself or your illness (something for you to work on), you should look for someone who's willing to help. See appendix I for referrals, contact local hospitals and universities, or use word of mouth.

Balanced, Holistic Health Optimization Plan

While I've written of the importance of integrating East-West healing, it may be hard for you to coordinate these efforts without doing a disservice to either the healing methods or to yourself. Fortunately, some programs offer FMS-comprehensive services. Experts working in these deserve thanks and credit for risking derision by their peers and financial cuts in exchange for acting on their Hippocratic oath. They've experimented and tried new approaches, a start in the right direction for treating FMS. These programs offer many types of health experts joined together to satisfy specific needs and custom-fit treatment for each client. They strive for a balance: of conventional and alternative methods; of activity and rest; of reality and hope; of support and autonomy; and of exercise and relaxation. Clients gain empathy, support, growth, and control, all of which are linked with pain and symptom relief, improved wound healing, and mind-body well-being. As yet no single treatment helps much more than one-third of FMS patients, and most of us try treatments falling well below this efficacy rate.

But a patchwork of remedies placed here and there doesn't get to the underlying problems. We need integrated treatment because we have fatigue and pain, both of which may increase after exertion. Our body's signal that we've overexerted ourselves doesn't work accurately. Also, our fibrofog means we must learn new methods of balance, time management, relaxation, mind-body awareness, and pain/symptom management. As most of us won't have access to integrated treatments, we must try to create something similar by seeking doctors knowledgeable about FMS who are willing to work with conventioanl and alternative health experts as well as ourselves. Tell your doctor about these multi-modal approaches and their relative success in treating FMS and strive to create your own multi-modal SHOC team. Contact people and organizations in appendix I to see if they know of any integrated treatment programs in your area.

Self-Management

As with other ARCs described here, you can refer to later chapters on alternative tools and coping and optimizing your efforts to work with chronic illnesses. Here you'll find specific methods of dealing with FMS to include in your toolbag. Conventional doctors suggest: medicine; regulated, sufficent sleep; gentle aerobic exercise; and pain management. I add: FMS education; stress optimization; relaxation training; cognitive tools; nutrition and supplements; coping, organizational, assertiveness, and communication skills; support network of doctors, health experts, families, friends, spiritual leaders, and support groups; chronic illness counseling; and, if necessary, eye movement desensitization reprocessing (with a certified mental health expert). In addition, biofeedback, massage (caution: read massage section in appendix II), acupuncture, acupressure, physical and/or occupational therapy, and chiropractic techniques.

Medications

Some medicines are helpful, but be sure to ask about potential side effects or interactions with other prescription or over-the-counter medications, herbs, and supplements. Be assertive in asking about effective medications, as many doctors are beginning to admit that their patients know more about FMS treatment than they do! You may be someone who steers clear of medicines. This is ultimately your decision, but you owe it to yourself to discuss all the options with your health experts. While medications don't yet solve the underlying problem, they may improve your lifestyle. Anti-inflammatories may be prescribed, but they aren't usually effective, as inflammation isn't central to FMS. However, they may help in treating headaches. Keep in mind that there are adverse effects from taking NSAIDs over time. Other headache medicines are Tylenol and calcium channel blockers. Muscle relaxants like Norflex, Flexeril, and Soma may give temporary relief, but they can make you sleepy and uncoordinated and interfere further with concentration and memory. If your doctor suggests these and you take them in small amounts, they shouldn't be a problem. (Note that Soma can be addictive.)

Antidepressants

For FMS imbalances in norepinephrine and serotonin, tricyclic antidepressants are widely prescribed, as they increase serotonin and the delta wave sleep phase. Elavil (amitriptyline) helps reduce pain and improve sleep in some FMS patients. Some feel groggy in the morning after taking it, so check with your doctor about taking half the dose early in the evening and the other half at bedtime. Desyrel (trazodone), generally prescribed in 25 to 50 mg, can be as effective as other antidepressants without as many side effects. Flexeril (cyclobenzaprine), another tricyclic antidepressant, may work as an effective muscle relaxant. It may be used in conjunction with Elavil and takes about ten to twelve days to reach maximum efficacy. The biggest drawback of tricyclic antidepressants is their side effects. While some don't experience any, others have dry mouth, headache, sleepiness, weight gain, morning grogginess, and heart rate fluctuations. Give these medicines several weeks to be effective and see if side effects disappear. If not, consult with your physician to explore other medications or avenues.

Those who can't tolerate tricyclic antidepressants may be given serotonin selective reuptake inhibitors (SSRIs), such as Prozac (fluoxetine), Zoloft (sertraline), Serzone (nefazodone, the newest), and Paxil (paroxetine), to increase serotonin and, with Serzone, norepinephrine as well. (Serzone causes far fewer sexual dysfunctions than the others.) Some FMS patients feel "revved-up" by these meds and require more sedating ones like Elavil or Sinequan (doxepin). SSRIs may be effective in reducing the depression that results from or is part of hormonal and neurotransmitter imbalances. Sleeping aids are of import in treating FMS given the central role of disturbed sleep. In addition to sleeping aids, tricyclic antidepressants like Desyrel (trazodone), Elavil, Sinequan, and Flexeril may help with sleep because they reduce pain and improve sleep and mood. One reason FMS patients have sleep problems is restless leg syndrome, or muscular spasms or jerks while falling asleep. Klonopin (clonazepam) and muscle relaxants can help here.

Pain Relievers

In terms of direct analgesics or pain-relieving medications, doctors prescribe Tylenol, Ultram, Tylenol with codeine, Darvon, Vicodin, or methadone. Use these sparingly; otherwise your body will adjust and no longer obtain pain relief. Work closely with your doctor with respect to which, if any, drugs are right for you. Doctors should know that chronic pain patients rarely abuse pain medications (Khalsa and Stauth 1999). However, you do need to monitor yourself to obtain maximum benefits. If anxiety and sleeplessness are severe, benzodiazepines may be briefly prescribed. These act to remedy anxiety and depression (Klonopin, discussed above, or Xanax [alprazolam]).

Other Treatments

Recall that FMS shares some symptoms with Hashimoto's thyroiditis even though tests may appear normal. However, some experts in the field have given thyroid hormone to their clients with some success. In addition, there are various theories claiming that people with FMS have a buildup of toxins in their muscles that is responsible for muscular weakness, fatigue, and the like. Dr. Paul St. Amand treats FMS patients with guaifenesin, an expectorant also found in cough syrup. He claims this element draws out toxic muscular buildup and has had some success. Guaifenesin also increases serotonin, so improvement may come from this effect.

If you want to learn about potentially effective medications, I recommend you read Dr. Goldstein's 1996 masterpiece *Betrayal by the Brain*, which offers thorough, scientifically based descriptions of medications he uses successfully to treat FMS and CFIDS. He often begins treatment with a client by giving sublingual nitroglycerin. Although headaches are a fairly common side effect, they often go away after several doses. A few headaches are a small price to pay, as Goldstein notes that 20 to 25 percent of FMS patients get pain relief from this treatment. He may also prescribe a type of antiseizure medication increasingly used by doctors to treat FMS. Goldstein uses lidocaine drips, which require time commitment and the ability to tolerate being hooked up to IVs, so they aren't for everyone. He has had good success with this method. (See appendix I to learn about his clinic.)

Trigger Point Pain

Trigger points are a source of great pain for those with MPS, FMS, and other musculoskeletal disorders. If trigger point pain is severe, your doctor may use a trigger point injection (TPI); they'll inject a numbing agent to make the procedure less painful and steroids to make the benefits longer-term. Much of the relief may come from the needle being placed in the trigger point area and being moved around to loosen up the generally tense muscle region. TPIs are temporary but can help. If your doctor uses steroids with TPI, don't have sessions more than every four months and do only one to three TPIs per session. Any more is over-doing it.

Buyer Beware

Many seeking alternative treatments believe that because they're "natural," they cause no harm. While these tools can be highly effective, you must treat them cautiously. As with conventional medicine, you must be active and respon-sible, and ensure you're working with trained professionals with proper certifica-tion, training, and experience. Find those with good experience in FMS. This is a basic element in the design and practice of your SHOC; you simply owe it to yourself.

Help Yourself Help Your Body

Recently, much has been learned of the impact of your work and life space on your mind-body health. You can make many changes at home, at work, and when traveling to reduce your pain and fatigue. These issues are relevant to ARCs in general, and you'll find a comprehensive discussion later in the book.

Alternative Techniques

The key lies in integrating appropriate conventional and alternative meas-ures. This is akin to keeping balance throughout your life, a key component of your SHOC. Extremes trigger relapses or symptom intensification. Moderation and balance take work, but they greatly increase your odds of living life to the fullest, obtaining most satisfaction, growing, and thriving. Learning to balance your life is one way of growth you derive from accepting the challenge.

Acupuncture, Acupressure, Massage, and Meditation

Appendix II explores these techniques—and when they're effective—in depth. My experience, that of many patients, and empirical studies confirm these tools can greatly reduce FMS pain, stiffness, and gastrointestinal distress, and

improve energy, sleep, and mood. The efficacy of therapeutic touch was discussed in chapter 6. The connection of touch with another person offers mind-
body healing. There are many techniques using touch that achieve specific goals,
like pain reduction, improved flexibility, opening blockages, realignment, and
reestablishing balance. Massage is one of these, and it's useful for anyone whose
movement is limited due to ARCs like FMS. If you're having a severe bout of
fatigue or pain, the manipulation and stretching act as passive exercise. Massage
offers FMS patients benefits at all times. It increases blood flow and oxygen to
muscles and tendons, which reduces pain and stiffness. Recall that hypoxia (oxygen insufficiency) in our cells is a major cause of pain and aches. However, you
must find a massage/physical therapist who's experienced in working with FMS
patients, because some types of massage may boost pain and achiness. Physical
therapists must be careful with deep, or neuromuscular, massage, as you may be
unable to tolerate anything but slow progress in probing tender and trigger
points. Talk to other people with FMS or see appendix I to find FMS professionals. You'll find referrals for acupuncture/acupressure in appendix I as well, and
appendix II explains more about these effective tools.

At this writing, there is excitement in the FMS community about a potential treatment, pulsed signal therapy (PST), which works on painful, inflamed
joints linked with chronic neck and back pain and arthritis. PST sends biological
signals on programmed frequencies through a magnetic field directly to certain
connective tissue and cartilage to boost your body's self-healing. There have been
reports of successful treatment of arthritis and other chronic, painful conditions.
Treatments last for one to two months, are painless, and haven't been found to produce any side effects. The treatment has been approved in some European countries, and it's still pending in Mexico and the U.S. Given the newness of PST and
the absence of many controlled studies, particularly for FMS, check with your doctor first.

Physical Therapy

Physical therapy can be controversial in FMS treatment. Reports range from
its being effective, to its having no discernible effects, to its actually increasing
pain and other FMS symptoms. This last experience can be avoided if physical
therapists use slow, graduated series of exercises and stretches, moving slowly
from simple moves to moderately paced, more challenging ones. This slow
approach, contrary to the "pain is gain" school of thought, should permeate the
entire therapeutic format. Physical therapists must be cautious about temperature
fluctuations when working with FMS patients, but you're the best judge of your
ability to tolerate cold and ice. Many people with FMS benefit from moist heat,
though recent studies show that alternating cold and heat can be effective. Also
be cautious of the room temperature; drafty, cool areas can trigger muscle spasms
and pain. I always take a sweater or scarf when I go out, even if it's hot outside. If
I end up in cold air-conditioning or if the weather turns cold, I can protect the
susceptible neck and shoulder muscles. If your physical therapist uses ultrasound, make sure she's experienced with FMS patitens, as some benefit greatly

but others report harm. Have her start at a low sonic level and format the treatment based on your reactions. Some benefit from work on the bursae of hips, knees, and shoulders.

Stretching is invaluable in reducing pain, releasing tension, relaxing muscles, and working against the unhealthy structural changes that occur over time. The "no pain, no gain" mentality has no place for people with FMS in stretching, weight lifting, or any exercise. Work slowly to increase flexibility through simple stretches; spread sessions throughout the day to maximize benefits. Start the day with a set of stretches to help you ease into the day. Mild aerobic activities and weight lifting, yoga, and Pilates are helpful. Hydrotherapy, in which your body is largely immersed underwater while you do stretches and movements to build muscle strength, allows you to take advantage of the supportive, weight-reducing qualities of water.

Nutritional Remedies

A diet replete with fruits, vegetables, nuts, seeds, whole grains, lean fish, and chicken and turkey without skin is ideal. It's hard at first, but you should do your best to avoid foods high in fats, like fried foods, some cheeses, and meats. If you have inflammation, fat increases it and thus causes pain. It's critical to avoid or minimize caffeine, sugar (including honey and fructose), and alcohol, which also increase fatigue and pain. Steer clear of preservative-filled foods and refined products like white flour. Many people with FMS find they need to eat smaller, more frequent meals, or else fatigue and greater muscle tension and pain result. The common adage to drink at least eight to ten glasses of water daily should be your credo. Having enough water in your body ensures your myofascia have enough moisture and don't "dry out," which would increase tightening and pain and disrupt communication around the body. Given the connection between immune system problems and chemical sensitivity, ensure you have clean, pollution-free, chemical-free water. You'll read about some supplements that can partially remedy the difficulty FMS patients have absorbing nutrients from foods.

Vitamins, Minerals, and Supplements

Antioxidants may be a current health buzzword, but they aren't just a trend—they are truly essential and include natural body substances, vitamins, minerals, and enzymes. They protect against free radicals that damage our cells and immune systems and are linked to infections, diseases, and aging. Some free radicals come from exposure to chemicals, cigarettes, radiation, excess sun, and natural body processes. In the body's wisdom, we also have free-radical scavengers that neutralize free radicals, preventing them from harming the internal integrity of the body. These enzymes are helped by vitamins, herbs, minerals, and hormones with antioxidant properties. As enzymes are critical in absorbing food nutrients, you may want to include the enzymes bromalain, papain, and chymotrypan. The following are also important in FMS.

Vitamin B complex, which boosts digestion (in this case, of protein), also maintains proper circulation, increases energy, builds stress tolerance, and boosts immune system functioning and energy. Take B vitamins together to maximize benefits. Some FMS patients obtain injections from their doctors. If you can't get these, find a sublingual form, as capsules may not work well since people with FMS don't absorb nutrients well. Coenzyme Q10 enhances body and brain circulation (reducing fibro-fog), boosts the immune system, reduces fatigue, and increases tissue oxygenation. Magnesium decreases pain and ensures good muscle functioning; it may be low in FMS patiients, particularly if they have muscle spasms. Take with calcium at a ratio of two to one (2,000 mg calcium/1,000 mg magnesium). Malic acid boosts energy and manganese influences the rate of metabolic activity. Also, 2,400 mg daily of malic acid, taken with magnesium, resulted in 100 percent of patients in one study reporting significant pain relief in forty-eight hours (Khalsa and Stauth 1999). The amino acid L-glutamine reduces mental cloudiness and forgetfulness associated with FMS. Take a free-form amino acid complex to get important amino acids to regulate brain function, rebuild muscle tissue, and supply protein. Each of these aspects is critical in decreasing FMS symptoms. (Don't take L-tyrosine, which can appear in amino acid supplements, if you're on MAOI antidepressants. Otherwise, it's a valuable precurser to dopamine, thyroid hormone, norepinephrine, and epinephrine. Insufficient tyrosine is linked to depression and "brainfog.")

Acidophilus reduces the candida infection damage that often appears with FMS. Garlic boosts immune system functioning and energy and fights parasites (two caps two to three times per day). Vitamin A, an antioxidant, improves immune system functioning, protein use, infection protection, and protection from free radicals. The maximum dosage is 15,000 IU per day (if pregnant, maximum 10,000 IU per day). Antioxidant vitamin E helps improve circulation, while vitamin C (another antioxidant) boosts key autoimmune components, stress tolerance, energy, and detoxification, and helps protect vitamin E. Zinc and grape seed extract, antioxidants, play an important role in keeping stable levels of vitamin C in the blood, help with vitamin A absorption, and improve immune system functioning. The antioxidant taurine maintains appropriate white blood cell functions in the immune system. Bee venom may boost immune system functioning (used for CFIDS/FMS). Melatonin can help sleep, but steer clear of it if you're on an antidepressant. Some users have dreams so vivid they prefer not to take this supplement but choose herbs instead (see below). Multivitamin/mineral complex is essential in ensuring that appropriate nutrients are obtained.

Smoking and frequent aspirin use deplete vitamin C and call for increased consumption. Recall that C also exists in herbs and foods including alfalfa, catnip, cayenne, dandelion, garlic, horseradish, kelp, plantain, papaya, raspberry, rose hips, strawberry, and watercress. Excessive alfalfa use may be linked to the onset of ARC symptoms in vulnerable individuals.

Collagen Formation and Tissue Repair

This is very important for FMS patients. See appendix II for details.

Herbal Remedies

Before taking herbs, check with a SHOC expert who's familiar with supplements, as they're not free of side effects and can interact with medications. Chinese herbal remedies, Qi Ye Lien and Xiao Yao Wan, reduce muscle pain, and the latter also reduces muscle spasms. Cayenne (capsicum) is a good pain-reliever as it disrupts production of substance P, the pain neurotransmitter. You can take cayenne in pill form or combine cayenne powder with wintergreen oil and apply it directly to the skin. To improve your sleep, try valerian and skullcap. To minimize fibro-fog, or memory and concentration difficulties, try ginkgo biloba. Chaitow's 1995 book (which I highly recommend) discusses studies showing that 120 to 240 mg per day for six months boosts memory and reduces symptoms of poor brain circulation. Ginkgo also improves the poor circulation we experience as cold hands and feet. Given the signs of immune dysfunction in FMS, you must ensure this system's health; two herbs beneficial for this are echinacea and astragalus. Take echinacea for limited periods only.

Homeopathic Remedies

These can be powerful tools for FMS patients. In a study of FMS, twice as many people improved using homeopathy compared to a placebo (Khalsa and Stauth 1999). Consider the following homeopathic remedies. Remember you must stop pain as soon as possible, as over time it becomes engraved into your brain and body. Arnica 6x can put a stop to this cycle; Chamomilla 3x helps with less intense chronic pain and is mildly sedating. Rhus tox 6x is great for FMS; Pulsatilla 6x helps PMS.

Progressive Relaxation and Deep Breathing

Progressive relaxation and deep breathing exercises should be central to your SHOC. Progressive relaxation allows your muscles to relax more than if you passively lie down and try to relax. This is particularly important in FMS, as our muscles become so tight and eventually shorten so much it's difficult to regain normal length and stretch. Deep breathing gives your muscles enough oxygen and releases waste.

Self-Bodywork and Trigger Point Relief

While touch, pressure, and movement greatly reduce FMS pain and boost relaxation, the reality is that many of us have limited, if any, access to massage or physical therapy. What could be a more central part of your SHOC than self-bodywork? There is no other way to derive such benefits whenever and wherever you need them, and by being able to reduce your pain and tension yourself, you gain a sense of control, which furthers your self-appreciation and mind-body health. See appendix II for examples and appendix I for referrals on bodywork.

Clients and research tell me an effective way to reduce trigger point pain is to press lightly and directly on the area for thirty to sixty seconds. You may move your hand around the "bump" or pain region, but try to keep pressure on the most painful, tightest spot. Including simple imagery will give you greater benefits. Marilyn, a client who has FMS, is an actress and quite creative in her imagery. While doing this exercise, she begins with an image of a tall, fiery volcano, under great pressure as it approaches eruption. She increases the pressure to the tender points while visualizing the moment of greatest tension, followed by a fiery explosion. As the lava flows down the sides, relieving the tension, she imagines the same happening in her muscles. Finally, the peaked volcano is torn apart and the area flattened, Marilyn's effort to transmit the sensation of release, lengthening, and relaxation to the muscles of the area. Move among tender points, becoming exquisitely aware of your body's habits, and do body scans through the day to ensure you're not tensing up muscles and retriggering the cycle.

And Now What?

FMS is an ARC that truly requires a mind-body approach if any significant improvement is to occur. While in many FMS cases, symptoms wax and wane or are present fairly continuously, the severity and frequency of pain, fatigue, infections, and feelings of helplessness and hopelessness can be reduced. Of course, this is just the case with today's treatments, and I expect major remedy discoveries in the next several years. Lasting can mean longer than the usual short-term approaches most of us have been given, such as pain medication and heat. For true mind-body healing, both conventional and alternative tools are key.

A "Sunny" Look at a Challenging Situation

Sunny is an outgoing, cheerful woman with grown-up children, recently remarried and retired. Although she was diagnosed thirteen years ago with CFIDS/FMS, some of her telltale symptoms go back much earlier. "I remember feeling pain and fatigue when I was in high school. It would come out of nowhere and I couldn't understand it. It was bothersome because I'd been an active tomboy as a child." It's surprising she was diagnosed with FMS as far back as she was. She'd seen a rheumatologist after her doctor couldn't understand her incessant pain, fatigue, headaches, and sore legs. She asked many questions when she got the diagnosis those years ago, when little was known of FMS. She was relieved to finally get a diagnosis, and also curious: "How did I get it? What do I do about it? How long does it last? " To every question, she got an "I don't know." She didn't return to these doctors.

Aspects of Sunny's conditions are seen by some as causes and by others as consequences of FMS. Some believe FMS results from toxin exposure; Sunny would qualify based on her toddlerhood, when she scuttled directly into toxic material. She'd had her stomach pumped, and her family and doctors were worried by the nature of the chemical. She also had candida dating back to her first rheumatologist visit. Candida, often manifest in FMS patients, has led some to view viruses, bacteria, fungus, and yeast as causes of FMS. Both CFIDS and FMS have been attributed to negative stress by some, while others see distress as just one trigger in an already predisposed individual. Sunny zeroed in on her first marriage: "It was a 100 percent negative stressor, and all bad news. Even without my illness, it was a bad scene." Researchers might see this long-term stressor as a primary determinant in FMS, but Sunny recalls CFIDS/FMS symptoms in childhood. Research sees distress as one factor switching the light "on" in those who are genetically predisposed. Genes certainly play a role in Sunny's situation, as her daughter also has CFIDS. Her symptoms weren't severe enough to disrupt mother-daughter bonding, and her daughter's condition didn't appear until long after she'd left the house. We discussed FMS patients' hypersensitive systems and Sunny agreed: "I respond to things others don't hear or feel. I feel like a receptive river runs through my body." I wanted to explore my ideas on personality and FMS and CFIDS as related to her achievement orientation, work relationship, and so on. "Yup, I was a 100 percent Type A. I've been called a perfectionist often enough. I know it was true and this added to my negative stress." She sees people's negative thoughts and pressured, stressed lives partly adding to these conditions. She believes FMS and CFIDS are akin to Gulf War Syndrome: "People are exposed to many toxins and some just have stronger immune systems than others."

What has she learned? "I've changed my behavior and thinking away from the Type A perfectionism. We create our realities. If you get something negative later, like an illness, it could be from suppressed thoughts that finally came out. But thoughts can be changed and miracles happen. I'm seventy and can say this is a good place, one that's changing for the better." The symptoms became noticeable enough to be truly bothersome some twenty years ago and she exclaims, "I've never given up hope yet!" She's tried many treatments. "It's taken a long time to get where I am. Doctors first gave me NSAIDs and drugs like Elavil to help my sleep, but they didn't help. I did learn I had multidrug allergies though. Sleep is still difficult. Also, I've had fibro-fog recently. During these times, I can't think, I lose things, I can't remember . . . things are fuzzy. I just remarried and moved into this house and can't find a thing! I take pure DHEA by prescription, which helps." Massage is effective, particularly craniosacral massage when the pain is intense. "I see an herbalist and take lots of nutrients like vitamins A and D, magnesium, selenium, boron, zinc, and calcium. It took a while to figure out, but my diet really helps. I eat green and yellow vegetables, but no tomatoes, which are too acidic. I eat fish once a week, rarely chicken, and get enough protein from tofu, nuts, seeds, legumes, and beans. I don't eat red meat, sugar, or dairy products." Is it hard to follow such an eating plan? Perhaps, but as I think about it, if it were to help reduce pain and fatigue, I'd opt for it! "My exercise is down a bit, but I do qi gong, which is great. My TENS unit didn't help, but I know it helps some people. Aquatherapy was amazing. I was in severe pain five years ago and the movements were basic but helped greatly! My new discovery is sulfur hot springs . . . wonderful!"

Personally, one of her best treatments is her new husband, who is "so understanding about FMS. He's thoughtful, believes me, and is caring." Given the importance of social relationships, particularly for women, it's understandable this is a potent curative! Words to share with other women with FMS/ CFIDS: "Women, get more than one opinion, as doctors have extreme tunnel vision for their own beliefs. Also, look into alternative treatments; groups for some of these are great. I also urge deep soul-searching of what you want from life and what you'll do to get it. Look at your spiritual beliefs and do what is right for you. Look around and see how bad others' lives can be. You think, 'This is terrible, it's ruined my life', but you're better off because you can have some control over it. Use it."

I'm thankful to her for the hope-inspiring words from seven decades of experience, aren't you?

CHAPTER 13

Chronic Fatigue Immune Dysfunction Syndrome

*I have always made a distinction between healing and curing. To me
'healed' represents a condition of one's life; 'cured' relates strictly to
one's physical condition ... there may be healed quadriplegics and AIDS
patients, and cured cancer patients who are leading unhealthy lives.
What this means ... is that neither my patients nor I need ever face the
inevitability of failure, for no matter how life-threatening their disease or
how unlikely a cure, healing is always possible.*

—Bernie Siegel, *Peace, Love & Healing*

CFIDS shares many similarities with FMS, leading some to question whether a
distinction is real. If you skipped chapter 11, refer back to the section called If
There Is No Such Thing, Why Do I Feel So Sick? One clear similarity between
FMS and CFIDS is, they're both the subject of contentious debate. CFIDS may
have had even more names than FMS over the years. It's been called chronic
fatigue syndrome, chronic mononucleosis, the "yuppie disease," neuromyasthe-
nia, chronic Epstein-Barr virus (CEBV) disease, persistent virus disease, myalgic
encephalomyelitis (Europe and Canada), and natural killer cell disease (Japan).
As with FMS, diagnosis is tricky, even though some tests can discern various
system abnormalities that suggest CFIDS. These tests, in conjunction with a

symptom history, are used to diagnose the condition (Hoffman 1993). Accurate diagnosis depends on the skill and education of the medical professional.

At this writing, there is an uproar among governmental agencies, medical groups, and CFIDS/FMS associations and their members with respect to finalizing a name change in the U.S. Many people are incensed that Americans don't use the term "myalgic encephalomyelitis," and they attribute the difficulties in legitimizing CFIDS to using the vague "chronic fatigue" term. Studies indicate that doctors take the former name more seriously and project less rosy outcomes than for CFIDS. The battle intensified when it was revealed in 1999 that millions of dollars allocated by the government to study CFIDS was shifted to research "really important" illnesses. This was yet another needless slight to the many frustrated CFIDS patients.

The CFIDS sex ratio mirrors that of FMS: nine women to one man. Until recently, CFIDS prevalence estimates have been as vague and diverse as have those for FMS. A 1999 community-wide study overcomes earlier biases in studies relying on patients referred by doctors or individuals already treated for CFIDS. Such "preselected" groups left out many CFIDS candidates who don't have access to such health care or who drop out of the system. The study provided valuable information beyond overall prevalence data. First, while earlier studies estimated anywhere fron two to 247 patients with SFIDS per 100,000 people (Friedberg 1995), this study indicated a more likely ratio of 813 per 100,000. Second, this so-called yuppie disease, ridiculed by many in the medical profession as a neurotic manifestation dreamed up by middle to upper class, educated white women, was actually found to be most prevalent across groups of minorities, and people with lower occupational and educational status (Jason et al. 1999).

What Causes CFIDS?

Research has shown that CFIDS has many possible causes. To be best able to make wise SHOC discisions, you should familiarize yourself with the possibilities detailed here.

Immune System Involvement

Initially, I included CFIDS in this book based on my suspicions of its auto-immune components. Soon after that, I learned that the AARDA had just categorized CFIDS as an ARC, a decision based on growing evidence. As some of its names indicate, CFIDS is increasingly believed to have an autoimmune component. Many people with CFIDS have antinuclear autoantibodies, and researchers now contend that they may have dysregulated immune systems. A study by Dr. Konstantinov and colleagues seen in the *Journal of Clinical Investigation* revealed that 52 percent of people with CFIDS have autoantibodies to components of the nuclear envelope protein (AARDA 1997). The new debate is whether such auto-immune disturbances are the cause or the result of CFIDS. Dr. Jay Goldstein asserts that immune system changes result from improper regulation by the brain. He contends that dysfunction in brain processes leads to increased immune response characterized by inappropriate B lymphocyte activity, causing antibody production in response to relatively weak stimuation. Further exploration is being conducted in this area and may lead to discoveries. Both FMS and CFIDS seem to involve elevated levels of cytokines (see chapter 1 to review cytokines and auto-immune dysfunction), while most ARCs involve decreased cytokine production. As discussed, cytokines are communicators in the immune system and play a critical role in ensuring this system's effective functioning. This disparity indicates how much more we need to learn about the complexity of ARCs. There are myriad empirical studies that have pinpointed various immune system abnormalities in CFIDS patients—the internet and support groups are good sources for more information on this topic.

Genes

There is recent, impressive work with respect to the role of genetics in CFIDS. Dr. Goldstein sees it as an illness arising from improper information processing (Goldstein 1996). The problem is misperception of both internal and external stimuli, with the main disruption involving the prefrontal cortex's errors in discerning what to allow (and what not to allow) in the body. The prefrontal cortex also manages neurotransmitter secretions, which stimulate glutamate (for proper cerebral functioning) and the release of sufficient norepinephrine (present in low levels in people with CFIDS/FMS). Such prefrontal cortex disturbances may arise from primarily genetic and secondarily developmental/environmental factors. With genetic predisposition, exposure to potentially infectious elements may affect your immune system at a particular time (exposure plus genetics plus situational factors). Goldstein believes that the nature and quality of a child's attachment and development within her environment play a part in determining her ultimate information processing. If a child grows up in a threatening environment, she can develop a hypervigilant style and place exaggerated importance on everyday situations. This is linked with CFIDS-related neurochemical changes like an increase in substance P accompained by a reduction in norepinephrine.

Goldstein adds that those with neurosomatic disorders (CFIDS/FMS) may have restricted brain abilities to adapt neural networks to shifts in external/internal situations. Restrictions in neural plasticity cause trouble today given the rate of change in our culture and the learning abilities this necessitates. Such limitations, plus the tendency to take in inordinate amounts of nonessential information, help explain why CFIDS patients are overwhelmed by sensory and intellectual information. You've probably had such experiences: "blasting" music others say isn't loud; moderate impacts feeling like strong jolts when we hit our hands, arms, or legs on yet another object; and sensitivity to smells, lights, chemicals, and the like. Simply put, we may be overly sensitive to unimportant or mild environmental information, have problems in learning and perceiving newness, and difficulties in effectively processing and thus performing typical, familiar activities in our lives. Genetics is also indicated in CFIDS because it often runs in families by itself, with FMS, or with other ARCs. Genetic predispositions may cause people with CFIDS to have detoxification enzymes that are more vulnerable to disruption by internal and external elements. Our bodies may be unable to tolerate today's stressors, chemicals, and pollutants (Ali 1994).

Infectious Agents

The idea that CFIDS results from viral infections has existed for some time, and many researchers endorse this notion. The nature of such a virus is unknown, though many have been suggested. The Epstein-Barr virus (EBV) was the first one to be linked to CFIDS; because tests available at that time to detect EBV often showed elevated Epstein-Barr antibodies in possible CFIDS patients, an oversimplified, inaccurate conclusion was drawn. Since the 1980s, we've learned that 97 percent of adults over age thirty have EBV virus in their systems—and CFIDS incidence is nowhere near that percentage. Elevated antibodies to this virus don't mean EBV causes CFIDS. Mono is caused by the EBV virus, and it involves extreme fatigue, though it usually lasts only weeks or months. Once the EBV is integrated and chronic, as it becomes in most people, the body adapts and fatigue ceases. At initial exposure or recurrence of EBV in people with ARC, other disorders can arise: mono (most frequently), viral encephalitis (rare), and, in those with compromised immune systems, non-Hodgkin's lymphoma.

Some believe several related herpes group or B-cell viruses may trigger CFIDS. Let's look at similarities and differences between the AIDS virus and EBV to understand the latter. One problem in controlling and understanding the AIDS virus is its rapid changeability; it mutates from 5 to 1000 times faster than the flu. Some types can't survive "in the cold," while others can survive outside the body from minutes to days. While the AIDS virus typically targets the immune system's T cells and EBV typically targets B cells, an HIV strain exists that works on the B cells, just like EBV. Both must be detected indirectly through elevated levels of viral antibodies, sometimes meaning the immune system isn't winning the battle (whether against AIDS, CFIDS, or other conditions). But a critical discovery is that these antibodies don't always indicate one is infected with the virus as healthy people also show elevated viral antibodies. The NIH used trials of acyclovir to interfere with EBV increases; however, this did not seem effective. The AIDS virus and other retroviruses lack something almost all of earth's organisms have; namely, their own DNA genetic "directions." They have RNA though, the product of DNA—a little backwards. This is more bizarre when we see how retroviruses like AIDS survive. With just RNA, the virus shouldn't do much of anything, but it does. When the virus attacks, it injects its RNA into targeted immune system T cells and emits an enzyme that picks up floating components, which go to making DNA. It uses these to help RNA create its own DNA, custom designed to produce copies of the very same RNA.

I've included this discussion of AIDS and retroviruses because researchers are studying a potential link between retroviruses (i.e., AIDS and leukemia viruses) and CFIDS. Researchers detected a retrovirus in 80 percent of a group of CFIDS patients and found similar results in 33 percent of those exposed to the people with CFIDS. However, an *unrelated*, healthy group had no evidence of the retrovirus (DeFreitas et al. 1991; Cheney 1991). Perhaps CFIDS arises from or is associated with a retrovirus' pirating of immune cells, assuming production control, and disrupting the modulation of the immune system. More research is necessary, as retrovirus transmission is thought to occur only through bodily fluids, and this transmission hasn't yet been found in CFIDS. Studies of other herpes-type viruses, such as oral and genital herpes, haven't yielded conclusive results. CFIDS expert Dr. Murray Susser believes it results in part from a combination of infectious conditions (Burton Goldberg Group 1997). He believes that people with CFIDS are often fighting obscure combinations of yeast, parasite, and viral infections resulting from weak immune systems. Other experts suggest that recurrent viral or bacterial infections, like sinus infections, cystitis, and acne, may trigger CFIDS.

Other suggest a causal link between persisting enterovirus and the chronic muscle fatigue of CFIDS. When CFIDS patients exercise, excessive lactate is produced and remains in the muscles. Such disruption in muscle energy metabolism has been linked with enterovirus (usually related to Coxsackie B subgroup) in the muscles. This may indicate a link between CFIDS, fatigue, and enterovirus, but doesn't support persistent enterovirus as a cause of CFIDS.

While many researchers believe the brain's hypothalamus and its chemical disruptions cause CFIDS, they don't suggest it works in isolation. They see the persistent viral infections discussed here as a potential cause of certain hypothalamus disruptions. Recently, CFIDS and FMS received a surge in interest due to their similarities to Gulf War Syndrome (GWS). Not surprisingly, many doctors doubt the existence of GWS as much as they doubt CFIDS/FMS. But, some believe the hypothalamus disruptions underlying CFIDS/FMS and GWS may be another example in which chemical exposure resulted in neurochemical changes. Other DNA viral agents tied with neuronal disruption, like herpes simplex, EBV, and adenoviruses, use chemical "tricks" to camouflage themselves from immune systems. Perhaps other viral agents that alter neuronal functioning and cause CFIDS can also camouflage themselves and remain undetected. Most recently, treating GWS patients with massive antibiotics has seemed effective for some, suggesting a possible bacterial infection. Further support for a viral/bacterial cause exists, as there have been outbreaks of CFIDS in small groups of people living or working together. Since CFIDS isn't highly contagious, genetics plus a specific agent may be necessary.

Brain Structures and Functioning

Several experts have been looking primarily at brain and neurotransmitter functioning in CFIDS. As discussed in chapter 12 on FMS, Goldstein used SPECT technology to examine the brains of CFIDS patients, half of whom also met FMS criteria. Results showed blood flow deficits in regions in the brain. Interestingly, results indicated blood flow restrictions were greater in those with both CFIDS and FMS (Goldstein 1993, 1994). Dr. Susser (1997) found decreased brain circulation after exercise in people with CFIDS, a pattern opposite to that found in healthy individuals. A PET scan study of CFIDS patients confirmed lower levels of activity in the frontal lobes than seen in "normal" and depressed subjects. These frontal lobe regions are important, as they're involved in expressive language, motor behavior, reasoning, concentrating, and time/place/person orientation. CFIDS symptoms often include disruptions in all of these elements.

Female Hormones

You'll read about the role of hormones in CFIDS in following sections, but you'll also benefit by refering to this section in chapter 12 on FMS as well.

Personality and Behavior

Some CFIDS/FMS patients describe themselves as having very high self-expectations; they tend to be perfectionistic, driven, and hard-working. Many of us in these fast-paced days feel stretched too thin, and this is so in particular for many women who are trying to fulfill multiple roles with often conflicting demands. We stand on stage trying to juggle all of our many balls, while naively, or because we've been taught, asking for or accepting another and another . . . But are we causing these conditions? Much has been said about the harmful results of distress on our mind-body health. Are women with FMS or CFIDS too stressed out or unable to cope with stress? Fred Friedberg comparied healthy people, CFIDS patients, and those with depression and found that people with CFIDS reported more stressors in the year prior to illness compared to the healthy folks. The depressed group, however, reported more stressors than the CFIDS group (1995).

Other researchers tie in personality through lifestyle factors like poor diet, lack of exercise, alcohol consumption, smoking, and leading pressured lives with no relaxation. As depression is seen in CFIDS, some believe depression's suppression of the immune system causes it. Fortunately, this view is waning, and the CDC notes that many CFIDS/FMS patients report depression and anxiety *after* CFIDS onset. This wouldn't be a surprising response to overwhelming fatigue, pain, loss, and disbelief by doctors and family. So while exhausting ourselves, overachieving, and leading negatively stressful lives may be a trigger for some, it isn't an only or sufficient cause. If it were, CFIDS would be today's plague and the country would grind to a halt!

Environment and Oxidative Molecular Injury

New evidence surfaced as I drew this book to a close. Researchers from around the world were arriving at a consensus: quite possible the first true neuro-chemical diffference between people with CFIDS and those without it had been found. It's believed that CFIDS patients can't break down or use glucose efficiently, allowing it to build up and act as a toxin in the body. It's too early to draw definite conclusions now, but further study is critical.

As mentioned in the genes section above, Dr. Majid Ali sees CFIDS patients' genetic makeup as creating overly vulnerable energy and detoxification enzymes, which causes accelerated oxidative molecular injury and thus CFIDS (1994). In essence, their systems can't tolerate the toxins and biologic stressors of our modern-day whirlwind society, a theory that aligns with the growing belief that CFIDS results from many influences plus genetics. Ali believes that CFIDS patients' molecular defenses are vulnerable to damage by allergies, pollutants, chemicals, personality styles like hostility, poor reactions to distress, and dietary factors like refined sugars, all of which generate a perpetual stress response. He sees chronic fatigue as the primary chronic health problem of the twenty-first century. While chronic fatigue can't be "fixed" by medicine, it's preventable and reversible through holistic approaches including nutrition, environmental changes, self-regulation, and slow, sustained exercise. Ali accepts other causes of CFIDS, like Lyme disease, though he thinks these are rare. His theory aligns with others that assert that the limbic system is involved in CFIDS, though he attributes different causal patterns to cognitive involvement. He believes loss of memory, confusion, and mood changes result from oxidative injury to neurotransmitter and nerve cell receptor molecules. The limbic system disruption may be involved at some level, but he doesn't agree with the typical drug treatments. To learn more, read his 1994 book, in which he says that decreased natural killer cells occur in the blood of CFIDS patients, but that this is a result of CFIDS, not a cause.

To learn more about this model, we would need to look at the factors that damage molecular defenses before individuals are exposed to or experience these other factors that others see as causally related to the onset of CFIDS. Ali's model aims to increase energy and detoxification enzymes through natural, nontoxic approaches involving nutritional changes (foods, IVs, oral nutrient therapies), allergy assessment, self-regulation, and slow exercise.

CFIDS/FMS expert Dr. Jacob Teitelbaum sees three chronic fatigue states, including CFIDS/FMS, which may or may not arise from the same cause but differ in severity and pattern (1996). Teitelbaum's first type, "drop dead flu," is probably most familiar. It starts with a bout of something flulike and gets more severe and disabling, with extreme fatigue. While viral infections contribute, brain and hormonal changes are also key in causing particular CFIDS (and FMS) symptoms. Viral infection underlying CFIDS may lead to brain inflammation that restricts hypothalamic functioning. Because of this gland's central role, its disruption means thyroid and adrenal glands no longer function normally and long-term hypothalamic-related symptoms arise. Teitelbaum asserts that treating CFIDS with adrenal hormones can be effective. He also sees adrenal and glandular suppression as leading to a second chronic fatigue subtype, the world of FMS. His third dynamic brings us back to the realm of ARCs, in which the body's immune system becomes confused and attacks parts of itself rather than an outsider. He sees CFIDS as an ARC in which the "attacked self" involves adrenal and thyroid glands and vitamin B12 absorptive cells. He brings up an issue that is crucial for you to remember. Despite how you feel, your blood tests may well look "normal," causing doctors to tell you that nothing is wrong. Medicine is a "show me" profession, and CFIDS/FMS don't play by the usual rules. While many conventional caretakers can be open-minded, it's essential you find CFIDS experts.

Multiplicity

Genes contribute to CFIDS and may be necessary but insufficient. Toxins (in air, food, water, medication, dental fillings, etc.), hormonal changes, viral/bacterial infections, immune system disruption from immunization, allergens, stressors, nutrition deficits, excess antibiotics, yeasts, and other conditions, combined with the genetic tendency, may trigger CFIDS.

Symptoms and Signs of CFIDS

While some see CFIDS as akin to FMS, different diagnostic criteria have been set forth by the National Institutes of Health (NIH) and the U.S. Centers for Disease Control and Prevention, including: clinically evaluated, unexplained, persistent or relapsing chronic fatigue of new or definite onset (not lifelong) that is not the result of ongoing exertion, is not substantially alleviated by rest, and results in substantial reduction in previous levels of occupational, educational, social, or personal activities; and the concurrent occurrence of four or more of the following symptoms: substantial impairment in short-term memory or concentration; sore throat; tender lymph nodes; muscle pain; multijoint pain without joint swelling or redness; headaches of a new type, pattern, or severity; nonrefreshing sleep; and postexertional malaise lasting more than twenty-four hours. These symptoms must have persisted or recurred during six or more consecutive months of illness and must not have predated the fatigue. People with CFIDS may also experience night sweats; allergies; hypersensitivity to temperatures, sounds, and sensations; confusion; GI problems; low grade fever; infections and autoimmune reactions; and frequent feelings of being cold.

As with FMS, one of the reasons the medical community has been reluctant to accept the legitimacy of CFIDS is the great variety of possible symptoms and their changeability. Also as with FMS, doctors and others don't accept our illnesses because we "look too good." Most people aren't told they look too good, but people with CFIDS and other ARC know what I mean by this statement. If it weren't for the pain, it might seem quite funny that for once looking good is actually a negative!

Related Conditions and Look-alikes

If you see your doctor in the early stages of CFIDS, you may have no idea you're opening Pandora's box with the complaint of fatigue; it's part of so many illnesses, and physical illnesses aren't the only cause of fatigue. When you mention fatigue, your doctor may look for immunologic conditions like severe allergies,

SLE, endocrine conditions like hypothyroidism or diabetes mellitus, severe ane-mia, drugs, or conditions like depression, anxiety, and stress.

Before looking at other conditions to consider when diagnosing CFIDS, let's look at mind-body unity and the persistent desire in our culture to classify so-called mental disorders vs. physical disorders. Fatigue is a central sign of depres-sion and if you have a thorough doctor, her data gathering won't look only at you or your family's physical history. She may ask about your current life, relation-ships, work, hobbies, and the like. If so, don't jump to the conclusion that she is either nosy or is about to give you the old, "You need to have somebody to talk to and I suggest Dr. Rebound, an excellent psychologist...." Do watch to ensure you're not being dismissed, but at the same time, realize that you could very well be depressed either as a result of CFIDS or because depression may be part of CFIDS (i.e., neurotransmitter imbalances). Be fair to yourself and your doctor in clarifying when depression, if present, commenced, whether there were major stressors, or whether it comes from your fatigue, pain, and inability to function as you did before. It usually won't take long to detect whether your doctor asks such questions as a result of being a conscientious assessor or because she doesn't believe in CFIDS.

There are a number of other conditions that appear in conjunction with CFIDS or cause confusion, because of shared symptoms and tests results.

Lupus

Localized joint pain, general diffuse pain, and fatigue call for differential diagnoses between SLE, FMS, and CFIDS. However, people with CFIDS/FMS can have SLE as well, so fatigue and high temperatures from SLE may cause your doctor to erroneously diagnosis CFIDS or vice versa.

Fibromyalgia Syndrome

There are substantial overlap in CFIDS and FMS incidence, which is described in chapter 12. Fifty percent of CFIDS patients have FMS, and vice versa.

Lyme Disease

CFIDS' central symptom—severe, chronic fatigue—is also primary in LD. Many doctors think people with CFIDS have LD, and such misdiagnosis inter-feres with proper treatment. CFIDS patients attending support groups may also have LD, and others with LD symptoms may not be diagnosed accurately (Lang 1997). See the discussion of LD in chapter 7.

Candidiasis

Often misdiagnosed as CFIDS, this disorder can often coexist with CFIDS.

Multiple Sclerosis

Though it differs from CFIDS, it shares extreme fatigue and relapsing/remitting periods. However, when MS bouts are over, one is generally worse than before. Other shared symptoms are extreme cold/heat sensitivity, clumsiness, numbness, and imbalance. Both conditions involve food, toxin, and mercury amalgam sensitivities and candidiasis.

Rheumatoid Arthritis

Because it causes muscle and joint pain, RA is often confused with CFIDS. If you have CFIDS, your doctor may erroneously diagnose you with RA or another connective tissue disease.

Thyroid Disease

In both Graves' disease and Hashimoto's thyroiditis, the immune system targets the thyroid gland. Thyroid hormones affect almost all body organs, including the hair, skin, nails, and muscles (muscle weakness in GD; muscle cramping in HT). CFIDS patients and GD patients may share anxiety, diarrhea, hand/body tremors, elevated body temperature, and sensation sensitivities. There are even more similarities between CFIDS and HT. The insufficient thyroid hormones of HT cause decreased metabolism and heat generation and feelings of perpetual cold often experienced by people with CFIDS (and FMS). Other shared symptoms are severe skin dryness; decreased nail growth and nail thinning; dry, damaged hair; GI distress and constipation, muscle pain and weakness, post-exertional malaise, concentration problems, problem-solving deficits, and depression.

By being familiar with these conditions, you'll be able to best direct your SHOC. The mere fact of taking an active role in your illness and care boosts your mind-body health.

The Courses of CFIDS

While there are common symptoms and signs, the courses of CFIDS vary greatly. One apparent consistency is immune system dysregulation. Due to the confusing array of changeable symptoms and the continued disbelief by some conventional doctors, many doctors see CFIDS patients after they've been bounced about and rejected by many doctors. Maoshing Ni, D.O.M., Ph.D., treats people with CFIDS by improving immune system vigor while reducing excess sensitivity and improving its healthy regulation (Burton Goldberg Group 1997).

Testing for CFIDS

There simply is no single test available tht everyone agrees is appropriate, valid, reliable, or even adequate. This is one of the reasons for the medical community's reluctance to accept CFIDS. The nature of the disorder is such that typical assessment techniques are often unable to detect real mind-body differences in people with CFIDS. CFIDS expert Leon Chaitow (1995) concurs that there is no one standard test but explains that certain diagnostic techniques, when combined, get closest to accurately diagnosing the disorder. He suggests basic steps doctors must take for any illness, like physical exams, lab tests, medical histories, and most importantly, studies of symptom patterns. The best approach is a complete assessment (see section on Testing for FMS, chapter 12).

Let's look at some specific tests to identify CFIDS and rule out other diagnoses. These descriptions can help you decipher your doctor's medi-speak (should it sound like a foreign tongue) and help you use jargon if necessary to ask questions and state preferences. You may need to educate and motivate your doctor to perform or refer for these assessments.

Blood tests can detect the presence or absence, as well as relative levels of, chemicals, nutrients, neurotransmitters, and the like. While general blood tests often appear "normal" in people with CFIDS, specific, targeted tests can be more revealing. Deficiencies in neurotransmitters, such as dopamine, neuroepinephrine, and serotonin, are often characteristic of CFIDS. Your doctor must explore such levels to gain an understanding of your condition and possible diagnosis.

Because 50 percent of CFIDS patients may also meet FMS criteria, it is helpful to look for characteristics of FMS as well. Some people with FMS have a problem with collagen synthesis. Collagen is used by the body to make connective tissue, which holds the body together. Blood tests can show a shortage of collagen in people with FMS. Other areas to explore include determining the level of GH (typically low in FMS) and substance P (pain neurotransmitter, usually high in FMS patients).

A manual trigger/tender point test should also be done before diagnosing either CFIDS or FMS. A major part of FMS' diagnostic criteria is that at least eleven of eighteen points are painful when touched with moderate pressure. Make sure your SHOC doc knows the potential points and has experience with CFIDS/FMS. If these criteria aren't met, you may have CFIDS alone.

Another important test for CFIDS involves checking thyroid hormone levels. While your test results may look "normal" to your doctor, this conclusion may be incorrect. Teitelbaum (1996) indicates that doctors usually judge TSH levels from .5–.95 as normal, but CFIDS patients may have lower levels (in the form of hypothalamic hypothyroidism) even when results seem normal. He suggests synthroid may prove effective when: TSH levels are below .95 or above 3.0 (or T3/T4 levels fall within the low normal range); FMS is present; hypothyroidism symptoms exist; and the client's average awakening temperature is below 97.4 degrees F. It's unlikely most doctors would follow up on a "normal" thyroid test, which is another reason you must be centrally involved in your SHOC and in selecting experts for your team.

Finally, brain imaging techniques add diagnostic information. One of the troublesome elements of CFIDS is that physicians have been unable to use many typical testing tools to find the hard evidence they're used to and want in order to decide whether or not CFIDS "really" exists and to differentiate CFIDS from other conditions. This arises because CFIDS and FMS are neural network disorders involving problems with circuitry throughout the brain. Most professionals look for structural changes or evident brain tissue damage to confirm that a true "physical" disorder is present. Given the nature of neurosomatic disorders like CFIDS, new brain imaging tools best detect functional brain differences. For example, SPECT, quantitative EEG (electroencephalogram), evoked response mapping, and positron emission tomography have been revealing in detecting real differences in the regional cerebral blood flow (rCBF) and activation of CFIDS/FMS patients' brains compared to such measures in "normal" brains (Goldstein 1996). By looking for specific patterns, brain imaging can help diagnose CFIDS. While rCBF typically increases when one exercises, such as during a treadmill test, the opposite occurs in CFIDS. Similarly, when people with CFIDS exercise, cortisone levels decrease, so tests like this can be helpful.

Other problems arise in diagnostic testing for CFIDS. When doctors attempt to detect CFIDS during its early stages, they may give SLE diagnostic tests, which may score positive. False positive scores arise because a type of autoimmune dysfunction exists, but it's not necessarily SLE. Such errors are frequent, and patients with this misinformation are subjected to unwarranted distress and inappropriate treatment. A newer diagnostic tool using the angiotensin-converting enzyme may come out positive in people with CFIDS, but confusion arises here as people with LD also obtain positive results and, as mentioned, LD can look like CFIDS. LD tests are weak in that they depend on finding antibodies rather than the infectious spirochete that comes from the tick.

Dr. Burke Cunha asserts that people with CFIDS have "crimson crescents," or redness of the tissues on the inner sides of the mouth, near the back molars, which can be reliable markers for CFIDS (Burton Goldberg Group 1997). He claims these marks redden as CFIDS worsens and become lighter as it improves. Replicating studies are needed, as Cunha found these marks in about 80 percent of CFIDS patients examined but completely absent in people with mono or strep throat.

What You Can Do

I have emphasized the great variety of individual CFIDS cases because I want you to be truly aware of your body's uniqueness. The last thing you should do is ignore symptoms or distress because they don't seem to fit with what you've heard or read about your condition. At the same time, don't just attribute mind-body changes to your CFIDS. Watch and listen to your body: What is it trying to say? Value your mind-body signals and educate yourself as much as possible, for the sooner you determine whether something is wrong and what it is, the sooner you can begin to form your plan, find kind, knowledgeable experts, change your attitude, reduce the progression or severity of your illness, and derive health-inducing meaning and prostress.

Your SHOC team will probably differ from those of others with the same illness because of the range of fluctuating symptoms and various systems involved.

Team members may include a family doctor, neurologist, ophthalmologist, psychologist, dermatologist, endocrinologist, or rheumatologist. The span of your SHOC team may widen based on your personal beliefs and values to include acupuncturists, herbalists, spiritual or religious guides, chiropractors, osteopaths, massage therapists, and so on. Whatever its composition, most important is that you feel good about the expertise, willingness to listen, cooperation, and respect of your SHOC team players. If you have people working for you who are demeaning or disbelieving and your reaction isn't misplaced anger or hostility at yourself or your illness, or some personal peeve you need to work on anyway . . . then kick them off the team. It'll be just one of many times you'll have to assume control, make decisions, and take action if you've decided on the path toward finding meaning and self-healing. Recall the potent role your mind and your resulting emotions and behavior play in improving your mind-body health and prognosis.

A Balanced, Holistic Health Optimization Plan

While most ARCs are complex, confusing, and not well understood, CFIDS is one of the least understood. Other ARCs now accepted as "real" diseases went through similar periods of suspicion and labeling as "women's psychosomatic" ailments until appropriate studies were funded and treatments showed some promise. However, I and the women with whom I work have strived to be pro-stressors and challengers by seeking some positive aspects of CFIDS/FMS. I know there is no way I can shut my eyes or suppress my memories of tearful faces; bodies hunched hopelessly; screams of pain and anger; beseeching prayers; accusations; shame; broken marriages, bodies, and spirits; and dreams swept swiftly away. This is a real side of CFIDS and FMS.

But there is another side awaiting you if you choose to travel its circuitous path, go new places, and try new things while making peace with your mind-body system and giving it what it needs to heal and grow. There can be some positives to these ills, such as increased patience and tolerance for ourselves and others, reducing our perfectionistic expectations of ourselves, learning balance is beauty, seeing ourselves beat situations we never would have believed possible, all while having an increased dependence on others for assistance but a decreased dependence on others for approval, self-esteem, and self-respect. Because our usual health caretakers can't offer easy remedies, we must expand our healing circles. This is a wonderful synchronicity, given our nature as women. We're free to look to new ways of handling our bodies, new ways of using woman's oldest remedies for relief, freedom, and growth. As importantly, we've gathered into groups to use the tradition of women exchanging words to be knowledge-holders, to communicate for shared purposes. This is a feminine strength and with it we can combine innovative, effective treatments and understandings of our health. We can be powerful individuals and also powerful groups. In terms of actual effective, holistic treatment programs, refer to chapter 12 and the section with the same title as this one.

Self-Management

What follows are specific recommendations for CFIDS as well as suggestions for readings in appendix II and referrals presented in appendix I. Among most conventional doctors, there is consensus that the following can help treat CFIDS: medications, good sleep, gentle aerobic exercise if possible, and cognitive behavioral therapy and pain management. I see the following as also essential: education; stress optimization and relaxation training; cognitive techniques; nutrition/supplements; organizational, coping, assertiveness, and communications skills; support network of SHOC members, families, friends, spiritual leaders; chronic illness counseling; biofeedback; massage (cautiously); acupuncture, acupressure, physical and/or occupational therapy, and chiropractic techniques. While not all of these tools may be necessary, you can use some as part of your SHOC tool kit. See appendix II for more on these tools.

Trigger Point Pain

Please refer to chapter 12 on FMS to learn about trigger/tender point pain. If you're one of many who have both CFIDS and FMS, it's important that you read this.

Medications

As with all the medications discussed in this book, you must refer to your SHOC doc before making any changes in your currently prescribed regimen. Medication prescription for CFIDS patients can be difficult due to chemical sensitivity and symptom variability. Many people with CFIDS experience low blood pressure, dizziness, and confusion. Reasons for this aren't well understood, though calcium-channel blockers that increase oxygen and blood to the heart can help. Your doctor may prescribe two such medications, Calan and Nimotop. Depression can be a result or part of CFIDS or any chronic illness, and while many medical experts believe depression causes CFIDS, an increasing number of studies show what some have suspected for years: depression is a consequence or a part of the illness. Various medications exist to redress norepinephrine and serotonin imbalances in CFIDS (see chapter 12 on FMS). Experts have had success in treating CFIDS patients with various serotonin-affecting antidepressants, such as Serzone, Zoloft, Prozac, and Paxil. As with FMS, sleeping aids can relieve CFIDS symptoms. In addition, tricyclic antidepressants like Trazodone, Elavil, Sinequan, and Flexeril may help reduce pain, increase sleep, and improve mood. Given the problem of fatigue, we must be cautious of sedative-type drugs.

Another common condition in CFIDS patients is headaches, for which anti-inflammatories may be prescribed. However, NSAIDs aren't usually effective in reducing body aches and pain, as inflammation isn't really the problem in CFIDS. Also, there are various adverse effects from taking NSAIDs over time. Other potential medications for relieving headaches include Imitrex, Tylenol, and calcium channel blockers. Muscle relaxants like Soma can provide temporary relief. However, they can be quite strong and make you sleepy, uncoordinated, and interfere even further with your concentration and memory. Refer to appendix II for a discussion of biofeedback, which can be invaluable in treating migraines and other headaches.

As discussed in the diagnosis section, thyroid hormones are often low in CFIDS patients, even though test results may look normal. Some knowledgeable doctors suggest a trial of thyroid hormone medication, such as Synthroid. In terms of dealing with this through nutrient supplements, manganese may help (Metagenics 1993) (see the following Nutritional Remedies section for more info). You really must work closely with your SHOC doc with respect to which, if any, medications are right for you. Women tend to feel happiest with doctors who are flexible and open in terms of trying different medications, and who haven't been needlessly concerned about pain medication abuse. Studies show that chronic-pain patients are unlikely to abuse pain medicines, and when one is experiencing the difficulties of a chronic illness, the last thing she needs is to experience unnecessary pain because of rigid, outdated thinking.

For a thorough exploration of effective CFIDS medications, refer to Goldstein's 1996 masterpiece, *Betrayal by the Brain*. This book offers thorough, scientific descriptions of medications he has used to successfully treat CFIDS. Goldstein uses a panoply of medications to accomplish his treatment goals. He finds drugs that increase norepinephrine to be effective in reducing CFIDS symptoms. While this may sound simple, he is aware of the trial-and-error approach to treating CFIDS, as represented by his wide-ranging protocols. These medicines are related to his theory about the cause of CFIDS, presented earlier in this chapter.

Before taking any medication, always ask about any potential side effects or interactions with other medications (over-the-counter or prescription), herbs, or other supplements you are taking. It's particularly important with CFIDS to be assertive in discussing possible medications you've learned about through your research. As with FMS, doctors are finally admitting that many patients know more about treatment than they do.

To date, medications have shown limited results. If little gain and strong side effects are the consequences, as they are for many, it's little wonder many of us turn to alternatives in seeking relief from fatigue, cognitive problems, and pain. You could be one of the fortunate ones for whom medications prove helpful. While they don't solve the underlying problem as of yet, they may allow you to return to a fairly active lifestyle.

Help Yourself Help Your Body

Much knowledge has been gained about the effects of our personal environment on our bodies. Many changes can be made at home, at work, and when traveling to reduce your fatigue and pain. Refer to the "Ergonomics and Body-Saving Techniques" in chapter 17.

Alternative Techniques

While alternative treatments are "natural," you must still treat them with caution. As with conventional medicine, you must assume an active, responsible role and ensure your SHOC members are properly certified, trained, and experienced with CFIDS. You simply owe it to yourself. The key lies in integrating appropriate conventional and alternative tools, akin to obtaining balance in your life overall. Extremes trigger relapses or worsen symptoms, triggering "stinking thinking." ("I knew it. I thought things were getting better. I was working a bit, playing with the kids. Now it's back. I just can't deal with this anymore . . . the pain, fatigue, forgetfulness, irritability, misery. Is this life?") It's easy to see how irrational thinking directly causes depression, frustration, and hopelessness, which directly interfere with a healthy immune system and other body functions. Moderation and balance take work, but they greatly increase your chances of leading the most satisfying life, growing, and even thriving.

CFIDS Treatments: Should They Stay or Go?

One useful study examined CFIDS treatments to determine if they made patients better or worse (Friedberg 1995). At first glance, a study of just under 100 CFIDS patients trying the drug Ampligen (an immune system modulator) offered what appeared to be the highest efficacy to date; however, a slew of recent studies did not indicate such efficacy and, at present, Ampligen can't be bought in the U.S. Anti-allergy diets were the second most effective, least harmful treatment. Moderate to major improvements were reported by 32 percent, with less than 1 percent feeling worse! Two other treatments, stress reduction/biofeedback and IV vitamins/injections, were promising, with 26 percent of people improved and less than 1 percent and 4 percent, respectively, feeling worse. Anti-yeast diets were as effective (27 percent moderate to major improvements) and not much more unhealthy (5 percent feeling worse). While 28 percent improved with antidepressants, 31 percent felt worse! Some of this may be due to our chemical sensitivity, while some may result from inappropriate types or amounts of medication prescribed by doctors unfamiliar with CFIDS. This doesn't mean you should refuse antidepressants but does mean you must ensure that your doctor is knowledgable about CFIDS. Other treatments that seem risky based on ratios of people improved compared to people worsened included: allergy shots (17 percent: 27 percent); gammaglobulin (16 percent: 20 percent); antibiotics (oral 14 percent: 36 percent or IV 16 percent: 39 percent); and nitroglycerin (9 percent: 25 percent). For more on this, I recommend *Coping with Chronic Fatigue Syndrome* by Dr. Friedberg. Some conventional doctors are now using infusions of concentrated IV vitamins and minerals. CFIDS patients may also be injected with Kutapressin to boost immune system functioning, or gamma globulin with blood antibodies to treat some symptoms.

Nutritional Remedies

Diets replete with fruits, vegetables, nuts, seeds, whole grains, lean fish, and chicken and turkey without skin are ideal for CFIDS patients, as well as the population in general. Given our chemical sensitivity and the possibility of compromised immune systems, we must avoid poultry treated with antibiotics and fish contaminated with mercury. Do your best to avoid foods high in fat, as fat increases any inflammation and thus pain. Avoid caffeine, sugar (including honey and fructose), and alcohol, which greatly increase fatigue and pain. If you have candidiasis, as many CFIDS patients do, you have all the more reason to remove these from your diet.

You don't have to cut out everything totally or immediately, as many of us become resentful this way and resume eating "forbidden" foods. The cycle is perpetuated if we see ourselves as "failures," feel out of control, and remain angry. Reframe this situation: It isn't a punishment, just as having an illness isn't a punishment for being a bad person. You do have a choice, even here, and you don't have to change your diet. But when you think through the consequences or have experienced them painfully enough, you'll probably *choose* to modify your diet to make yourself feel better. Remind yourself that this is something you want to do for yourself and see it as a challenge, one that is difficult but offers potentially great rewards. Secondly, tell yourself these changes aren't only due to CFIDS, as most are recommended for everybody to improve mind-body health. Thirdly, to see this as a challenge and maintain motivation, create goals and choose rewards to give yourself. Be creative about your new way of eating. These days there are so many fat-free, sugar-free, preservative-free, and such foods that your palate may not even discern most changes. As you learn about new fruits, vegetables, seasonings, and low-fat cheeses and other protein sources, you can build a sense of mastery and turn all of this activity and knowledge into an enjoyable hobby. Eating is certainly one of the great pleasures of life. You're already experiencing enough "loss" (i.e., change), so make this a positive area of growth and fun.

The anti-allergy diet discussed above was effective for CFIDS patients and may be a good place to start your SHOC. Consult with your doctor or allergist about problem substances and how to systematically remove items to pinpoint your body's sensitivities. If you have many allergies, you'll want to learn about new varieties of foods and how to prepare them. While you may have to change your eating, you don't have to live on a regimen of boring, rigid meals. Many clients have new interest in nutrition as a result of CFIDS and are surprised that a "chore" can be a prostressor. Activities you didn't have time for before may be of great interest to you now. This is a good example of how your SHOC can work; namely, taking what seems to be a distressor (food restriction) and changing the perspective to see a challenge turn to a prostressor (learning about new foods, new ways to cook, etc.).

Of course, there will be times when you're so fatigued or pained that the last thing you want to do is cook. Let's use this example to see what you've learned about how your thoughts determine your feelings and behavior. You've become interested in cooking, purchased some books, and feel good about your abilities . . . when out of the blue comes a bout of fatigue and you can barely move. You suddenly remember you've invited friends over to sample a new creation. Put yourself in this scene and without censoring, note the thoughts that come up. Anything like, "Not again, not another day of hell. I can't take this anymore. I invited everyone over to show them what a great cook I've become and that because I'm not working, I'm not totally useless. I can't win. So much for any progress I thought I'd made with this life or growing with this damn sickness! I'll just call while they're at work and leave some excuse." Yes, this is very negative self-talk, but can you relate? Any emotions like frustration, depression, hopelessness, guilt, or self-loathing? What about resulting behaviors: withdrawal, sulking, bad habits? Maybe this is totally off and your self-talk is quite different: "Oh, I'm feeling kind of fatigued today. I'll take it easy, have a warm shower for the aches. It's a good day to hang out, maybe read a bit. I invited some friends for dinner and wanted to show them my food skills. They keep asking what I'm doing and I say, 'Oh, just some cooking.' Well, I'll delay it for now, maybe build up the anticipation. I'll call to tell them tonight isn't great; they're good friends who'll understand. If I'm up to it later, I'll have them over for pizza. It's good for me just to be with them."

The common reminder to drink at least eight to ten glasses of water each day should become your credo. Given chemical sensitivity and immune system vulnerability, ensure that you have a chemical- and pollution-free water source. Some of you may find that you do best with smaller, more frequent meals throughout the day, which can help reverse fatigue, muscle tension, and pain caused by heavy meals.

Antioxidants

These aren't just current health buzzwords—they are truly essential and include natural body substances, vitamins, minerals, and enzymes. They protect against free radicals that damage your cells and immune system and are linked to infections, diseases, and aging. Some free radicals come from exposure to chemicals, cigarettes, radiation, excess sun, and natural body processes. In the body's wisdom, we have defense components, free-radical scavengers, to neutralize free radicals that would harm the internal integrity of the body. These enzymes are helped by vitamins, herbs, minerals, and hormones with antioxidant properties. Vitamin A improves immune system functioning and protein use, and protects against infection and free radicals. The maximum dosage is 15,000 IU per day (if pregnant, maximum 10,000 IU per day). Vitamin E helps improve circulation, while vitamin C boosts key autoimmune components, stress tolerance, energy, detoxification, and helps protect vitamin E. Zinc and grape seed extract play an important role in keeping stable levels of vitamin C in the blood, help with vitamin A absorption, and improve immune system functioning. Taurine maintains appropriate white blood cell functions in the immune system.

Other Supplements

CFIDS patients must also get the most absorbable type of multivitamin/ multimineral supplement with enough of certain trace minerals. Essential are: beta carotene, 15,000 IUs per day; vitamin C, 3,000 to 5,000 mg per day; pantothenic acid, 150 mg per day, though not at bedtime; zinc, 15 mg per day (picolinate form). For CFIDS, we look for elements to maximize immune system efficacy, increase energy levels, and improve mind-body health. Bee venom may boost immune system functioning. Vitamin B complex maintains proper circulation, increases energy, builds stress tolerance, and boosts immune system functioning and energy. Take B vitamins together to maximize benefits. Some benefit from injections; your doctor may give you additional B6 injections, which enhance B12 absorption, and extra B12 to increase energy and prevent anemia. If you can't get these, find a sublingual form, as capsules may not work well for CFIDS patients who don't absorb nutrients well. Coenzyme Q10 enhances circulation (reducing mental fogginess), boosts the immune system, reduces fatigue, and increases tissue oxygenation. Magnesium decreases pain and ensures good muscle functioning; it may be low in people with CFIDS. Take this with calcium at a ratio of two to one (2,000 mg calcium to 1,000 mg magnesium). Malic acid boosts energy production, including in the muscles. Manganese influences metabolic activity and is essential if there is an indication of hypothyroidism or secondary hypothyroidism.

The amino acid L-glutamine helps reduce mental cloudiness and forgetfulness. However, it's best to take a free-form amino acid complex to ensure you're getting all of the important amino acids, because they play a central role in regulating brain functioning, rebuilding muscle tissue, and supplying necessary protein. *Note:* Avoid taking L-tyrosine if you're on an MAOI antidepressant. It's important to include at least the following: leucine, taurine, isoleucine, valine, lysine, and tyrosine. Acidophilus is important, particularly in decreasing candida damage; it comes in pills or in supplemented milk (the latter may not be best for people with CFIDS). While I include acidophilus in my regular regimen, I increase the dosage if I'm taking antibiotics and try to keep antibiotic use as low as possible. For those of us who are plagued with infections, this can be difficult. However, acidophilus helps replace the good bacteria that are killed along with the bad bacteria.

Talk to your SHOC doctor about: adrenal extract, one to two tabs three times per day; thymus gland extract, one to two tabs three times per day (Burton Goldberg Group 1997), and possibly spleen glandulars. Evening primrose oils, fish oil, magnesium-potassium aspartate, and magnesium sulphate injections have been suggested (Teitelbaum 1996). Magnesium-potassium aspartate can increase energy levels of some people with CFIDS (1 gram twice per day with efficacy as soon as two weeks), while intramuscular magnesium sulphate can reduce severe aches and pain. As such injections can be painful, some combine them with novocaine. Teitelbaum notes that some doctors add B vitamins and calcium and reduce the amount of magnesium. This IV combination is known as a Myers cocktail and may help those with severe pain, migraines, or asthmatic conditions.

Oxytocin is a hormone and neurotransmitter that may be deficient in CFIDS patients; it helps with short-term memory disturbance and cold extremities. DHEA is another hormone deficient in some people with CFIDS. Refer to chapter 6 on MS for details, benefits, and risks.

Collagen Formation and Tissue Repair

This is very important for CFIDS patients. See appendix II for details.

Herbal Remedies

Before taking herbs, check with your SHOC expert for side effects and drug interactions. You can boost immune system health with echinacea, maitake, and astragalus, but take echinacea intermittently, as rest periods are necessary. Pau d'arco in caps or tea, goldenseal, and Saint-John's-wort protect against infections, with the last helping ward off viral infections. Dandelion, red clover, or burdock root tea (four cups per day) cleans the blood and boosts immunologic functions (Balch and Balch 1997). Chinese herbal remedies, Qi Ye Lien and Xiao Yao Wan, reduce muscle pain, and the latter reduces muscle spasms. Cayenne (capsicum) is a good pain-reliever, as the capsaicin in it disrupts the production of substance P (pain neurotransmitter). You can take cayenne in pill form or combine cayenne powder with wintergreen oil and apply it directly to the skin. To improve your sleep, try valerian root and skullcap, and to reduce memory and concentration difficulties, try ginkgo biloba. Chaitow's 1995 book (which I highly recommend) discusses studies of ginkgo showing that 120 to 240 mg per day for six months boosts memory and reduces symptoms of poor brain circulation. Ginkgo also improves the poor circulation we experience as cold hands and feet. Melatonin can help you sleep, but steer clear if you're on an antidepressant. You must be patient when using herbs, vitamins, and minerals as they're typically slower acting than man-made medications. Be patients and stick with these for several months . . . you'll find it worthwhile.

Heat and Cold

Both are useful remedies for the muscle pain and achiness associated with CFIDS and FMS. Many benefit from heat, though some prefer cold. I use heat regularly, in particular moist heat, to reduce pain and spasms. There are many varieties of heat wraps and pads on the market, and they mimic physical therapy treatments using heated, moist towels. There are also patches lined with medications that adhere to your skin's surface and produce a sensation of heat, which disrupts pain signals. Hot baths also decrease muscle tension and reduce pain. In general, heat is important for many of us because we're often overly cold sensitive, and cold can intensify pain and muscle tension. Keep your house warm enough for you—your partner may complain, but probably doesn't have increased pain from being warm. Some CFIDS studies indicate that cold showers at a determined frequency reduce CFIDS symptoms but more research is needed. A recent discovery is that chronic pain may be most effectively diminshed with alternating heat and cold applications. As with heat, many cold products exist, ranging from specially designed ice packs for the body to using ice cubes wrapped in some thin outer covering. (I sometimes borrow my three-year-old's lunch box freeezer pack, for his rental rates are quite fair!) Check with your SHOC experts before using heat or cold treatments.

Acupuncture

The approach of using acupuncture to treat CFIDS is not so different from that of other tools described here, including some conventional ones. Chinese medicine and acupuncture experts suggest treatment that focuses on regenerating or strengthening the immune system. As with other theories, it's thought that the immune system is engaged in fighting some disease or infection and has become weakened, allowing the rest of the body to become vulnerable and fatigued. The needles are traditionally placed in acupuncture points associated with the autoimmune system and the meridians of the body. True Chinese medicine experts don't address CFIDS solely through acupuncture, but also use herbs, meditation, simple foods, and exercise. Results reveal equivalent and sometimes superior recovery rates as compared to conventional treatments (based on using qualified experts). Appendix II has more on acupuncture.

Progressive Relaxation and Deep Breathing

Both techniques can help some people with CFIDS. For further information on the benefits and details of these techniques, see chapter 14.

Self-Bodywork and Massage

The reality of the matter is that many of us will have limited, if any, access to professional massage or physical therapy because of the cost. For many of us, touch, pressure, and movement are very effective in reducing pain and inducing relaxation. No way other than self-bodywork offers the benefits of massage and touch whenever and wherever you feel you need or want it. Specific methods are discussed in appendix II. Some of you may be fortunate enough to have the services of a masseuse or physical therapist. Just as with FMS, the type of massage is critical, because some types can increase your pain. Again, your SHOC must include an expert who is knowledgeable about CFIDS. See appendix II for more on bodywork and massage.

And Now What?

Much has been said in these pages about the importance of using holistic techniques, establishing balance, and using your mind-body perspective to optimize healing and growth. From the interviews I've conducted, informal talks in our doctors' waiting rooms, and the many women with whom I've worked, I've seen again and again that those who make the most progress in accepting, growing, and healing are women who are committed to these techniques. Some have ousted their CFIDS, while others remain with CFIDS in their life. From either group, these women have surpassed the temporary approaches typically used (which can be of some help) and reached freedom and release by balancing alternative and conventional modalities.

Given the variety of symptoms and courses of CFIDS, it may well be that the best treatment depends on your particular case. Certainly medications or other treatments may be found that can treat certain symptoms or improve overall health, but the nature of CFIDS is such that I believe a holistic, balanced approach synthesizing and thus optimizing conventional and alternative methods will remain most effective.

PART III

Coping Strategies

CHAPTER 14

Mind-Body Techniques

I.   I walk down the street. There is a deep hole in the sidewalk. I fall
     in. I am lost . . . I am helpless. It isn't my fault. It takes forever to
     find a way out.

II. I walk down the same street. There is a deep hole in the sidewalk
     I pretend I don't see it. I fall in again. I can't believe I am in the
     same place. But it isn't my fault. It still takes a long time to get out.

III. I walk down the same street. There is a deep hole in the sidewalk.
     I see it is there. I still fall in . . . it's a habit. My eyes are open.
     I know where I am. It is my fault. I get out immediately.

IV. I walk down the same street. There is a deep hole in the sidewalk.
     I walk around it.

V.   I walk down another street.

—Portia Nelson, "Autobiography in Five
Short Chapters"

Here you'll find techniques you may not have seen elsewhere. They all involve
using mind-body methods to achieve relief from fatigue, pain, ARC symptoms,
stress, depression, anger, and other factors that can make life with chronic illness
difficult. These aren't cure-alls, but they will greatly reduce your pain, boost your
energy, and improve your mind-body health, life meaning, growth, and joy. Use

these to make a good, different, and better life . . . a life of thriving rather than just surviving.

Stress and Your Personality

Every ARC can be worsened by distress. Negative stress is so pervasive, and research so consistent in showing its link with mind-body problems and disease, that it's essential you address distress if you have an ARC. You must be aware of certain facts before you can make inroads against distress. One of these is the subjectivity of your response to stress. Two people exposed to the same situation can have completely different experiences: one may experience distress, anxiety, and fear due to her perception and self-talk while another may feel excitement and challenge due to seeing the situation as a challenge rather than a threat. Her self-talk is not full of "I can't do this. I'm going to fail and people will see how bad I am," but instead goes, "This is a challenge. It's new, but I'll try my best. The end result may not be perfect, but at least I'll learn something and maybe do better next time." Such disparate thoughts cause different reactions.

Depending on who you are or strive to be, you can worsen or improve your mind-body health with respect to stress. If you're a "threat-seer," you'll create much unnecessary distress in your life, and your reactions can harm your health. For example, do you ever find cookies and potato chips more tempting as your distress increases? Many of us respond to distress by soothing ourselves with food. While this isn't healthy for anybody, it can be dangerous for those of us with ARCs. Another unhealthy distress response is to "freeze," or stop activities and thoughts by numbing out or procrastinating. We need to be active, do light exercise and stretching, stimulate our minds with learning, and change negative, irrational thinking to realistic, rational thinking. Avoidance becomes habitual and causes us to see ourselves as helpless people in hopeless situations. We don't realize the true control we can have. Let's look at positive, healthful characteristics to incorporate into our SHOC. Studies show that patients with active, assertive attitudes before surgery or while hospitalized do better than passivists. Patients who depend on others for motivation and self-esteem do worse than those with internal motivation and self-esteem. Self-esteem and ego strength also reduce distress and boost prostress, thus helping your immune system and health. This supports what you've read throughout, that assuming responsibility and control in your SHOC is critical. Feisty people fare better healthwise. Take the challenge and keep on fighting!

People who regularly give and receive affection live longer, are healthier, and report less distress and better life quality. This doesn't mean it must be a sexual relationship or even that your partner has to be human! Widows and singles with pets live longer and are happier and healthier than those without. It also doesn't mean you must have a large circle of friends, as even one or two good friends offer the same protective benefits. Recall this as you go through the lows of your illness and your pain makes you irritable, angry, and likely to lash out at everyone. To whatever degree possible, try not to take things out on others. When you do lash out and it isn't deserved, be the strong one and apologize.

Take the advice of folk tales, empirical research, and Norman Cousins' wisdom and introduce humor into your life. Read funny books, watch funny movies, and take a lighter view of life. When you're in what you see as a distressing situation, evaluate how serious it really is. Is it truly the end of the world? Is it bad enough to ruin your whole day, week, life? Okay, go with the negative forecasting and look at the situation in the worst way possible. How likely is this worst case to happen? You have some control over every situation, for as your mind makes something seem terrible and catastrophic, it can also make it ridiculous, funny, and absurd. Add comedic twists to your interpretations and laugh at how seriously you take some minor things. A positive mindset spreads: It makes you see things more positively and recall more positive events.

Another distress reducer is the ability to empathize. Maybe the nurse, collections agent, or family member who is being "rude and obnoxious" is feeling ill or having a bad day, or maybe that's just the way they are. Don't take it personally. Put yourself in this person's shoes and recall that you've had days like that yourself. The ability to empathize and give others a break changes your view and can stop an escalation in distress and hostility. Being kind to the offender makes you feel even better.

Let's take a close look at forgiveness. I don't follow the school of forgive and forget, and I don't believe this is healthy or even possible when someone has really harmed you physically or emotionally. Forgiveness doesn't require that you forget a wrong someone did you. It involves remembering, placing responsibility where due, and then letting go. After all, when you let somebody's actions keep affecting you negatively, you're giving that person control rather than having it yourself, even thought a sense of control is central to healthy ARC living. You also can't afford to harbor negative thoughts and feelings, which suppress your immune system and interfere with your health. Acknowledge the problem, attribute responsibility appropriately (not only on yourself, as so many women do), confront the person if it helps resolve the situation or allows you to work through it, and then move on with your life. I work with many clients who have experienced such heinous, traumatic violations (rape, incest, physical and emotional abuse) that letting go and moving on is incredibly difficult. If you've had such mind-body damage, you might benefit tremendously from working with a psychologist or mental health expert.

Exercise: Are You in Control?

Take out some paper and respond to these questions. How do you rank on assertiveness and your sense of control over your life? Do you feel too passive? Recall that stress management is self-management. Take charge of the way you live your life, and you'll benefit mentally and physically. Do you see your illness as a threat and major loss or can you see it in some ways or at some times as a challenge?

When and how? Are you committed to improving your health and life by learning and taking action? Do you feel you have control over your life—and do you exert that control—or do you feel victimized and immobile? While you may not be able to directly improve your immediate health, finances, and so on, you do have control over your thoughts, emotions, and behaviors. By exerting control over these, you'll more easily resolve these other areas. You'll learn many mind-body tools later in this chapter.

Pleasure, Prostress, and Mind-Body Healing

Prostress is the term I use to refer to positive stress. You typically experience prostress when you are in a situation that's important to you, believe you have some control, believe you have the abilities or resources to meet the demands, and see the situation as a challenge that offers growth and positive benefits. Obviously, prostress is largely personal, and what might be prostress for one woman could be distress for another. Prostress is very important for people with ARC, given its positive effects on mind-body health and the evidence that it boosts immune system functioning (Ravicz 1998). In addition, prostress gives the doer a sense of control and increased life pleasure, both of which have been shown by studies to be linked with improved mind-body health.

Lest we think science should exist in an exalted realm by itself, we must accord attention to the fact that science often trails culture in accepting certain truths. For example, a cliché, "laughter is the best medicine," appears to hold true. Deepak Chopra, the doctor who helpfully unites Eastern and Western traditions to prevent and treat illness, asserts that different emotional states produce different effects on the mind and body (Chopra 1993). Love, hate, and excitement all activate the body in a variety of different directions. While you laugh, your body is aroused, but after you stop laughing, there is an overall healthy net decrease in your body's arousal and blood pressure. Laughter's positive state of mind affects your immune system by decreasing certain neuroendocrine hormones and stimulating killer cells that are central in preventing and combating disease. Laughter exercises your lungs, relaxes your diaphragm, increases the oxygen in your bloodstream, improves your mood, increases relaxation for more than thirty minutes ... and, just as importantly, doesn't cost much! You can't truly laugh and enjoy yourself while feeling anxious and distressed—so which would you prefer?

Prostress and Psychological Benefits

How does prostress affect you psychologically? One of the benefits of prostress is that it increases satisfaction and pleasure with life and social interactions.

In turn, this motivates us to maintain or develop our social networks. Having a strong social support system has been touted as a great distress-reducer for years. Even just *believing* we have a good support system reduces the negative effects of stress.

As I'm sure you've gathered by now, one of the most important characteristics determining whether you'll perceive an event as threatening or challenging is the degree of control you believe you have over it. True prostress and its benefits arise in situations when we feel involved, active, and in control to some degree. This was clearly shown in a study comparing people who engaged in two different types of pleasurable activities: *positive origin events* were those in which the person was actively involved in initiating and carrying out the pleasant event; *positive pawn events* were those in which the person experienced a positive event but was only a passive recipient. A positive origin event might be going out and making a new friend or learning a new sport, while a positive pawn event might be your finding five or ten dollars on the ground. The results showed that those who experienced positive origin events in which they had control and actively participated reported a better quality of life and rated various events as more pleasurable than those who experienced positive passive events. In fact, increasing the number of events that were pleasurable and positive but passive did *not* increase happiness or satisfaction. Negative events were linked with distress and lower life quality (Zautra and Reich 1980).

Scheduling Your Positive Stress

The positive results of prostress are linked with the frequency of prostress experiences, not their intensity. Many people complain that they lack time for positive experiences, though once they start including them in their lives, this problem often vanishes. As an ARC patient, you may feel that your losses are overwhelming but instead of focusing on loss and letting the void grow, replace these with new actions, beliefs, interests, and attitudes. While nobody wants to be so ill they must stop working, a positive by-product is increased personal time. Some of this is spent on recovery and healing, but some can be spent on getting out of yourself and doing positive things for others. This doesn't mean to the exclusion of paying attention to your needs, growth, and healing, which many of us have done previously.

Chronic illness shakes up our beliefs about ourselves and our relation to others and the world. We may lose any sense of joy and pleasure in our lives, making prostress more essential than ever. People with ARC who can still work and maintain busy lives must find time for prostress. It doesn't have to be a major undertaking . . . just learn a new hobby, buy a foreign language tape, join a social group, get a walking buddy or walk on your own, learn how to use a computer, or write poetry. Do whatever it is you want to do. At first, it's best to schedule prostress into your life. That's right, jot it down in your calendar with your other activities. Make sure you set time aside for prostress and follow through. Like any new behavior, it may be hard at first, but stick with it. Before long, the benefits will keep you going. Prostress involves positive thoughts, which lead to positive emotions and improved health, which allow you to do more prostressors, and so on. You can also increase prostress by stealing it from the distress side. This includes all the situations you've been seeing as threats and responding to with distress. Use cognitive restructuring and reality testing to change what you initially see as "terrifying" events, situations, or people into challenges instead. As you find you have control over your thoughts, feelings, and behaviors, you'll experience fun, excitement, joy, and even peace instead.

Now we'll look at holistic mind-body techniques that harness the power of thoughts, feelings, and actions to reduce pain, symptoms, and distress and improve energy and healing. The physical response to stressors, the fight-or-flight response, involves an elevated heart rate, increased blood pressure, disruption in digestive functions, release of various hormones, muscular tension, and other bodily changes. If this arousal goes on for too long or too frequently, physical disorders arise and existing ARC conditions worsen. For example, distress increases blood glucose, and as people with TID must keep glucose in a limited range, this is harmful. Distress also increases muscle tension, thus perpetuating the vicious cycle of pain for people with FMS and others with musculoskeletal problems. Many doctors give drugs to deal with the physical problems that arise from stress; however, this is just a temporary measure. Prolonged arousal from distress also causes irritability, frustration, depression, anxiety, and other psychological upset. Often what needs to be changed to combat the situation can be done only by you. This is one of many entry points for designing your SHOC. Your goal is to change your thoughts and learn relaxation and healthy ways to cope with pain, stress, and negative feelings. The tools are proactive so you can change root causes rather than using "fix-it" approaches.

Take a Deep Breath

Central to stress reduction and healing is the simple art of proper breathing. Most of us don't breathe in such a way that energy is effectively brought in and waste expelled. Experts aren't sure why, but focused attention on breathing reduces mind-body tension. To tell if you're breathing in the proper, deep, diaphragmatic way, try this exercise. Put your hand below your rib cage and above your stomach and inhale deeply. In proper breathing, your hand moves out as you inhale and in as you exhale, and the abdomen moves out as the movement flows up toward your chest.

Visualize air entering your body and moving up from the bottom to the top of your lungs. Deep breathing (DB) is a simple route to relaxation. When you do these exercises, inhale for five seconds, hold your breath for twenty seconds (or less at first), and exhale fully for twice as long as your inhalation, in this case, ten seconds. Exhalation should be twice the duration of inhalation in order to favor the parasympathetic system, which is linked with relaxation, over the sympathetic system. As you exhale, visualize ridding your mind-body system of its tension, toxins from your illness, mutinous autoantibodies, or your own representations of your disease.

Why is proper DB important as a foundation for all we're going to do? During the distress response, your breathing is shallow and rapid and your heart rate increases. Also, when you're in pain, you may hold your breath or breathe shallowly. However, when you're relaxed, your breathing is deep and your heartbeat slows. Breathing is an easy physical system to control, and by breathing the deep, slow breath of relaxation, you become relaxed. Schedule at least thirty-five to forty deep breaths each day in your journal. Annette, a client who has TID, does her DB exercises each time she measures her glucose. She finds this relaxing, as the measuring routine initially bothered her. Jamie, who has SLE, links her DB to red lights she encounters on her way to work or her medical appointments. I told her DB was a great stress reliever, but didn't mention the other benefits. At our next session, she wanted to be sure I knew DB wasn't just for relaxation but also boosted energy and reduced pain.

Exercise: Setting DB Goals

Use the suggestions below to design a system to track your deep-breating practice in your journal. I'll use the following situations as cues to practice my deep breathing:

1. Stopping at red lights

2. After taking my morning, afternoon, and evening medications

3. When the commercials come on the TV, etc.
   (Come up with ideas that best suit your lifestyle.)

I met my goal for DB today (Y or N):

Day 1 _____ Day 2 _____ Day 3 _____ Day 4 _____
Day 5 _____ Day 6 _____ Day 7 _____

Progressive Relaxation

Another tool that brings relief from pain, muscle tension, and distress is progressive relaxation (PR). While there are many types of physical relaxation, PR has been widely studied and found effective in reducing body tension. When people try to just relax their muscles, tension is reduced, but residual tension remains. PR achieves greater muscular relaxation and thus mental relaxation because after a muscle is tensed, it's automatically more relaxed and less painful. Also, as you focus on the difference between muscle tension and relaxation, you feel even greater relaxation. Remember, being relaxed is incompatible with being tense and anxious. Since stress and anxiety directly increase your pain, use your body tension as a cue to relax and inhibit pain and distress. We can't afford to hold tension and stress arousal in our bodies as it causes further damage, pain, and immune system disruptions. To get the most from PR, find a quiet place where you won't be disturbed. As you become PR proficient, you'll be able to relax and obtain benefits even with some noise or distraction. Wear loose clothes and lie down or sit in a comfortable chair. Taking time out for yourself may be the hardest part of this for you, but giving yourself permission and feeling guiltless are essential goals of your SHOC. If loved ones interfere, you need to establish limits. Enter into this with a calm, detached attitude, not asking yourself, "Am I doing this right or not?" Just go through the motions, follow the directions, and let what will happen, happen. Some clients like to read my directions aloud and record them to play back while doing PR. Use a calm, even voice and add soothing music or sounds of the ocean or rain if you like.

Instruction for PR

(Begin recording here:) *Start by taking three deep diaphragmatic breaths. Place your hand on your lower belly and inhale slowly and deeply for five seconds, making sure that your hand is pushed outwards. Hold the breath for twenty seconds and exhale completely for ten. Imagine as you do this that each inward breath brings purifying, nourishing air into your body and each exhalation expels your tension, stress, pain, and illness. Second and third breaths . . . in and out. Take a moment to focus on your body's inner sensations and feelings. Pay attention to the places where your body is touching the floor or chair . . . your head, your shoulders and back, your behind, and your legs. Feel a sense of relaxation flowing smoothly throughout your body. Now, attend to your right hand. Tighten it as hard as you can and hold it for eight seconds. Attend to the feelings of tension in the muscles of your fist and forearm. Now, quickly and completely relax this area for ten seconds. Enjoy the relaxation and limpness and notice how it differs from the previous feeling of tension in your hand. Repeat and again notice the difference in the feeling. You may feel some tingling or heaviness in this area. Feel the warmth as the blood flows into your hand and into each finger . . . these are natural relaxation responses and are signs you're letting go of tension. Inhale deeply, feel the relaxation, and exhale . . . letting all of the tension flow out with your breath. Now we go to the left hand and repeat the sequence. Tense your hand and fist for eight seconds and then relax them completely for ten. Feel the feelings of relaxation and how they differ from those of muscular tension. Don't forget your breathing . . . breathe in deeply and hold it, then exhale completely. Let all tension in your muscles flow out with your breath. Repeat the tensing and releasing of your left hand and fist. Attend to the warmth and tingling of relaxation. If you become distracted and have thoughts other than your inner sensations and feelings of relaxation, let those thoughts drift away easily. Imagine them as clouds being blown away by the wind.*

Now, we'll move to your biceps. Bend both of your elbows, and raising your hands up toward your shoulders, tighten your muscles. Hold this tension for eight seconds and then release both biceps and let your arms fall downward.

Feel the soothing comfort of relaxation. Breathe in deeply and exhale, letting all concerns and worries flow outwards with your breath. Enjoy the relaxation of your muscles for ten seconds. Repeat tensing for eight and releasing for ten. Notice the relaxation, tingling, heaviness, or warmth. Now, we'll focus on a different area of the arms—the triceps or the muscles on the back of your upper arms, behind the biceps. Stretch your right arm straight out in front of you as far as you can so that it forms a right angle to your body. Stick out your fingers and spread them widely, now tighten your fingers, hands, and triceps as much as you can. Pay attention to the feeling of tension in your muscles of your triceps. Do this for the usual count of eight seconds. Let your arm totally relax and drift down to your side, hanging loose and limp for the count of ten. Remember to keep taking the slow, deep breaths in and out. Repeat the same movement. Again, pay attention to any tingling feelings, any warmth or heaviness. Now, shift the focus to the same exercise with your left arm. Stretch out your left arm as far as you can in a right angle to your body. Stick out your fingers and spread them . . . tighten your fingers, hands, and triceps as much as you can . . . feel the tension in your triceps muscle for the count of eight. Now, let your arm totally relax and drift down to your side, hanging loose and limp for ten. Remember to keep taking slow, deep breaths in and out throughout this relaxation exercise. Repeat with left arm. You may have a strange feeling that your arms are longer than before. In fact, your muscles do become longer following the relaxation.

Now, we're going to work on your legs and feet. First, take some time for deep diaphragmatic breathing . . . breathe slowly and deeply and imagine letting the tension flow outwards as you exhale. Okay, let's focus on your right foot. Tighten your toes by bending your foot backwards, toes up towards your ankle. Hold the tension for eight seconds, paying attention to the sensations in your toes, foot, ankle, and calf. Remember to keep the rest of your body relaxed while you're working on each particular muscle group. We tend to tense areas completely unrelated to the area we are working on tensing. Your awareness of this pattern is very important in healthy responding to stress. You'll learn to keep the tension only in the area of your body that needs to be activated, and when the arousal is no longer needed, you'll be able to relax completely. Now, let go of the tension and pay attention to the difference in the sensations. Relax for the count of ten. Repeat the exercise. Keep breathing regularly, slowly, and deeply. Now, move on to the left foot and do the same exercise. Bend your foot backwards and feel the tension in your toes, foot, ankle, and calf. Hold it for eight and release for ten. Do this again, remembering to breathe slowly and deeply. If any distracting thoughts should intrude on your serenity, you can easily let them float away like clouds as you return to focusing on the soothing relaxation and peace within your body. Now, let's move up a little higher in the legs. Tighten your right thigh and knee area. Hold the tension for eight. You can build the tension in your thigh by pushing your heels down on the ground if you are sitting. Now relax for ten counts and pay attention to the difference in the sensations. Does your leg feel heavy, tingly, warm? Okay, one more time with the right thigh and knee. Let's move over to the left leg.

Tighten the left thigh and knee area, hold the tension for eight and now relax for ten, nine . . . all the way down to one. Does this leg feel heavy, tingly, warm? Okay, one more time . . . tighten the left thigh and knee and hold it for eight. Release the tension and relax for ten seconds.

Moving upwards, we'll work on your stomach, chest, and shoulders. Beginning with your stomach, tense those muscles . . . try for the sensation you feel when you're doing sit-ups. Hold this for eight, focusing on the tension. Now release the muscles and feel the relaxation for ten seconds. One more time for eight . . . tense only your stomach muscles and make sure you're not tensing any other areas in your body. Now relax for ten, nine . . . all the way down to one and remember to keep breathing deeply and slowly . . . in and out . . . Now let's move up gradually to your chest, shoulders, and neck, where we tend to hold much tension. Here I want you to build the muscle tension by pushing your shoulders up and back and tightening your neck muscles. Lean a bit forward if you're doing this sitting in a chair. Hold this for eight seconds and feel the entire line of tension from your upper back out to your shoulders and up to your neck. Now release the muscles and feel the relaxation all the way from your upper back, shoulders, chest, and neck. Scan the area, searching for any residual tension, and focus on releasing any tightness you find. This is an area of chronic tension for many of us and you may find it difficult to completely relax these muscles at first. As you continue to practice, you'll relax this region. One more time, push your shoulders up and back and tighten your neck. Feel the tension for eight seconds. Now, completely relax your neck, shoulders, and chest and feel the difference . . . you may feel some tingling or some warmth or heaviness for ten, nine . . . all the way down to one. Remember to keep breathing in and out, deeply and slowly. Feel the peaceful relaxation in your whole torso and in your limbs. Try to recall those areas that were particularly tender or sore as you worked through your body. These are the areas that are staying tensed unnecessarily throughout the day and which you will need to work on when you begin to experience negative stress.

Time now to proceed to your face and head. Most of us have no idea how much tension we hold in these areas when we're negatively stressed. First, let's work on the forehead. To tense the muscles in your forehead, raise and hold your eyebrows up as high as possible. It's generally quite easy to feel the tension we hold in this area. Hold this for eight counts and then completely relax for ten counts. Okay, one more time—raising the eyebrows and tightening the forehead for eight. Now, remembering to breathe deeply and fully, relax the eyebrows and feel the comfortable sensations in your forehead for the count of ten. The last area on which we are going to work is the face. Here, you will build the tension by clenching your eyelids shut and opening your mouth as wide as possible. Hold for eight and release for ten. Okay, one more time. Feel the tension for eight and let all of the tension go. Keep your eyes shut and notice the areas around your eyes and mouth feeling loose, smooth, and relaxed. Make sure you aren't clenching your teeth. You may let your mouth remain slightly open and relax your jaw. If you're seated you may also let your head hang forward if that feels more relaxing for you.

At this point, your entire body should feel completely relaxed. Your legs and arms will feel longer, as your muscles have elongated after being tensed and then relaxed. Relax in an enjoyable heaviness and feel the warmth spreading throughout your body. Inhale and exhale several slow, deep releasing breaths. Just relax and enjoy this pleasant, calm feeling and keep your head clear. Should any thoughts come into your mind, just imagine them floating out and away like clouds. Now, gently open your eyes. (End recording here.)

Sample PR Worksheet

If you practice even once a day, you'll quickly be able to master this exercise. Make some sheets like the following in your journal and record your sessions. If you skip a day, still fill out the third and fifth lines around the time of day you've been doing PR. You'll notice a difference!

1. Practiced PR today (Yes or No)

2. Date & Day (Monday through Sunday)

3. Tension level before PR (scale of 1 to 100, with 100 being very stressed and tense and 1 completely relaxed and peaceful

4. Tension level after PR

5. Any symptoms of tension (neck pain, back pain, headache, etc.) before practice

6. Tension symptoms after practice (scale of 1 to 10, with 10 being extreme pain or tension and 1 no pain or tension).

Guided Imagery

Another relaxation method to use by itself or as a PR supplement, guided imagery (GI) uses visualization and imagination to obtain relief from pain, negative stress, tension, and anxiety. If you don't have time or the right place for PR, this method is ideal. One imaging technique I've found effective for myself and my clients proceeds like this: Close your eyes and take several deep, relaxing breaths. While inhaling and exhaling deeply and slowly, imagine yourself descending in an elevator or escalator. Count slowly backwards from ten to one for each "floor" you descend. To increase your peace and serenity, decorate your path of descent in a way most pleasing to you. My client Megan imagines everything cloaked in white with soft billowing fabrics, ribbons, and soothing music. Descend as many "floors" as feels comfortable, imagining as you go that all tension, cares, and worries leave you as you go to a calmer, peaceful place deeper within yourself.

A GI Journey

Here is one of my personal favorites; many of those whom I've taught this feel the same. Select a scene that's particularly pleasing and relaxing for you that is your own temporary escape when pressures or pain become excessive. I used this technique while giving birth to my son (which included twenty hours of labor ending in a rushed C-section) and felt increased calm and decreased pain and anxiety. In designing your personal escape, involve all of your senses . . . smells, sounds, touch, sight, even taste. Below is an example you can try, but GI works best when you personally create your private place. If you want to try my imagery first, it's a good idea to read it aloud on tape so that you can play it back and more easily enter relaxation. Start by making yourself comfortable by sitting in a chair or lying down.

(Begin recording here:) *Close your eyes and take several deep breaths. Pay attention to any areas in your body that feel tense and take a moment to relax them. Visualize areas of tension as tight knots slowly unwinding and releasing. Now imagine that you're sitting on a beautiful, tropical beach and feel the slight balmy breeze caressing your skin, ruffling your hair. The sun gently warms your skin as you hear the rhythmic, slow crash of the surf followed by the soft sound of water rolling back over pebbles and sand out to the ocean. In and out . . . in and out . . . a soothing, even pattern. You have no cares or worries and are at peace and at one with the world around you. You decide to take a stroll. Rise slowly, stretch luxuriously, and feel the warm grains of sand giving way beneath your feet and rising between your toes. The sun gently warms your skin and you notice that the warmth soothes any pain and makes it drain from your body. You can see it melting off of your body and into the sand below as you stroll along the shore. A seagull calls and wheels lazily from view. You look out to the clear blue sea and notice the silver diamond flashes of sunlight dancing on the water. The sky is a beautiful light blue and a few white, wispy clouds drift easily above. You take slow, deep breaths of the clean air. As you inhale, you feel joyous and relaxed, at one with nature. Utter comfort and peace fill your mind and body and you realize this is the truth . . . the here-and-now. You, simply* being. *Any stressors or problems worrying you are now unimportant as you stay in the present in this place of beauty and calm. Your muscles feel relaxed, yet you feel inner energy pulsing. Your mind is clear and sharp. You look around, appreciating the peace of nature. This is your private place to which you can return whenever you want to regain this feeling of utter relaxation. Now, slowly open your eyes and return to your surroundings. Take a moment to calmly adjust. You still feel the sense of peace and relaxation you felt on your beach. Minor problems, worries about juggling doctors' appointments, and financial pressures are no longer as disturbing, and you realize you can and will approach them in a calm, organized, and effective fashion.* (End recording here.)

Exercise: Personalized GI

Now that you're familiar with GI, create your own special place. Think back to places and events that have made you feel the most relaxed and peaceful. Write a script in your journal you can easily run through in your mind or play back from a tape recorder. To make your escape most realistic and effective, include all of your senses: sounds, scents, visuals, touch, taste. Remind yourself to relax several times throughout and feel your pain and tension leave the areas where you habitually hold it. Remind yourself several times that all your daily concerns and worries float easily from your mind and away. You can stay in your scene as long as you like; tell yourself that the blissful relaxation and calm will carry over into your daily routine. Believe it or not, it will! It may seem counterintuitive that taking time for these techniques actually increases your productivity and energy. The fact is that when you're calm, focused, and centered, your pain decreases and your increased energy and productivity more than compensate for the "time-outs." You can also use PR and GI to help you fall asleep, a problem for many ARC patients. You know that insufficient sleep increases pain, depresses the immune system, and worsens symptoms. As you'll read, GI can specifically target illness and pain.

Exercise: Tracking Physical Responses

A critical way to short-circuit the buildup of distress is by listening to your body. We're so often caught up in rushing from task to task or thinking about the future or past that we ignore our body's messages. Then "all of a sudden" our bodies scream at us through migraines, neck and back pain, blood sugar surges, and GI problems.

For this exercise, take a breath, close your eyes, and find any body tension. Now that you're listening, you may be surprised at the number of tense, painful areas. Common areas of tension are the forehead, neck, shoulders, chest, and stomach. The following tool helps you track which distressors elicit mind-body tension. When you feel irritated, anxious, tense, or pained, jot down the situation and your mind-body reactions. More than 90 percent of the time, we misperceive harmless situations as dangers or threats. As you become aware of your triggers, you can use your self-talk and PR to drastically reduce this tendency. Do several journal entries of this daily. When you make your entries, be sure to list your extreme, irrational thoughts first, followed by the emotional and physical events such unhealthy events cause.

Sample Tracking Worksheet

DATE _____   DAY _____

Time	Stressful Situation	Mind-Body Symptoms and Thoughts
1. 7:30 A.M.	Late to doctor	"I can't stand this pain." Neck/shoulders tense and painful, breathing shallow. Getting very irritated.
2. 10:30 A.M.	Late to work because of doctor appointment—again!	"He thinks I'm making this up. My illness is ruining my life." Stomach tight, achy. Anxiety, anger at boss, hopelessness.
3. 6:00 P.M.	Have to meet friends; tired but will keep up the front.	"Life is no fun. It'll never be fun again. All I have to look forward to is sickness/pain." Headache, neck tight. Irritated, depressed.

Biofeedback

See appendix II for a detailed discussion of biofeedback and how it can help people with CFIDS.

Meditation

As more research is dedicated to studying meditation, even the skeptics are being convinced of its value. But the millions who've practiced it over the centuries haven't needed studies to convince them of its efficacy. You can use meditation as a systematic technique to obtain balance within and between your inner and outer worlds. By increasing understanding and acceptance of your true inner self, you're less likely to be negatively buffeted by symptom changes or external events. Proficiency in meditation is linked with decreased physical stress and increased psychological stability. Of special import for you is that meditation can boost immune system functioning and reduce chronic pain. (When I'm experiencing severe pain, meditation rapidly helps with the pain and makes me feel calm and sometimes euphoric.) With continued meditation, self-confidence and acceptance increase. As you read about mindfulness meditation, you'll see why it's suited to those with chronic pain and illnesses.

There are many types of meditation belonging to either the mindfulness category (vipassana or insight meditation) or the concentrative category (samadhi or one-pointed meditation). The first example below is a concentrative type, with both relaxation and effortless concentration used to obtain a meditative state. The latter arises when you aren't actively trying to maintain concentration. When starting to meditate, you'll probably find it hard to concentrate on inner objects, images, or sounds and avoid distraction. To get an idea of this, try right now by selecting a word upon which to concentrate. Allow only that word into your consciousness and see how long you can do this. Your mind will probably start wandering or you'll be distracted by a noise or sensation quite soon. Don't let this disturb you, but simply release the thoughts or sensations and return to focusing on your word. With practice, such distractions decrease dramatically. This type of meditation, in which thoughts or feelings are viewed as distractions and in which focus on a word, object, or one's breath is central, is one-pointed meditation. Importantly, remind yourself you're not wasting time by sitting and not *doing*. Meditation often increases productivity and focus overall. Be patient and know this will improve your health and well-being. Practice daily in a quiet place and at a set time so your meditation becomes habitual and the time associated with peace and relaxation.

Exercise: Concentrative Meditation

Begin by sitting in a comfortable, straight chair or erect on a pillow with your legs crossed. Start to breathe with the DB you learned earlier. Commence this exercise with the intent that you won't let your mind take you on its usual twists and turns. Of course, this is exactly what your mind will do until you gain expertise in this practice. Your mind is used to functioning through free association and always being busy as a bee. You'll learn to discipline your mind by focusing and attending to one single point. Attend to the feel of your breath during your inhalations and exhalations. An essential part of this process is focusing upon a single point, your breath, an object, or frequently a word called a mantra. After you have calmed your mind, inhale and focus on a selected space within your body. Introduce your mantra and silently repeat the single word, a sound, or several words (perhaps "heal," "peace," "light," etc.). You may prefer focusing instead on an object like a candle or on your breath. My clients find meditation to be a valuable stress-optimization tool as they use their newfound mental control to focus on positive images or thoughts and let go of the negative ones. Try to meditate twice daily, working up to fifteen to thirty minutes. You deserve and need this quiet time for your healing. Put it in your calendar if necessary and give it top priority.

Exercise: Mindfulness Meditation

You begin the second meditation form, mindfulness meditation (MM), as before: sitting, relaxing, and then focusing on a single word, image, or place. Here this form departs, for when the inevitable feelings and thoughts arise, you simply let yourself be aware of them and don't try to get rid of them. Observe them objectively, avoiding the usual judgment of your thoughts and feelings. See them as an interested voyeur rather than doing your typical multiple role-playing as the director, lead actress, nervous stand-in, and critic. MM gives you the skills to achieve inner clarity and balance. Many of us with ARCs were (and may still be) overly controlling and perfectionistic over-doers. Now use your strength and will to follow the prescriptions of this technique. Of course you have to act and be directly involved in the world to get what you need and want. That is the very reason why meditation is so essential. It offers a respite from such behavior and thought and so balances your life. MM is ideal for people with ARC as it creates balance, for it generates a mind-body connection and an ability to truly live in the present moment, whether it be joyful or painful, prostress or distress. All emotions and thoughts, good and bad, are accepted as parts of ourselves, which helps us accept the harshness of what life dishes out. It makes us aware of our physical pain, depression, or rage. Why be aware of such things? The goal of mindfulness is for you to be aware of what is happening in and around you *as it is occurs throughout the day*. You work to accept what is happening to you and within you at any moment. Devoid of our typical judgment and criticism, we are able to accept. Accepting communicates the bounds of reality but then sets you free to move on, make the changes you desire, and grow in ways you choose.

There is a very important adjunct to the meditative practice of mindfulness. This is the informal practice in which you go about your day, checking in often to ensure you're in synch and aware of the here and now. Ask yourself, "Am I operating totally in the present right now? Am I paying attention to what is going on here and now? Am I working, playing, loving, crying here in the present?" You'll learn to forestall the immediate, typical negative responses to stressors and will feel more calm and at peace. The informal practice helps maintain that sense of peace and balance throughout your days.

Mindfulness is a pain management tool as well. While the relaxation of MM helps reduce pain, as you know by now, pain is subjective, tied up with your emotions and thoughts. Mindfulness goes beyond relaxation to reduce pain because by experiencing and attending to the pain rather than running and hiding, you'll learn much about your pain experience. As you become one with it and relax through observing it, you'll separate actual physical pain from the negative feelings and thoughts linked with it. In fact, *it's these feelings and thoughts that make your chronic pain even worse than the mere physical sensations*. Listen in and you may hear yourself: "I can't stand this pain anymore! I can't live like this another day! This pain is constant, there is no relief! Life isn't worth it!" I'm sure some of these will sound familiar. I've found myself thinking them many times. Now, though, when I tune in and hear this, I challenge what I'm telling myself: "I can't stand this!—Is that really true? Am I going to explode here and now because of this pain? I am standing it right here and now. I've made it through before and I can make it through now. It's not always this bad, sometimes there is relief." You'll get a boost in your self-esteem as you realize that you have at least some control over your pain. See this as a challenge to experience the immune system help of prostress. Studies confirm that meditation results in great decreases in symptoms, anxiety, and depression, plus increased self-confidence lasting up to three years after termination of the studies (Kabat-Zinn 1993).

Hypnosis

To the many who practice hypnotherapy or self-hypnosis, this technique is miraculous, and a number of studies support its therapeutic and medical benefits. There is strong support for using hypnosis to manage chronic illness through reducing pain (and pain medication use), learning to modify autonomic functions (like blood pressure), and reducing fear and anxiety. Hypnosis was really the first anesthesia used during operations (with the exception of getting patients drunk on alcohol). However, many still see hypnosis as "fake" and an "entertainment trick." Some researchers believe hypnosis works in the same way as acupuncture, by activating nerve connections in the brain that release our body's natural pain-killers, endorphins and enkephalins. Studies show that during the hypnotic state, brain waves indicate deep relaxation with wave patterns differing completely from those that happen during sleep. One study explored hypnosis and pain. People hypnotized with the suggestion that their arms were injected with anesthetic were then given mild shocks. There was less brain activity in response to these shocks during hypnosis than when the subjects weren't hypnotized.

These brain wave changes aren't particular to hypnosis, since states with the same characteristics, namely relaxation, calm, and focused attention, produce similar brain changes. For example, yoga, PR, daydreaming, and listening to certain music can all produce brain wave changes like those of hypnosis. These activities also yield similar benefits including reduction of pain, anxiety and stress. Despite the differences between meditation and hypnosis, both reduce pain, manage stress, enhance one's sense of self-control, and decrease anxiety.

Can hypnosis improve immunological functions as meditation does? Karen Olness (1993) presents several studies suggesting this is the case. Children were divided into three groups: one group was taught to use self-hypnosis through imagery to relax; one group was taught self-hypnosis involving the hypnotic suggestion to increase certain salivary immune substances; and one group was told just to talk to one another. Groups one and three showed no changes after the study, while group two (using active suggestion to produce a particular change) showed a great increase in a particular immune substance in the saliva! Another study of adolescents found that with training in self-hypnosis, the subjects could make significant changes in white blood cell activity.

A good imagination is essential, as hypnosis is based on the ability to imagine and involve senses, like hearing, seeing, tasting, and smelling. You must be able to imagine situations based on your own suggestions or those of a hypnotherapist who would first teach you to relax through the means most effective for you, whether PR, music, or imagery (a peaceful ocean scene). When you're relaxed, she may "take you deeper" by telling you that as she counts, you'll become more and more relaxed, or as she counts from ten down to one, you see yourself going down an escalator to a lower, deeper floor.

If the goal were to stop smoking, the hypnotherapist would offer suggestions like having you imagine being in a small, crowded, smoke-filled room. She might tell you, "Imagine yourself in this horrible room. You're feeling smothered by the close air, your chest is tight and your lungs ache, your nostrils are filled with the overpowering stench of smoke, your eyes are stinging, and you feel a quick burn as somebody flicks an ash on your arm." Then she might say, "Now, feel yourself lying in your bed in the morning and just beginning to awaken. You have that typical foul taste in your mouth and it's dry as the desert, you try to lick your lips but your tongue is thick and dry. You sit up and reach for a cigarette. As usual you can't find any matches, which infuriates you. You get up and search furiously, getting more and more upset. Finally, you go down into the cold kitchen for a light. As you walk up the hard, cold steps you feel winded and have another coughing fit. You have an important business meeting this morning and, as you take out each suit, you panic because they all reek of cigarette smoke. You feel a knot in your stomach and the old headache starting as you realize you don't have anything to wear that doesn't reek of smoke." After this, she might present different hypnotic suggestions: "Now imagine your goal: your life now that you've stopped smoking. You wake up early, take a deep breath in, and feel the clean air of your room rushing into your lungs. You remember how you used to be able to inhale only a bit, to avoid triggering your hacking couch . . . you're pleased with yourself for having quit. You jump out of bed, with great energy, and run to the window to greet the sunny, clear day. You recall that you used to drag yourself into a sitting position and light a cigarette right away. Your lungs start to ache, but you realize you've freed yourself . . . and you feel cheerful and clean. You open your closet to choose a suit for work, your favorite, the new one you bought with the money saved by not buying cigarettes and not having to dry-clean your clothes so often. You smile and feel pleased as you think about your accomplishment. . . ." You get the point.

The way you perform the relaxation and hypnotic suggestions is important, but most important is your true desire to change your behavior and your ability to imagine your life with less pain, more energy, and "downtime" spent in a way you feel better about. For pain, you might visualize muscular pain and tension as huge ropes tied up in knots. With each exhalation, these knots loosen until they're free and your muscles themselves are relaxed, and less painful. An image I use with patients is: "Imagine you're in a large room with many switches on the walls and each switch is labeled as part of your body. As you turn off a switch, no more pain is felt there. Feel this part becoming numb, as if anesthetic had been injected. When you open your eyes, you'll still feel this peace and relaxation, and your pain will be replaced with slight numbness or tingling. You tell yourself the pain won't interfere and see yourself getting up from the couch and going outside to visit and laugh with your family." (This is just a brief version).

Just as with all of the treatments I've discussed, it's important you work with a well-trained, licensed hypnotherapist who preferably has a graduate degree in psychology, psychiatry, dentistry, or medicine. See appendix I for referral sources. You may want to have a few sessions with a trained pro and then try self-hypnosis. There are many tapes and books out for self-hypnosis, but check on their quality. As always, check with your doctor before starting.

Traditional Chinese Medicine

A basic introduction to traditional Chinese medicine (TCM) and its views on health, illness, diagnosis, and treatments will help you understand the hows and whys of alternative tools you are already using or may be considering. There has been much research on the efficacy of alternative methods, and many have stood up well to such scrutiny. Our country's reluctance to accept this mode of healing is perplexing, considering that it's been used by Chinese healers for at least 5,000 years. It's unlikely that such techniques would be used for so long if they didn't produce some beneficial effects! There are still those physicians who don't believe acupuncture helps, but fortunately the number of health care experts who endorse acupuncture's efficacy is increasing at a good clip due to consumer inter- est and the limits of typical treatments. However, people who use alternative methods without considering their type of illness, its severity, or the reality of other effective techniques available (i.e., surgery, drugs, or chemotherapy) are taking unnecessary risks. There is no clear-cut answer as to the best treatment overall, because all ARCs and individuals require different healing modes. Again, balance is the name of the game. We'll examine some acupuncture-responsive conditions and their explanation by TCM experts.

Many Westerners see acupuncture as a nonscientific, even fraudulent, prac- tice. If somebody reports it has worked for them, nonbelievers conclude that it was merely coincidence, the placebo effect, or that the person's illness wasn't real but was an all-in-your-head variety. At the other extreme are our fellow citizens who see TCM as ancient, mysterious, and spiritual and therefore more real and accurate than Western practices. Neither of these extreme views acknowledges that TCM is based on critical thinking, practice, and testing over hundreds of years. Neither the Western or Eastern system is more "right," because each is based on different assumptions and beliefs about health and sickness, and each is more effective in treating certain conditions. Western medical thought subscribes to the linear germ theory of disease; namely, where there is a symptom, a single underlying cause is not far behind. Also, the focus is often restricted to the one or more affected organs or systems. On the other hand, TCM includes a holistic mental and physical assessment of the person with no search for a particular dis- ease or germ, but a consideration of the whole person in disharmony or imbal- ance. Our medical field's endless search for linear cause and effect is replaced with understanding the *relationship* among "causes" and "effects" and among mind-body *patterns* at a point in time (Kaptchuk 1983).

Many of you have heard the Chinese terms, yin and yang. They represent different aspects of the same phenomenon, with yin associated with passiveness, darkness, cold, and the internal, and yang associated with activity, light, heat, and the external. Yin and yang exist necessarily only in relation to one another; both are changeable and include aspects of the other. If both are balanced and harmonious, there is health, but if there is imbalance or a deficit in one and excess of the other, there is sickness. Strong disharmony means the deficiency of one can't maintain the excess of the other: for example, if a sick person has a high fever and much sweating (excess of yang) she may suddenly go into shock (reassertion of strength of yin). The three possible outcomes of sickness are rebalancing through healing and medication, transformation into opposites like shock as mentioned, or death (Kaptchuk 1983).

Another concept central to TCM is qi ("chee"), translated in our country in a simplified way as "energy." Qi plays essential roles in our bodies, as it protects the body from external invaders, maintains body heat, transforms nutrients into energy, and prevents excessive loss of body fluids. Disharmony or illness in the body is traced to the status of one's qi.

There are various mind-body methods that work in similar ways to reestablish balance and healthy qi, thus allowing you to select those with which you're most comfortable. The following comes from a study of various methods (Goleman and Gurin 1993). Appendix II offers greater detail on these, and referrals and resources are available in appendix I.

Transcendental meditation (TM) decreases oxygen consumption, breathing rate, heart rate, and blood pressure in those with high blood pressure. It increases alpha waves (brain waves when you are awake but relaxed) as well. Progressive relaxation decreases muscle tension. Hypnosis decreases oxygen consumption, breathing, and heart rate. Zen and yoga decrease oxygen consumption, breathing and heart rates, and blood pressure in those with high blood pressure. They also increase alpha waves. As for massage, remember that some ARC patients must avoid certain types. If you have high blood pressure or another vascular disorder, you shouldn't let anyone practice deep massage with strong pressure on your body. Other situations in which to avoid massage include the presence of infection, malignancy, or inflammation. See appendix II for more on massage. Qi gong helps with mind-body integration and helps you gain control over pain and symptoms. See appendix II.

Chiropractic Treatment

I've seen an interesting pattern involving chiropractors: Clients either love them and can't brag enough about them, or they hate them after one visit and never return again. While such reactions are extreme, you must follow the same procedures and use the same selection guidelines in choosing a chiropractor that you would use in choosing any of your SHOC members. Make sure your chiropractor is well-trained and experienced in your ARC, or you run the risk of worsening your condition. Check with your doctor for referrals or contact local hospitals, clinics, and associations. Friends and family often provide the best referrals, for beyond telling you about the expert's education and experience, they'll tell you about the chiropractor's personality, healing approach, openness, and how they treat clients. For information on specifics of chiropractic technique, refer to appendix II.

Homeopathy

In many countries outside of our own, homeopathy gets top billing when it comes to public usage and prescription by health care professionals. Some may be surprised to learn that it doesn't come from the East, as it was Hippocrates, to whom we owe so much of our modern-day thought and philosophy, who noticed that if people ingested moderate to great amounts of certain substances they would become ill while those who ingested small amounts experienced symptom remission. Thousands of year later, in the late 1700s, a doctor tried to use Hippocrates' theory by using bits of toxic substances on himself and others. Lo and behold, symptoms of the diseases developed, but when he then administered infinitesimal amounts of the same substances, these symptoms would remit. Mainstream Western medical science has a problem with one of the central tenets of homeopathy—the fact that homeopathic substances have so little of the select substance present and are so diluted that the supposedly active ingredient often can't be chemically detected. True to form, conventional medicine concludes that if you can't see or measure it, it doesn't exist. On the other hand, homeopathic practitioners maintain that while they're perhaps not detectable, these substances do affect the human body and stimulate the immune system.

Even if this were untrue and the substance didn't have the ability to cause benefits, the most traditional allopathic experts would still have a hard time denying these remedies have positive effects. This is due to one of the most interesting and telling aspects of the mind-body phenomenon, which nobody can refute; namely, the efficacy of the placebo. Story after story and study after study reveal its incredible potency. Simply stated, when people believe a substance has a curative effect, it can and will! One famous story is that of a woman with extreme nausea and vomiting for whom no medicines helped. Finally, her doctor gave her a medication known to cause nausea and vomiting, but he told her this was the most recent innovation in combating these symptoms and that if anything would help her, this was it. She took the pill and, lo and behold, she stopped vomiting and was freed from the terrible nausea. The lesson: Mental beliefs are so powerful that because of mind-body unity they can change physical symptoms and systems. Even if homeopathy were ineffective based on its proponents' claims, we could still see benefits based upon the placebo effect.

As was briefly explained above with respect to a typical acupuncture session, let's take a look at what you might find if you visit an osteopath, a healer who prescribes homeopathic remedies. The osteopath will assess you in a way that is quite different from that of a typical allopathic doctor. The examination will proceed slowly and in great detail. In a way comparable to Chinese medicine, osteopaths believe symptoms have more to do with the specific individual than with the specific illness. Also as with the Chinese approach, a much more holistic perspective is used. You will be asked about all areas of your life, including work, family, play, problems, personality, family history and patterns, diet, exercise, and so on. In general, osteopaths prefer to prescribe you only one substance at a time, although they have a huge number of substances from which to choose. Their version of the *Physician's Desk Reference* used by allopathic doctors is the *Homeopathic Pharmacopoeia*, published a century ago and continuously updated. Osteopaths have a point in their decision to generally prescribe only one medication, for as many as one-third of today's hospitalizations result from toxic reactions, often from interactions among the many medications people use these days. Osteopaths can help you rid yourself of some of these excess toxins. What are the tools used by osteopaths? They include a panoply of seeds, roots, berries, salt, snake venom, vegetables, flowers, roots, and many substances. While osteopaths claim they can treat almost any illness or problem, such as arthritis, diabetes, rashes, PMS, allergies, and pain, they still offer a healthy, balanced perspective in that they maintain that certain treatments should be handled by allopathic physicians.

Osteopaths assert that although the substances they use may be weak in terms of concentration, they are quite powerful in providing the immune system with what is necessary to defend the body. Those who are skeptical of the process of homeopathy say that there is a dearth of strictly scientifically conducted research studies. However, several studies appear to pass muster in the eyes of these individuals. For example, one study was published in the well-respected medical journal *The Lancet*. The study compared the use of a homeopathic remedy to that of a placebo in treating individuals with asthma. Compared to individuals taking the placebo, those who had taken the homeopathic remedy had a 30 to 40 percent improvement in respiration (Rosenfeld 1996). There have been some other studies indicating that homeopathic substances are superior to placebos, although this has not necessarily been the case across the board. What this means is that further research into the efficacy of homeopathy is necessary. This is particularly the case when so many people rely on this type of approach. It has long been popular throughout the world, and it has hit the U.S. fast and furiously. With so many of us frustrated and angry at doctors and the medical system, and disappointed with medications and treatments that don't work, we are turning in record numbers to alternatives, such as homeopathy. In 1996, Isadore Rosenfeld asserted that sales figures for homeopathic remedies were increasing by 27 percent each year.

For some situations and women, homeopathy can be helpful. Particularly if you have tried traditional, allopathic approaches and haven't found relief, it may behoove you to try homeopathy. As the ingredients are natural and the treatment substances present in minimal amounts, the risk may well be far less than with medicines. However, I'm still urging my flexible, open-minded, and holistic approach here. Don't treat a serious illness or injury without at least giving some conventional interventions a try. When you and your SHOC team have determined the safety factor (i.e., that a new technique or substance won't interact negatively with what you're already using), you may well benefit by adding tools like homeopathy. It's clear we must allocate more resources toward researching and understanding the benefits of homeopathy and then incorporate these into a holistic SHOC.

CHAPTER 15

Enhancing Your General Coping Skills

As I've allowed myself to feel a little at a time, I learned that the valve to feelings was neither totally open nor totally shut—totally overwhelming or totally suppressed. I could feel bad without wanting to kill myself. I could be scared without being terrified ... a whole range of gradations. Once I stopped trying to rein my emotions in, I had more control than I thought."

—*The Courage to Heal*, by Ellen Bass and Laura Davis

With the armamentarium of tools you've gained for your SHOC, you can build on this foundation to make changes in more complex thought-behavioral patterns, such as coping skills. If you've done your best to incorporate the techniques presented so far into your life, you'll have gone far in learning to cope with your particular ARC, pain, and illness in general. But just as I define healing as more than a return to your previous level of functioning, coping can mean more than "getting by." It can open the door to enlightenment, growth, and thriving rather than surviving. This chapter is icing on the cake of the many coping methods you've learned from this book. Progressive relaxation, breathing, meditation, massage, nutrition, Eastern philosophy, cognitive work, social skills, knowing what you can control and letting go of what you can't, the pursuit of purpose and meaning, and a desire to stretch your mind-body limits are the keys. I hope you see a meaning in your illness, as I do and as so many of my clients have over time. All isn't dark, and as Nancy Mairs states, "a life commonly held to be insufferable can be full and funny" (1996). Recall this, because it will open your eyes to the light rather than only darkness and loss.

How Do You Cope?

If you see your ARC as the enemy and focus only on completely controlling it, you may be applying problem-focused coping erroneously, and you risk worsening your mind-body health. If you can talk and express your feelings about it, accept the illness, and still challenge yourself to improve your situation (i.e., emotion-focused coping), you'll fare much better in terms of mind-body healing. In dealing with ARCs, women's greater flexibility gives us an advantage; we're able to combine the two coping approaches (problem- and emotion-focused), as required by the situation. Think about each phase and situation you are going through and what type of coping would be best for dealing with that particular issue. This is one of the ways in which you can maximize your coping abilities, become more flexible, and even grow in abilities and knowledge.

Coping involves much more than whether you choose problem- or emotion-focused coping. It means your ability to choose the means to deal with the reality of your losses and restrictions, to experience the natural consequences of sadness and distress, and then to move on in an unfettered way, which allows you to grow and develop. A gentle reminder, folks: We're all going to die at some point. This is a fact of life and whether you are ill or dying in no way indicates you're a failure. You may be fortunate enough to be able to use your illness to derive life meaning and learn how to live more fully, freely, and joyously. Coping techniques help us deal with the facts of day-to-day pain and increasing losses of mobility, abilities, skills, or cognitive faculties without becoming paralyzed or losing ourselves within these losses. When we can admit to certain changes and somehow continue to stand strong, we will live life finally with truth and sincere appreciation.

Focus on minimizing extreme, irrational thinking to avoid perceiving minor life events as catastrophes. Negative stress levels will decrease greatly and formerly squandered mental and physical energy can be freed for healing purposes and to react to "real" traumas appropriately and effectively. Here you'll hone your skills to uncover your negative, irrational thoughts. Based on your increasing familiarity with your own particular irrational, dysfunctional thought patterns and with your growing ability to challenge and disprove these downers and replace them with positive, rational thoughts, you will access a reservoir of both more positive and more realistic self-talk to get you through sticky, potentially negatively stressful situations. Remember, we want to minimize our experience of negative stress because of the damage it causes to our pleasure, satisfaction, self-esteem and physical growth, repair, and immunity.

About Acceptance

If you recall, one of the stages of mourning and loss (the final phase in most models) is acceptance. I certainly don't see this as a final phase, but as a phase opening on to many other future possible journeys. What can acceptance do in terms of coping? Firstly, for you to truly be able to make changes in yourself and move on, you must start from a position of acceptance. This must come after a search of your inner beliefs and values, as discussed earlier in this book. Of course you're not pleased to have a chronic illness, but in order to move forward, it's imperative that you accept your mind-body situation. You have the greatest chances of success if you mourn your losses up front, look at them realistically, and then move on to seeing what you can improve and change in your life to make it an even better, more satisfying one. How to accept yourself when you may be feeling extreme guilt and like a complete failure? You need to do everything in your power to understand that you didn't cause your illness by yourself and that it isn't a punishment based on what a bad person you were.

If you continue to use the same expectations and judgments about what you "should" be able to do in order to be a worthwhile person and gain respect, you are not going to move forward in the direction of growth, satisfaction, and wellbeing. After acceptance, you need to give yourself what every child needs from the very beginning of her life: unconditional positive regard simply for being a human being—one with strengths and weaknesses. As you work to reclaim the lost legacy of all human infants, unconditional positive regard, any changes you want to make in your life or regarding yourself will be made out of a positive concern. You'll feel you have much more choice in the matter and that you are choosing to make certain improvements rather than just reacting with imperative changes because you're a bad person who is doomed to suffer. Recall from the mindfulness meditation that one of the goals is to realize, acknowledge, and accept the pain. This objectivity has been shown to actually lead to a decreased experience of pain. Thus, the ability to accept your current situation will help ease your physical pain and emotional trauma.

Secondly, once you're truly able to develop this central acceptance, you're ready to start making some changes. You need to continue to work on valuing yourself throughout this process, because you're going to be accepting the loss of certain important elements in your life. However, to balance this out, and very possibly to gain much more than you've lost, you're going to be searching for and exploring new ways of doing your favorite things, or learning and developing new skills, talents, hobbies, and relationships. Perhaps you were a career woman who worked a sixty-hour week, volunteered at the church, raised your children with a bit of help from your husband, exercised, and did all of the right things. Well, some of these things may have to go, or at least be greatly modified. This is a chance for you to truly get in touch with your values and what you want from your life. Did you really want to be working sixty hours a week, or was it something you'd been caught up in as a result of being sold the superwoman myth or because your self-esteem required the external admiration of other women and men? What about volunteering? Did you have to be the chair of the committee or could you have given just as much by being a general volunteer? You will find that while your life will undoubtedly change, this isn't inevitably bad. We tend to jump into thinking that if we have to change this or can no longer do that, we're losing out and are losers. However, many of my female clients have turned their lives into something they enjoy more and find much more valuable than what they had been doing previously.

Thirdly, you may want to recall the essence of the serenity prayer. Frequently remind youself that you want to cultivate the serenity arising from acceptance, the strength to realize in what areas you can make changes and then go through with implementing them, and finally the wisdom to realize the difference between situations and things you can control and those which you cannot. This is one of the best coping tools that anyone could ever have. It takes some time to develop, like most things that are very worthwile. It promises you great relief, decreased tension and pain, perhaps a reduction in symptom severity, and the wonder of seeing that your life isn't necessarily restricted and negative but can be full of movement and joy.

Exercise: Watch Out for the Big Fifteen

Whenever you dig beneath feelings of distress, depression, and anxiety, you'll find particular irrational ways of thinking that cause or worsen your mind-body state. Check and see how many of the following types of unhealthy, distorted thinking you use. Initially, you might say, "This is too extreme, I don't think like this. It doesn't even make sense!" This is your personal journey, so there is no need for defensiveness here; just be honest in asking yourself whether you, like many of us, use some of these ways of thinking (McKay, Davis, and Fanning 1981). Circle those most characteristic of your thoughts:

1. Filtering: using tunnel vision to perceive and process only one part of a situation. Involves magnifying negatives and ignoring or minimizing positive elements. Depressed people focus on aspects that suggest loss; anxious people focus on things that could suggest danger; angry people focus on injustice. Incessant thought: "I can't stand it."

2. Polarized Thinking: perceiving everything in extremes, in black and white. You think about yourself, your health, your job, your husband, your friends, your life . . . as all good or all bad. With respect to your health, the most dangerous element is applying these errors to yourself. Each single thought causes you to conclude that since you aren't perfect, you're a complete failure and loser.

3. Overgeneralization: taking one or two minor events to draw an irreversible, negative, all-encompassing generalization. One of my clients recently told me, "My Mom and now my best friend have let me down . . . I'll never depend on anyone else again. I'll have to be completely responsible and do everything by myself."

4. Mind Reading: using guesses, vague feelings, or limited experience to draw arbitrary (ironclad in your eyes) conclusions about others' motivations, particularly with respect to yourself. Mind readers are so sure they're right that they don't test their conclusions, which are so often wrong.

5. Catastrophizing: just as it sounds: "I'm a day late with the rent and know my landlord will kick me out on the streets." "My boyfriend broke up with me; nobody will ever love me again." Catastrophizing is a favorite of many clients who eventually love catching other people doing this.

6. Personalization: another big-time favorite that involves interpreting everything around you (experiences, other people's conversations, other people's feelings) to yourself and ultimately to your self-worth. "My boss chose four people to work on a new task force. They're all from a different division than mine, but he should know I'm interested in that. He just thinks I'm not smart enough."

7. Control fallacies: believing that you're a helpless victim with an external locus of control, or else that you're in control of or responsible for everything and everyone. We've discussed much about how the former view increases your helplessness, poor health, and distress. It can also be paralyzing, because if something else controls your life, why try to change anything? The latter extreme view also harms your health. Imagine how difficult your life would be if you really were responsible for everything and everyone around you. This is irrational, and your energy is better spent focusing on your needs and wants. From this healthier place, you can more efficiently and effectively care for others if you desire.

8. Fairness Fallacy: this is a dangerous mode of thinking because each person's definition of fairness is subjective, and expecting others to behave by your view of fair brings frustration and distress. My client Laura had a deep belief that things were supposed to be fair, and when she was diagnosed with lupus, she simply couldn't accept this or move on because "it wasn't fair." I had to ask her "Who said life is fair?" many times, and explore this reality with her before she could begin to accept and then strive to heal.

9. Emotional Reasoning: thinking that whatever you're feeling is the final, unquestionable truth. "If I feel stupid, I am. Since I feel bad about being sick, I am a bad person." Remember that it's your negative thoughts that cause negative feelings; emotions per se aren't inherently realistic and often stem from illogical or myopic thinking.

10. Change Fallacy: believing that you can change others so they'll perfectly meet your needs, take care of you, and make you feel good. The problem is that you can't really change other people; they'll often end up being angry or resenting you, and you'll resent them. Don't place your hopes

of salvation in others—you're the only one who can finally heal and satisfy yourself.

11. Global Labeling: going overboard and exaggerating (typically negatively) in perceiving a situation, person, or yourself based on one tiny fact. "My so-called friend didn't return my call, she obviously thinks that because I'm ill, I'm worthless."

12. Blaming: attributing problems, your emotions, failures, and disappointments either completely to others *or* to yourself. The first method is ideal in absolving yourself of any responsibility for changing yourself or your life. The second approach, often used by women, leads to similar results as the first one; namely, since everything including your illness is your fault and you're a complete mess, there is really nothing you can do to change anything.

13. Shoulds: using your own values and beliefs to judge how the world and everybody in it, including yourself, should function. Like blaming, shoulds can be used against external events, people, or yourself. "I'm stressed out and now I'm really in pain because if he really loved me, he should know I wanted to stay in tonight." "I shouldn't lay around, doing nothing (i.e., resting, taking care of myself, healing), it just means I'm lazy." Clients eventually become proficient at catching themselves using this word frequently and eventually steer clear from using such critical judgment on themselves and others.

14. Being Right: needing to appear omniscient drives your life; you must prove to everybody that you're always right, know more than anyone else, and do everything right. Because you ignore any information that's not perfectly aligned with your views, you stay stuck in a rigid pattern and can't let down your guard to relax, enjoy, share, and heal. This directly suppresses immune system functioning and increases pain.

15. Heaven's Reward Fallacy: you do as much as you can for others while ignoring your own needs and feelings because you know that if you just keep working hard enough and sacrifice enough, you'll eventually be rewarded for being the truly special person you are. This directly hampers your health, increases your stress, and interferes with heeding your mind-body needs.

Reading about these dysfunctional thought patterns makes it easier to notice their irrational, judgmental, and restrictive nature. The more "stinking thinking" patterns you exhibit, the more often you're journeying to the land of poor health, distress, and pain. As you self-monitor such thoughts in your journal, you'll be surprised about several things: 1) you'll find it difficult at first to catch these lightning-speed irrational thoughts (IRTs); 2) their relentless frequency will surprise you; 3) tracking your internal dialogue will really let you see how powerfully and directly your irrational, unhealthy thinking causes much of your pain, distress, depression, and the like; and 4) when you learn to confront and modify your negative automatic thoughts (ATs), you'll be very pleased with your improved mood, energy, and pain.

Exercise: Daily Mind-Body Monitoring

Use a form like the following to monitor your negative thinking, resulting emotions and pain level, new rational thoughts (RTs), and new emotions and pain level. The general form comes from the work of cognitive scientists, but I've modified it for my work with ARC patients. The following is homework done by my client Brandy, recently diagnosed with CFIDS and FMS.

Brandy's Mind-Body Self-Monitoring Sheet

1. Situation	Automatic Thoughts	Emotions and Physical Sensations	Irrational Thinking Style
Friend got job promotion	I used to be her boss. ↓ It's so unfair I'm so sick I ↓ can't work. I'll never work ↓ again. Everybody thinks I'm a ↓ loser, and I am. My life is worthless	Resentment, anger, disgust, headache Neck pain, fatigued Depressed	Fairness Fallacy Overgeneralization Catastrophizing Emotional Reasoning Polarization Filtering/ Polarization

2.	New Rational Thoughts (New RTs)	New Emotions, Thoughts, and Physical Sensations
	Life isn't always fair; besides, she's a hard worker. I'm unable to work now, but it doesn't mean I'll never work. People do respect me. I'm working now . . . on healing. Life is about much more than a job.	Acceptance, happy for her Hope, headache/neck pain is reduced, feeling better about myself Proud, feelings of control

It's important to realize that when you're negatively stressed, your beliefs become more rigid than usual. You'll actually look for evidence confirming your unrealistic beliefs while ignoring information that disproves them. When you notice you're feeling tense, stressed, anxious, or depressed, briefly jot down the situation, your feelings, and those destructive ATs that are directly causing your negative mind-body state. Try to make several entries each day, as the more you practice this journaling, the sooner you'll catch your irrational ATs and replace them with realistic, moderate ways of thinking. Just how do you replace irrational thoughts with rational, positive ones?

Here are some other tools to reduce excessive stress, worry, etc.

1. In your journal, write down which of the big fifteen irrational ATs you're using when distressed; list them under Irrational Thinking Style on your worksheet.

2. Ask yourself if rational reasoning underlies your negative ATs; in most cases the answer will be "no." Recall that your perceptions of yourself, others, and the world are all subjective and biased based on your expectations, fears, beliefs, and experiences. You'll need to hold up your irrational thoughts to the light of day and ask for evidence supporting beliefs and evidence against beliefs. Confront irrational thoughts. Not doing one task perfectly doesn't mean you're an unlovable failure; such a conclusion is based on negative ATs that you must be perfect so others will value and accept you. Remember, women are often overly dependent on feedback from others to bolster our self-esteem. You'll feel great relief and less distress when you free yourself from this irrational, demeaning way of thinking. Also check to see if you're using catastrophizing, fairness fallacy, and other cognitive errors that increase distress and pain.

Taking It Off the Page and Into Your Life

Once you're proficient at catching and modifying your negative ATs with your journaling, you'll be able to consciously detect your ATs before they've done their typical mind-body damage. You can decrease the frequency of your writing, but don't discontinue it altogether. With a little more practice, you'll be largely able to prevent ATs from warping your reality and your thinking will be much healthier, more flexible, and more realistic. You'll feel happier, more energetic, tolerant of yourself and your life situation, in control, and able to change those things you can. Also, when stressors arise, you'll be more able to experience them as challenging prostress rather than the threatening distress of old.

When your reasoning isn't faulty, you can decrease your distress by accepting the fact that life isn't perfect or even fair sometimes but that you can choose how you think about this reality and thus how you react to it. By accepting the reality of the situation and taking steps to control and change what you can while letting the rest go, you largely free yourself of mind-body distress. By taking the steps or making changes you want, you'll experience prostress' benefits like better self-esteem, energy, pleasure, and growth.

Another step to reality-test your thinking and thus feelings is to ask yourself two questions: A.) *What is the worst thing that could happen to me?* Unlike the usual half-formed catastrophic expectations zooming through your mind, by forcing yourself to realistically appraise the situation, your expectations will be more tame, true, and less distressing: "I may learn I have an area needing improvement; someone may not believe I'm sick; I may feel discomfort or inconvenience." But, you'll survive it! B.) *What positive things could result?* Think about how a distressor could become a prostressor: "I may boost my confidence by meeting an unexpected challenge; I may become more patient; I may learn new skills; I may boost my self-esteem by making it through a trying time and realizing I don't have to beat myself up or become stressed out." Along the same lines, use this quick tip to put things into perspective. Do you find yourself obsessing, "What if this? But what if that?" Add the simple word "so" to defuse the negative power of such ATs. Instead of worrying, "What if I can't finish all this work before I go home? What if I commit and am then too tired or sick?," simply say, "So what if I don't finish it all" and "So what if I can't go after all." Will you definitely be fired? Will all your friends decide you're lousy, lazy, and selfish? Will the world end in a fiery explosion? I think you get the point.

Some Powerful Coping Tools

Finally, you'll be learning a powerful technique created by a leading cognitive therapist, Donald Meichenbaum. He has designed a pwerful technique that improves one's coping abilities, thereby reducing distress, anxiety, and the like. Besides looking at the presence and effect of negative beliefs, he also focuses on the absence of positive thoughts and responses and on how to reinforce adaptive coping. Meichenbaum's focus on cognitions and self-talk actually arose from his early work with hyperactive children who were cognitively impulsive. He found that what he learned was transferable to adults. When children are learning, they go through a three-stage process of verbal control. Initially, their behavior is controlled (or is attempted to be controlled) externally by the statements of parents, teachers, and others. After this, the child begins talking to himself or herself out loud in directing behavior. Finally, the child's internal, silent self-talk guides his or her behavior. Adults follow a similar pattern in learning a new behavior or response. Meichenbaum focuses on the internal speech of the adult in order to improve the ability to cope with negative stress and learn to change behaviors.

As you've read, your irrational thinking and negative automatic thoughts will lead you to interpret events as threatening and negatively stressful, which will then cause you to feel distressed, anxious, and angry. Donald Meichenbaum's technique, presented in his 1985 book, *Stress Inoculation Training*, attacks the problem at the core by helping you take control and change your self-talk. Basically, you learn to say positive self-statements at each of four phases when you are feeling negatively stressed and are facing a negative (according to your interpretation) situation. Meichenbaum's self-instructional approach is oriented toward having people: 1.) Observe their responses to distressors and, 2.) Use self-talk to select adaptive coping responses. Having completed the earlier assignments, such as the Daily Mind-Body Monitoring, and familiarized yourself with your favorite cognitive distortions and irrational thinking, you have already completed step 1.

Step 2 involves coming up with positive, more realistic self-statements, which may be difficult at first but gets easier over time. Meichenbaum has broken the entire process of dealing with a potential stressor into four phases: prepping, doing, dealing, and rewarding. What follows is a brief description of these stages and examples of helpful distress-reducing and even prostress-increasing self-talk. The extra lines are provided in case you want to write down some self-statements in your own words to make it more user-friendly and thus more effective. To generate some of your own ideas, it can help to think about something that is going to happen in the near future and is "making you" feel negatively stressed (of course, we know it's not the situation that is making you stressed, but your expectations and self-talk). In using this technique, it's best to start with an event that is minimally stressful so that you can practice this method slowly at first.

Description of upcoming stressful situation: I'm going to have some tests at the doctor's office next week. Then we are going to discuss my diagnosis and where we're going from here. I'm so anxious that I don't think I can stand it.

I. **Prepping**
You are preparing and planning. For example:

1. I'll write down a plan of the test times, dates, and a list of questions to help me get organized; 2. Why should I worry? It's a waste of time and doesn't do anything but hurt me; 3. I'm anxious but that's natural. I'll use this extra energy to take this challenge; 4. I'll read about my condition first and I'll go in there prepared and more in control; 5. _____ .

II. **Doing**
While doing the task, focus on controlling your stress reactions through relaxation, breathing, using positive thinking, and telling yourself this is a chance to challenge yourself (prostress). For example:

1. My body's tension is my cue to start the relaxation; 2. If I feel anxious, I'll take a break and focus on breathing and relaxing; 3. Take one step at a time; 4. I'll do the best I can and then reward myself for that!; 5. _____ .

III. **Dealing** (Note: This step doesn't always happen).
Stay in the here-and-now and remember that you have some control, even if the worst happens. If you're very distressed, think realistically—what is the worst that could happen? For example:

1. I'm going to relax my mind-body now; 2. I've finished most of this . . . only a little more to go; 3. If I can't remember all of it, my partner will help me; 4. _____ .

IV. **Rewarding**

Assess how things went, how you coped, and what things you want to change. Reward small steps as much as big steps. Focus on the positive and what you learned. For example:

1. That was easier than I thought; 2. That was worse than I thought but I made it through so it will be easier next time; 3. I confronted the fear and made it through by relaxing and focusing; 4. The stress and anxiety I felt and the worrying I did was worse than getting the physical and meeting with the doctor; 5. I learned _____ ; 6. _____ .

Make sure you have a copy of this list of stages and sayings available when you start using this technique. Carry it around in your purse or leave it where you'll often see it on your desk, bedside table, or car seat. Once you're comfortable with the process, try it with events of greater potential distress. The exposure to increasing levels of stress explains the name Meichenbaum gives the process: "stress inoculation training." By practicing on less stressful events, you're exposed to limited amounts of the harmful agent (negative stress) and are able to develop antibodies (stress management, coping skills, changing distress into prostress), which boost your resistance to greater levels of stress. Remember, it takes practice, practice, practice but you'll find it pays back over and over.

Journaling and the Art of Life Enhancement

There are many ways to journal. Recent studies show that journaling actually improves immune system functioning! My clients who do their "journaling homework" inevitably report that it clarifies their thoughts and feelings, brings up old memories and new understandings, and reduces the intensity of negative emotions. One fairly free-form way to journal is to jot down entries—from a few words to a pages—as you desire. A second type of journaling (as shown on forms A and B, below) is more structured and helps you understand your personal experience of illness, the dynamics of its symptoms, and factors that increase or decrease pain. It can also highlight decreased pain ratings as you gain control over your thoughts, emotions, and behaviors. The more often you journal, the more rapid your insight about symptoms, pain, automatic negative thoughts, and triggers. Then comes the hard part . . . change. I can't tell you the number of clients who tell me, "I just don't understand this. I mean I know all of this stuff in my head, and what you tell me makes sense, but I can't make the changes we've talked about. Maybe I'll never be able to." What these women lack is an organized, complete understanding of their negative cognitive styles and why they developed, techniques to challenge irrational thinking and replace it with realistic, positive thinking, and a venue to express and work through emotions. I find that a synthesis of cognitive-behavioral and psychodynamic approaches plus the invaluable EMDR technique offers the best method to move realizations about unhealthy thinking and behavioral patterns from the "head" to the "heart," bridging the gap between knowing intellectually what to do and feeling and doing what it is we finally want to do.

It's also necessary to engage in a lot of soul searching to truthfully answer questions like "Do I have anything to gain from holding onto my symptoms? How would I feel if my symptoms were suddenly gone? Who would I be?" You may initially think, as many do at first, that this isn't applicable to you, because you'd give anything to be rid of illness and symptoms. You probably would, at least on a conscious level, but on a deeper level that requires effort, time, and tools to access, these questions may well make sense. This isn't to say that you (or anyone) becomes sick for some gain or that it's the only way for a weak person to get attention and a self-identity. However, once a person is ill over time, certain factors can and do take hold. I've seen many clients who are becoming healthier when "out of the blue" they're hit with severe anxiety, dread, or depression. Again, the issue is about change and change can be frightening. When we've restructured our lives, our family's life, our work, and our self-image to include our illness, having to change this all over again and accept complete responsibility for our actions can be frightening. Psychologists (and people with ARCs themselves) must be cautious of destroying all habitual, defensive thoughts, beliefs, emotions, and behaviors without having healthy alternatives to put in their place. Otherwise the foundation, devoid of its support structures, can collapse or the old, treacherous support blocks will be re-erected, the whole structure weakened by the change. By using cognitive tools and challenging this fear of fear, developing new coping skills, thoughts, and behaviors, and replacing unhealthy ones, you maximize your ability to break away from the familiar but unhealthy.

As mentioned, frequency of monitoring is key so add to Form A each time you use your tools each day. (All the techniques listed here are described in individual chapters or in appendix II.) Form B helps you learn how to deal with pain and distress arising from one or more particular distressors you experience in a day.

Form A

Use this format in your journal when you practice your techniques at points throughout the day, not necessarily linked with a distressing event.

I. Rate your pain (on a scale of 1–10) a) before and b) after each of the following techniques. (1 = no distress to 10 = most distress imaginable) On the next line, describe specifically what you did, on what date, and at what time.

Meds   a) ____ b) ____   Meal/Snack a) ____ b) ____

_____   _____

Exercise   a) ____ b) ____   Sleep   a) ____ b) ____

_____   _____

Physical Therapy a) ____ b) ____   Massage   a) ____ b) ____

Acupuncture   a) ____ b) ____   Acupressure a) ____ b) ____

Chiropractic   a) ____ b) ____   Progressive Relaxation a) ____ b) ____

Deep Breathing   a) ____ b) ____   Cognitive Work a) ____ b) ____

Imagery   a) ____ b) ____   Prostress   a) ____ b) ____

Form B

Use this format in your journal when you choose to practice certain techniques as a result of your perception of a disturbing event. Use the same 1 to 10 scale as in Form A.

Date and Time	Situation	Thoughts	Emotions, Stress Level, and Pain
12/20 8 A.M.	Family reunion tomorrow	I don't want them to see me ill. They'll think I'm lazy or faking.	Stress 8 Anger 6 Pain 7

New Ratings

Because of this incident and my resulting painful reactions, I am using the following tools:

1. Progressive Relaxation 8 A.M.	2. Imagery 10 A.M.	3. Cognitive Techniques 2 P.M.	4. Other technique _____
Stress 5 Anger 5 Pain 4	Stress 1 Anger 2 Pain 3	Stress 1 Anger 1 Pain 2	Stress ____ Anger ____ Pain ____

Another way to check your automatic thoughts in is how you perceive and react to stress. Your personality characteristics, belief systems, self-esteem, and other aspects of your "self" are central in determining whether you'll experience a situation as a distressor or prostressor. The previous chapters taught you to get in touch with your body's responses to illness, pain, and stress and gave you tools to change your body's habitual responses to avoid the harm of further weakening your immune system, and increasing pain and distress. Now, you'll learn to detect harmful ways of thinking and to change these to assist your mind-body self-healing.

How often do you say or think things like, "He made me so mad," "My co-worker makes me feel stupid," or "My illness makes me feel worthless"? Such statements suggest that other people and external events control and dictate our emotions. This is way off base, though it's often easier to blame others than realize that it's our *interpretations* of events, others' behavior, and our own behavior determining our mind-body reactions. Look at the statement above: "My co-worker makes me feel stupid." Perhaps you're talking about a co-worker who seems to effortlessly zip through her work and is always prepared to spout off the right answer to all questions. Meanwhile, you're engaged in a woman's favorite way to put herself down; namely, by comparing yourself to others and seeing yourself as wanting. Realize when you're being your own worst enemy: *you* make yourself feel this way through the words you use to talk to yourself. Reconsider the statement about your co-worker. It's highly unlikely that this woman never makes mistakes. She may be better than you at certain things, but is she really a better person than you because she may be more organized, well-prepared, or whatever? Are you really a "fool" compared to her, or is this a somewhat irrational, extreme label?

Remember, we're usually much more harsh and judgmental about ourselves than about others. Women are especially critical and tend to blame themselves for situations. Let's look at another example. Take an event like the offer of a job promotion. One woman might be ecstatic about the opportunity. She has many plans she wants to implement, believes she can make important changes, and feels energized and excited. Another woman might feel tense and anxious and spend her time thinking about how hard the new position will be and how her illness and deficits will cause her to fail to live up to her superiors' expectations. The situation, an offer of a promotion, is the same for both women, but what differs is how each thinks about it. One woman views it as a challenge and a chance for growth, and healthy feelings of energy and pleasure, as well as productive thought processes (creativity, organization, planning) and behavior, arise from this positive interpretation. The other woman sees it as a threat and tells herself that because she has an illness she will screw up in the new job, even though it won't be any more taxing than it will for the first woman. Accordingly, she will experience the mind-body drawbacks of distress. Because she is anxious, her thinking process will suffer, and increased pain will interfere with her ability to be creative and focused. What is important to realize is that each woman created her own reality. Her interpretation of the events determined her reactions and behaviors, thereby creating a self-fulfilling prophecy. The following exercises will help you discover and change your unhealthy thinking.

Stop the Vicious Circle

While your thoughts determine your emotions and behavior, emotions and behavior then feed back to influence thoughts (see diagram below).

Triggering Event   ◄────────►   *Perception/Self-talk /Interpretation*

Behaviors (Feelings, Actions, Physiological responses)

Diagram 15-1

Here's an example of a self-fulfilling prophecy: You've avoided doing presentations at work for fear your illness will act up and you'll be too tired or pained that day. When the dreaded time for you to speak arrives, you've been too anxious to sleep, so you're exhausted and in pain, which then does interfere with your presentation. This confirms your initial belief that your illness means you're no longer a competent worker. This pattern is the reason I have clients challenge irrational, fearful beliefs by engaging in the feared situation. When expected crises don't occur, they see the fallacy of their irrational thinking, but without such evidence, they have no reason to change their negative beliefs.

Exercise: Playing Center Stage

Another effective tool to destroy unrealistic negative views of yourself and your illness, as well as the resulting rigid behavior, is to journal about the woman you'd like to be and then play the role of this person's life for a specified time. Borrow values and traits from anyone you respect, even fictional characters: "What is this character like? What activities does she do? How does she handle social interactions?" You may want to add the fact that this character has your ARC. "How does this affect her? Is she any different, and, if so, how? What does she do to cope with pain and symptoms? Does she continue to work or spend all of her time at home? How does she express her feelings and beliefs?" I work collaboratively with a client on this in a question-and-answer session, and I then have her go out and have a week of great fun being a temporary actor and behaving as her "ideal" would: she will talk, walk, eat, and dress the part. She'll change parts of her routine that she doesn't like, and she'll take better care of her health so she can go out and attend music or art events, go to movies, research in the library, go to restaurants or dance, attend exercise classes, approach people she's been afraid to before, and do what she has wanted to do but has felt too sick or scared to do.

This is your assignment: Please remember to have fun with it. The idea that you're playing a role lets you break free of habitual, limiting preconceived thoughts and rigid behaviors. One of my clients, Margaret, couldn't grasp her automatic thoughts or how such thoughts could increase her pain and other symptoms. All she knew was that life was no fun, and her reactions to her illness made her question living at all. After doing this exercise, she was exuberant, saying she'd never realized the power her thinking had in determining her feelings and behavior. She was delighted because she'd been able to act as a challenge-seeking, friendly, energetic person, and the low self-esteem caused by her illness had fallen to the wayside. Her irrational predictions were negated, and she saw that she could use her thoughts to positively affect her emotions and actions.

Exercise: Two Lessons in One

At first, you may think this technique is too simple to work. Yes, thought stopping (TS) is simple, but it's very effective in ending disturbing thoughts. Stop your ruminating by saying—out loud or silently—"Stop!" This disrupts unhealthy images and associations and lets you regain control and focus on something else. You then de-catastrophize and replace negative ATs with the new RTs, positive statements, and "so-what-ifs" you practiced above. Let's use a common example: It's the night before a doctor's appointment and you're obsessing about the results. By dwelling on the negatives and all that could go wrong, you're intensifying your pain, physical symptoms, distress, and anxiety. You have something important to do tonight, but you can't focus on it because your arousal isn't the kind that improves performance—it's the extreme kind that shuts it down. By using TS, you'll interrupt the negative, self-sabotaging thought-behavior cycle. It takes practice to completely eliminate negative ATs and images with your stop signal and replace them with positive, assertive statements or a distracting activity. Some clients like it when I give them a "worry time" at first that lets them indulge in their negative ATs and imagery for a set time, like five to fifteen minutes a day. Then they use TS and replace the negative ATs with positive or new RTs. For our example, rather than ruminating on all the negatives you expect tomorrow, tell yourself that worry does nothing constructive now, but only adds to your anxiety. You'll deal with whatever comes up tomorrow *then*, and for now you'll focus on doing a good job on your work (*then* visualize yourself doing this in an assertive, efficient way).

Do you tend to obsess over all of the activities you "must" or "should" accomplish day-to-day? Because my client Cindy had forgetfulness and attention-span problems caused by the recent onset of MS, she became obsessed with planning, scheduling, and rescheduling what she had to do daily, when to start each activity, how long it would take, what to start first, and what might go wrong (forecasting and catastrophizing) that by the end of the day, she'd accomplished little and used this fact to confirm to herself "how sick, worthless I really am." She created a subjective "reality" that couldn't help but drag her down. If this pattern sounds familiar, use TS, as Cindy did to stop obsessing and to rationally and calmly plan her day. In the morning, when her confusion and obsessions were worst, she'd shout "stop" and then get busy writing down her day's schedule. If you do this, you'll find it frees you from ruminating about everything you must do. When worries crop up, refer to your schedule and move on to the next activity. It's wise to check off completed tasks so you feel a sense of accomplishment and disprove your beliefs that you never get anything done. (Also use this as a chance to grow and develop "thriver" qualities, which counter distress.) Unexpected events will inevitably prevent you from following your schedule "perfectly." Use these incidents as opportunities to develop your flexibility by telling yourself change is inevitable and you'll find a way to eventually get things done. Situations like these offer you a chance to grow and learn to thrive in our 120-mph lives these days. Organization and scheduling are central to stress optimization as you'll be reading.

TS is also very helpful for those of us who ruminate about past events, especially those for which we blame ourselves. If you belong to this club, stop here for a brief self-talk: "What is the benefit of replaying past events? They're in the past and I can't do anything to change them now. What I *can* do is learn from them and move on." A number of my female clients enter therapy struggling to let go of past events or relationships. They feel stuck in their lives and unable to grow and accomplish things. A big part of their stagnation comes from this constant rumination on the past, the self-imposed shame and guilt, and their frequent companion, self-sabotaging behavior. Chronically ill clients are often unable to let go of the past and tend to blame themselves for causing their sicknesses. The usual refrain goes like this: "If only I'd eaten a better diet, I wouldn't be punished by having this illness. I should have exercised, but I was always too busy doing things for other people. I guess I shouldn't have put my career first or made it so important . . ." Women also obsess over intimate relationships that turned out to be unhealthy for them and often for their children. Who among us hasn't made mistakes, great and small, in relationships? You only compound the problem by replaying ITs like, "If only I had . . ." or "I should have . . ." Your rational response is "Well, I didn't, and all I can do is learn from it!" Remember, hindsight is truly 20/20, and most of us make the best decisions we can *at the time with the information available.* Of course, anxiety, low self-esteem, and past trauma interfere with healthy coping and decision making, and if you find yourself repeatedly involved in harmful relationships or situations, professional help from a psychologist or other health expert can be useful. Working through your emotions, gaining feedback from an objective observer, and acknowledging that you rarely can change other people or even situations, will all help you to let go and move on.

The cognitive tools you've learned here can truly change your ways of thinking, perceiving, feeling, and behaving. I've little doubt that the change will be welcome and healthy. Cognitive tools allow you to have some control over your thoughts, feelings, and behavior in the here-and-now, and over planning how you'll think and be in the future. Because those of us with ARCs are faced with many uncontrollable dynamics, this gift is profound.

Let's look briefly at some tools to reduce the hair-pulling, nail-biting, teeth-grinding attacks known as "I-can't-cope-itis." To use these coping skills, you'll need the progressive relaxation, deep breathing, guided imagery, and cognitive techniques you learned earlier. First let's look at one of my clients who faced a chronic, potentially fatal, illness. Gina represents the ideal when it comes to moving forward through pain, fear, and distress. She ended up focusing on the positives in her life, her gains since her illness, and the growth she was able to obtain because of her condition. Gina had been diagnosed with the third recurrence of a life-threatening illness when she came to see me. She was confused and hopeless given that she'd been doing "everything she was supposed to" (i.e., meditation, eating a good diet, exercising, trying to balance her life) and still she'd gotten sick again. Her beliefs and hopes had been blasted apart. We worked together, discussing the previous episodes of her illnesses, her upbringing and personality characteristics that could be associated with the onset of the illness, continued unhealthy patterns I pointed out of which she'd been unaware, and her perpetual feelings of unworthiness and intense need for approval from others. While she had made progress after her second bout with her illness, she had indeed continued pushing in her career, striving to be perfect and please everybody, and convince everybody else that she was healthy. So, while she'd paid lip service to practicing mind-body techniques, she remained focused excessively on externals and hadn't made the necessary real underlying changes in her thoughts and behavior. After our intensive work, she changed on many levels: she was able to go for days without thinking about the illness or the possibility of its recurrence; she now truly led a balanced life, listening to her body when it needed to rest, listening to her inner child when it wanted to play, satisfying her own needs and wants rather than only those of others; and finally communicating openly and assertively with others. She finally approved of and loved herself *internally* rather than depending on validation from others, which had always caused her to ignore her own needs to satisfy those of everybody else in her life. Now she can see the gains from her illness and she feels a sense of gratitude. Not only does she no longer spend her time worrying about the return of her illness, but she actually believes that should it return, she would again be able to cope with and grow from it. This is a wonderful, inspiring story but I don't mean to say that these changes are easy. It takes a lot of legwork, faith, courage, and soul searching.

Refer back to the exercise, "Your Coping Style," in chapter 4 to remind yourself about your way of coping. This will give you some guidance about your areas of strength, as well as the areas of improvement that are awaiting your intervention. Ask yourself some other questions: 1) Do you strive to get involved, learn, adapt, make changes, consider alternatives, and communicate your needs and wants in potentially stressful situations?; 2) Do you prefer to avoid conflict, and potential stress by allowing others to control your decisions and life?; 3) Do you hold in your feelings rather than expressing them, possibly hoping that if they aren't stated out loud, they'll go away or cause no harm? Think about these questions before going on with your reading, because you truly need to know your coping style—it has both direct and indirect impacts on your illness, its severity and progression, and your mind-body health. Remember those who actively seek information about their illness, follow SHOC doc guidelines but also ask questions, search for alternatives, and make necessary changes in their thoughts and behavior tend to fare best. If you answered yes to question 1 above, your coping style is a healthy one, while if you answered yes to question 2 and/or question 3, it's time to strive to model yourself after question 1.

One way to improve coping with situations that are traditionally distressing and anxiety-provoking for you is to practice going through them in your mind while you're in a relaxed state. This is a safe place where you won't be at risk of experiencing the array of dreaded consequences (generally unrealistic) you've conjured up in your imagination. For more information on expectations and unrealistic thinking, refer back to the first part of this chapter. Also recall that relaxation and anxiety are opposing reactions, so when your body is relaxed, you can't simultaneously experience negative stress. A useful technique is to use PR to relax and then imagine the feared situation in your mind. If you become anxious and your body tightens, replace this image with a positive, relaxing one. Then, when you're ready, imagine the feared scenario again. If you feel tension returning, shift your image to the peaceful one. Practice until you imagine the feared scenario without any increased tension or pain. Then you begin to work in the same way on a scenario that is a bit more distressing than the one you just completed.

Be Your Own Writer and Director

The principle behind the stress hierarchy is also applicable to events other than those that occur regularly in your life. If you're experiencing significant anxiety and distress about an upcoming one-time event, this technique can prove invaluable. My client, Ava, a lovely, warm woman, had sought therapy prior to attending her son's wedding across the country. As the months dwindled and the time drew near, she became more and more anxious about the event and began experiencing increased pain and symptoms from her rheumatoid arthritis and type 1 diabetes. She explained to me that the wedding would be her first meeting with her ex-husband's new wife. While obviously there are some potentially painful emotional dynamics that could arise, her fearfulness and feelings of intimidation were excessive and unhealthy. She was unable to concentrate or make decisions and awoke each day intensely anxious. Any joy that the upcoming event would typically have offered her was nonexistent. There was obviously something wrong with the way Ava was thinking about the upcoming meeting. I asked her to describe her thoughts about this meeting, to tell me in detail the horrible story she had written and was replaying over and over in her head. She said, "I am standing face to face with her. My heart is pounding and I'm weak. I say hello but then I can't think of anything else to say. I feel like everyone will know I'm sick and see me as weak; they'll think my husband was right to leave such a physically ill person. I feel ashamed, rejected and terrible. My ex-husband and sons are watching me make a fool of myself." I challenged the inevitability of this scenario and asked her if it was, maybe, just a little bit exaggerated. She laughed for a moment, which gave me some hope that she would be able to modify her heretofore rigid expectations.

I first taught her DB, PR, and visualization skills, and then introduced her to the assumptions and techniques of cognitive therapy. Our next step was to create an alternative scenario (to the terrifying, humiliating one she'd created by herself) to practice and visualize after her PR. In her new story, Ava sees herself dressed in her new, beautiful outfit, walking with poise toward the woman, extending her hand, and calmly saying hello. Ava expresses her pleasure at meeting her, speaks briefly about the wedding, and moves off with energy and purpose to meet other friends. The exact nature of her revised story wasn't as important as was the fact that she could see herself being calm and in control of the situation. Her anticipatory fear was greatly minimized, because she realized how irrational and distorted her initial forecasting had been. The more she rehearsed this, the less distressed she felt. We also used cognitive techniques (see chapter 14). For example, we examined her negative, extreme thoughts, like "I'm going to hate her and she'll be rubbing it in my face that she's married to my ex and can take care of him in a way I couldn't because of my illness" and "She is intruding on this wedding" and revised them to moderate RTs like "The fact that my husband couldn't deal with my illness is his problem; I still tried to do as much as I could in the marriage" and "I'm here for my son's wedding, not to see my ex-husband and his wife." After this preparation, Ava was minimally nervous meeting her ex-husband's new wife and instead completely enjoyed the celebration, her sons, and her relatives and friends. As a result of the work she'd done, Ava had developed coping skills so she could easily manage the situation.

Exercise: Writing Your Own Script

You'll find this technique very helpful for a variety of situations that cause you significant distress. *What we anticipate will happen is generally much worse than what usually does happen.* Our extreme thinking causes us to feel extreme emotions like distress, anxiety, rage, and depression. Below you will find a series of comments and questions to complete. Add the following format to your journal and fill it out diligently. (Refer back to the description of Ava's dilemma if you have difficulty filling out the form.) Use any event coming up within a few weeks or months that is causing you distress and anxiety. The last set of blank lines allows you to symbolically take control by revising what you tell yourself is going to happen. Then practice your success scenarios while maintaining a relaxed state, as you did in the earlier stressful events hierarchy exercises. You'll find your distress will greatly diminish while your ability to function calmly and effectively and to experience the pleasure of prostress will greatly increase.

Describe upcoming stressful event:

_____

What is it that I fear will happen? What is the scenario in my mind?

_____

Is my thinking about this event rational? How is it faulty?:

_____

This is my revised scenario in which I am calm and controlled. the outcome is a positive one (you can create several):

_____

As an additional note, it's essential to reward yourself once you have made it through the initially feared situation. Things may have gone completely smoothly or there may have been some mishaps and remaining distress. What is important is that you took the steps to develop your coping skills. This is something to celebrate, so reinforce it by rewarding yourself. You deserve it! I repeat: Reward yourself! In my experience, no other group of people is so poor at and conflicted about reinforcing themselves as are women. Just do it! Remember, the more challenges you allow yourself to meet, the better your self-esteem will be and the greater the amount of health-inducing prostress in your life.

CHAPTER 16

Working with Others

I have beautiful things and people in my present. I have beginning friend-
ships with women who understand from inside what I'm going through ...
I do not have to lie to them. I do not have to keep up appearances for them,
I do not have to regain perspective (their perspective). I am not alone.

—Ely Fuller, in *The Courage to Heal*

ARCs involve multiple unknowns in multiple areas, but ARC patients can say
one thing with complete certainty: Illness causes myriad changes in our relationships with family, friends, acquaintances, co-workers, supervisors, and many others. This chapter explores some changes you can expect, how to make some of
them pleasurable for you and others, and how to avoid or minimize typical pit-
falls and problems (also known as challenges!). Chronic illness can be a tremendous stressor on any relationship and even the best can end in breakups, divorce
(73–80 percent in multiple sources claim this), or with major losses in intimacy
and connection. Avoiding this is goal number one.

As this book is based on an undeniable gender difference in ARC prevalence
rates, I'd like to bring up another difference relevant to this chapter. Most people
in our culture see women as more nurturing than men, and scientific evidence
suggests this is true (at least in our culture). Much data indicates that men suffer
more than women after losing spouses or partners. While married men are
healthier than unmarried men, women don't always derive such consistent,

health-enhancing benefits. One reason posited for this is that women must give much more support in relationships. Dr. Laura Glynn and co-researchers (1999) compared physical negative stress measures in both sexes. Subjects were put in a stressful situation with either a male or female observer. The observers acted in one of two ways: they responded supportively by smiling, nodding, etc., or they responded unsupportively by appearing bored. Subjects placed with supportive females showed the least physical stress, while those with unsupportive females showed the highest stress. Being with a supportive or unsupportive male didn't have a significant effect in reducing stress. What does this mean? Am I saying that if you're ill, you won't benefit from support from male friends or partners? Absolutely not! Social support from men or women is beneficial in many different ways. It does highlight the importance of maintaining friendships and relations with our female family, friends, and acquaintances.

I bring this issue up because it relates to a behavioral pattern that many of us with chronic illness and pain experience. Sometimes we get to a point where we just want to withdraw from everybody and everything. This is natural, and you do need time alone to do as you wish: rest, think, plan, dream, create, heal, and visualize. But we can get so tired of having to depend on others, answering questions about how we feel, defending ourselves, or just plain feeling irritable that we just want to shut down. I often hear, "I'm so sick and tired of being sick and in pain that I don't want to think or talk about it. I'm bored with it and I'm sure everyone else is too!" While some time off is good, danger comes when withdrawal or not talking become your long-standing strategy. You take a risk when you choose to stay away for long periods, lose out on essential social support, and suppress feelings. This becomes unhealthy and further interferes with your immune system and pain relief. As usual, the answer lies in balance. Take time for yourself and draw healthy boundaries. Also, spend time with loved ones and friends, share feelings, listen to their stories, get objective advice, and get out of your own head.

There are many challenges that await families with chronic or long-term illness. Why do I say "challenges" when potential incidents can be devastating, frightening, and so sad? I'm not taking this lightly, as I know through many interviews, research, work, and my own life how easily things can go awry. In fact, it is often easier to see them as threats and problems, become defensive, and stop communicating, because if we use words like challenge and try to keep positive attitudes, what happens when we're let down and our expectations are dashed? Many of us try to avoid positive expectations because, as I often hear, "That way I won't get hurt. I'll be prepared." This is a normal human defense and has its value, but as usual, a balanced view is more healthful. Your expectations need not be black or white, as many shades fall in between.

From all you've read and experienced, you know the incredible power of your mind and positive thinking, and you must use this force to self-heal. By creating prostress in your life, challenging yourself to meet your goals, serious and fun, and focusing on all you can do (much more than what you can't), not only are you going to enjoy your life, yourself, and other people more, but you'll also optimize your mind-body power, the strongest "medicine" of all. Share this with people in your life and tell them you're surrounding yourself with positive things, thoughts, and people and that they have to join the bandwagon if they want to go along for the ride. Okay, you might be thinking, this positive stuff is good for you, but what about the terrible, painful things that happen? What do you do then? Quite simply, you do the best you can at the time. By using tools from this book, having a strong support network, forming a SHOC team you trust, and using your incredible mind-body healing power, you'll be prepared should these "terrible, painful" things happen. By feeling constantly anxious or depressed, expecting the worst, spending life worrying, giving up, or not striving for growth or meaning, you're also preparing yourself for these things to occur. In fact, as a payoff, you may be able to say, "See, I was right; there's no reason to be positive about anything," but the losses you've created overpower any glory of "being right." You'll have lost days and months of joyful time with others, learning new skills, feeling your positive power, and healing yourself. Don't let this happen because after all, when we look back on our lives, most distress comes from regrets for the things we didn't do.

The Hard Job of Caretaking

As you may have guessed, women are the primary caretakers (73 percent are female). The number of caregivers is three times greater than it was a mere ten years ago, and the value of caretakers' contribution to society ranges from $113 to 286 billion (Sobel and Ornstein 1998). Caretakers greatly lower societal costs overall, but they often end up shouldering a heavy financial and emotional load. One fact is certain: caretakers save society a lot of money. Unfortunately, little attention is given to the critical role of carertaker, and I again wonder whether this results from the fact that women predominate in this area. What do you think?

Family, Significant Others, and Caretakers

Chronic illness affects family relationships, roles, and responsibilities. People differ greatly in their ability to adapt to and accept changes, but most have some difficulty and conflict with these areas of life with a chronic illness. The more difficulty you and/or your family have, the more distress and symptom severity you'll experience. Please know that some of these changes are normal, predictable, and often necessary parts of a family's efforts to reestablish a new equilibrium. This knowledge will prepare you and even help you gain some control over certain situations; however, realize that neither you nor your family can completely control the situation or prevent necessary changes. Your second goal is to be informed as to what to expect, how you can influence how things proceed, and how you can control the only things you truly can—your thoughts and deeds. Also, while change is inevitable, realize that you can aim for positive goals around your family's shifting dynamics. Many of us with ARCs look back regretfully, comparing the past with the present. While some differences are true, watch for the human tendency to glorify the past and recall only the best times: past comparisons such as "I used to have enough energy to work for hours, then go out, play, exercise. I needed little sleep but when it was time to sleep, I easily did so. I got so far because I pushed myself. I did so much for myself, which is the only way to really get things done right"; and current negative thinking like "I can sum it all up easily: I can't . . . I'll never again . . . I'll always be in pain; I can't stand it anymore. Why me? I must have been so bad or life is so unfair, what's the point of living?"

We like to see ourselves as independent, strong, healthy, intelligent, and productive. When illness strikes, we often think we're no longer any of these things. There are obvious losses when you develop a chronic illness or pain, and grief is a normal, natural response. Refer to chapter 5 for more on typical reactions, like the model of denial, anger, bargaining, depression, and acceptance. How we feel affects our relationships with others. If we're in the denial stage, our family may become irate with us for stubbornly trying to act or do as much as before. We may forget medications, keep pushing and working, eat what we aren't suppposed to, and so on. Recall my TID client and how close she came to death on several occasions due to denial. Her husband was furious and terrified about losing her, but began to think he might have to leave because he couldn't bear seeing what she did to herself. We're not the only ones who feel a sense of loss. While it's difficult, a great way to beat depression and reduce pain is for us to get *out* of our heads and focus on others, our third goal.

In addition to sadness, we're also going to experience and exhibit much anger. In fact, for some of us, it's easier to express anger than to admit sadness. Also, we're often very angry at what "fate has dealt us" or at ourselves for somehow "causing" our illness. The anger reaction is quite hard on your family. When you're in pain or feeling a bit sorry for yourself, your fuse is understandably much shorter than usual. Anything a family member or friend does or says can trigger an outburst of rage, causing them confusion if they're unaware that it isn't them or their behavior that is causing your rage. You yourself may not realize it until later. Get a head start and avoid much shared pain by understanding that your anger can stem from suppressing sadness, blaming yourself, and ATs like "it's not fair." It's a threat to your ego integrity (and possibly your life) to be diagnosed with an ARC. What is a response to a threat? One is anger and attack. Of course, running and hiding is preferred by some and comes into play in the denial stage. It's hard to control yourself from lashing out and being irritable when you're in pain or distressed, but such behavior certainly doesn't help your victim, and if the pattern continues, you're increasing the risk of losing the relationship. Your fourth goal, then, is to communicate with your loved ones and friends. Tell them what you're thinking and feeling and explain how this affects your actions. Reassure them that it isn't them or their behavior (unless it is and your anger is warranted). Your fifth goal is to stop lashing out, making others furious with you and increasing your self-anger and self-loathing. To change your behavior, start by examining your thinking and resulting feelings with your cognitive tools. Don't suppress your feelings, but get in touch with them, label them, and express them in ways that aren't harmful to yourself or others.

I've noticed a mirroring of phases of feelings by patients and their loved ones. You feel a loss of control over your body, your health, and your doctors, and your family experiences a loss of control over their ability to help and protect you and over their power to keep things the way they were. Denial is also shared by you and your family. It's difficult—if not impossible—for you to accept in a brief period the many meanings of being diagnosed with an ARC. Your family also may be unable to grasp the whole meaning or even aspects of the fact that you, a beloved family member, has "this thing." Sometimes a family's denial is more complete and long-lasting than an ARC patient's. Anger, another phase after diagnosis, may be directed at yourself, family, friends, doctors, God, and your ARC itself. Instead of taking it out on others, take it out on your pillow, write or draw your anger, or scream at the top of your voice. Your family may also feel irrational anger toward you, so be prepared to talk about it. You and your family may also share shame. You may be ashamed of your ARC or what you perceive as weakness, of not being the perfect, invincible person you portrayed, of no longer being the caretaker but now needing care while your family may be ashamed when the going gets hard, as it inevitably does. They're exhausted, and wish silently that they could escape. Some family members may be ashamed if they first reacted like so many do; namely, by denying the condition and seeing it as being all in your head or as a way to shirk responsibility. Finally, thoughts and feelings about your own mortality will arise. The same issue comes to the minds of your family. People don't like thinking of such painful things, and you may find your family or friends pulling away. Just when you need them most for support and assistance, they may withdraw, stop speaking, or become busy with outside activities. Bring it out into the open and talk about it. With your knowledge of what is going on, you can speak to them from a point of understanding and awareness.

Sharing Knowledge

There are several other goals to pursue to help you and your family/friend caretakers anticipate and defuse potential conflicts. One of these is the sharing of knowledge. One of the most useful exercises you and your family can do is to develop an appropriate understanding of feelings, beliefs, expectations, and experiences on both sides. For example, sharing with your family the stages you're likely to pass through helps reduce their self-blame or guilt if they mistakenly think they're to blame for your anger, depression, and the like. They'll also be more likely to let you take things at your own pace when they know denial is a normal part of reacting to news of your chronic illness or constant pain. You'll also benefit from learning their fears, expectations, and frustrations. This isn't a time to engage in mind-reading, as there is too much potential pain and too much at stake.

Communication

Communication is another controllable aspect of the chronic illness experience that, if not dealt with directly and purposefully, is a frequent causes of breakups, divorces, and lost friendships. By developing your comminication skills, you can draw your family closer rather than further apart, as often happens when communication fails because of changes in family members or family dynamics. Let your loved ones and friends know what is going on with you at different points in your life. If they're behaving in ways that are truly disturbing to you (and you've determined that this isn't part of your shorter-than-normal fuse), you must talk to them about it. How you talk is very important, as you don't want to put others immediately on the defensive. A good way to ask for changes on their part without their feeling attacked is: "When you do _____ , it makes me feel _____ . If you could do _____ , this would benefit you by _____ as well as me by _____ ."

Let's take a concrete example. If your husband's concern is manifested by constantly checking your medications, or repeatedly reminding you about your doctors' appointments or doing your physical therapy, you may begin to feel angry, controlled, and resentful. Rather than suppressing these feelings until you explode over a minor issue, handle it early. You might say, "When you keep checking up on me, it makes me feel like a child and as if you're trying to control me. If you could ask me once a day about these things, I'll be less resentful and angry and won't lash out at you as I have lately. I'll appreciate your caring and it will make both of us feel better." Also encourage family and friends' efforts to communicate by listening closely and verbally expressing your appreciation for their efforts. You may not always agree with what they're saying, but show them that you'd rather hear this than nothing. Watch for warning signs of withering communication: prolonged silences, superficial talk, withdrawal, spending more time away from you, and/or tendencies on both parts to get defensive. Communication can worsen during chronic illness if those close to you don't understand your disorder or what you're going through and you choose not to share such information.

Sometimes communication is so poor and inflexible it's advisable to seek professional help. A psychologist or other expert can listen and watch your family's communication and areas of blocked communication. She can point out what the errors are as they are occurring, act as a mediator, teach family and friends to declare a "time-out" when things are heading toward an argument, and offer specific suggestions and reinforcement in "real time." Another way to increase the likelihood that you'll communicate is to schedule a "talk-time." Establish simple rules, such as no interruptions, cross-talks, or personal attacks. Everybody gets a turn to speak and the mediator, who may change each week if desired, makes sure no single person dominates the session.

Communication can also go awry if someone doesn't want to speak about events or feelings that frighten them or they mistakenly believe will frighten the other. My client Irene is terrified about the need for another operation, but each time she tries to speak of it to her husband, he withdraws or becomes angry and leaves the room. Irene is bewildered, tells herself he no longer loves her due to her illness, and has become severely depressed. At the same time, her husband is berating himself for his behavior. He is so anxious about Irene's health that he can't tolerate hearing about it, let alone about operations! Trained by parents, schools, books, movies, and other sources that men don't express emotions, he is too frightened to listen to his wife for fear he'll "break down" and let his emotions get the better of him. Furthermore, he has always had good health and hasn't thought about his own death. Irene's condition keeps bringing this issue to mind, and he becomes increasingly focused on his own mortality. Of course, this fear-based scenario can work in the opposite direction. The ill individual may be so fearful about her health and future that even when loved ones want to share her burden and give her support, she withdraws and tells them it's not their business. Inside, though, she's torn by maintaining denial and her desires to accept the help and concern of her family and friends.

Are you ready to talk yet? It's hard, but the benefits greatly surpass the efforts. Since you know the other best yourself, you can arrange an appropriate time for talking, present information in a way this person can comprehend, share your feelings and thoughts, and elicit as much from them as possible. Use behavioral examples of what they're doing or how they've changed and what admittedly are your perceptions and feelings about this. Ask for clarification. Be slightly confrontational if this is how this person operates. Tread gently with those who are shy.

Division of Labor

Another change better addressed than left to work itself out involves division of labor. Many ARC patients pride themselves on autonomy and their ability to function well by and for themselves. I'm not saying this inevitably disappears when an ARC develops, but based on the severity and type of ARC, you may not be able to do as much for yourself or others as you did before. It's tempting to keep trying to carry most of the load around the house, with the children, at work, and so on, as this helps us maintain the image of ourselves as healthy and independent. However, when we do this, we often end up paying the severe price of increased pain, fatigue, symptoms, and even injury. What to do? Ask for help. These three simple words cause many women unnecessary agony. Give it a try and you'll see your fears were extreme. Kids, spouses, partners, and friends are often delighted to help, so this can be a win-win situation. It doesn't mean you're lazy or trying for a free ride, nor does it mean you'll become spoiled and lose all interest in doing anything for yourself. It does mean you're serious about taking care of yourself and want to lead a satisfying, healthy life. If those whom you ask are resentful or berate you for exaggerating your symptoms, they may need some education about your ARC. If this doesn't help, this person isn't the supportive, empathic individual you need in your SHOC. This is a source of negativity you can control, and while it's very hard, it's important for your healing and growth to do so. The strength to let go of those who aren't supportive or helpful is mentioned often by women as one of the greatest lessons learned from their ARCs.

Issues on the Job

For some, the decision about working is straightforward. If you're greatly incapacitated, if days go by when you can't get out of bed, if you can't sit for more than ten to fifteen minutes, if you can't stand for more than a few minutes, if your job is labor intensive and requires physical strength and endurance you don't currently have, if you have significant cognitive disruptions, if your manual dexterity is no longer sufficient, if you're overly sensitive to chemicals or other stimuli in your workplace, or if your so depressed or anxious about your condition and life that your functional impairment is severe, you're decision about taking time off or leaving your job will be more clear. I'm not saying your decision will be any easier or less painful, but there will be greater restrictions on the likelihood of your ability to continue working. This is especially true if your employer isn't willing or able to make changes to the work environment or your job so you can keep working while still being "cost-effective."

For others, the decision is very difficult given the fluctuating nature of many ARCs. One day we feel hopeless, helpless, and as if we can't continue another day, and the next we may feel we've been given a pardon and our energy and old productive selves have returned. It's sad that social institutions like social security and disability and the business world still secretly hang on to Theory X when it comes to humans and work. Theory X purports that people are basically lazy and must be prodded to work. Most ARC patients who turn to such institutions couldn't be further from thoughts like how to take advantage of the system and how to avoid working for as long as possible. When we must turn to such designated places for services, we're repeatedly up against cold, uncaring employees of huge organizations who want to provide as little as possible. Payments are inevitably late, often wrong (underpaid), phone calls aren't returned, and efforts are to make us feel guilty and needy . . . who in their right mind would voluntarily choose to go through this type of torture? If there were some way to put legislators, attorneys, social security workers, and the like into our lives for a few weeks, even a few days, I'm sure most social programs for the physically and emotionally disabled would be quickly and completely changed. Those on the other side simply don't believe that most of us who don't work want to . . . desperately. I try to help such clients watch for irrational ATs: "It's not fair. I didn't choose this. First I can't work and now they put me through this?" or "Maybe I do deserve this kind of treatment. After all, I can't even do a day's work anymore. What use am I?" If you have such thoughts, use your cognitive tools to squirrel them out and subject them to scrutiny, looking for any evidence to support them. For example, recall the danger of thinking "it's not fair." No, it may not be fair, but the world isn't a "fair" place; sometimes you're on the upswing and sometimes you're on the downswing. Okay, so it's not fair and you didn't ask for your illness and related losses. But here they are. It's time to accept reality, stop wishing for the past, and look for ways to grow, thrive, and make your life better in any ways possible.

Many employers are biased against hiring those with disabilities because they're unaware of their many benefits. Share these with them: 1) many employers think such employees will often be sick and miss work, but in fact evidence show the opposite is generally true; 2) such workers are often more loyal, and when they see that a company values them for what they *can* do, they're more dedicated and perform better than others; and, 3) such employees have better organization and time management skills, greater societal responsibility, and more flexibility.

If I Stay or If I Go

Careers are a part of our lives we use to understand, create, and communicate "who we are" to ourselves and others. Chronic illness may cause vast changes in this realm of "self" based on illness type, severity, beliefs, personality, financial issues, job type, and workplace flexibility. Given these factors, there may be work options to ask, negotiate, or fight for (part-time work, job-sharing, different type of work, ergonomic changes). If such chances don't exist at your workplace and you wish to keep working, you must search for or create your own.

Many ARC symptoms, pain, and fatigue, even if intermittent, will be noticeable to others at work. You may struggle with whether to keep hiding your condition or "confess." You may well have to speak to your employer about physical and mental changes and tolerances if they truly disrupt your performance. Hopefully this won't jeopardize your job; while there are certain legal protections, there are also unscrupulous people. You may do well to see a specialist who helps people cope with job demands based on the type and degree of impairment. Occupational therapists watch you in your work environment and make suggestions about your workplace layout, timing of job duties, and tools or ways to improve your productivity while reducing excess stress and physical strain. Physical therapists can design treatment plans with specific exercises to boost your strength, mobility, and endurance on the job. Your SHOC doc can help by suggesting medications to improve sleep, decrease anxiety or depression, reduce pain, and achieve other changes that will help you to optimize your work abilities. Don't forget the value of consulting with alternative health experts who may suggest or offer services like massage, biofeedback, vitamins and herbs, acupuncture, and so on. Of course, remember that you are the most powerful source of tools—practice your meditation, hypnosis, imagery, positive thinking, humor, and so on. Recall that you optimize your abilities by maximizing your mind-body health and following a holistic approach.

Your illness, symptoms, work environment, or job type may be such that you can't remain at your job. This situation and self-perceived failure, loss, and low self-esteem can trigger severe distress. As you know, long-term arousal and tension from distress can permanently alter your mind-body state. While it may not be feasible to stay where you are, it doesn't mean you must give up work altogether, although if this is the case you must be honest with yourself and accept this for whatever time period is necessary. You'll find there are always things you can do to contribute, learn, and grow. Your challenge will be different; namely, to search out areas of interest and find ways to use the abilities and talents you have. The inability to work may hit women in their mid-forties and younger more forcefully. These are the generations who were told they could and should have it all. Many of us have incorporated into our selves external expectations that we must marry, raise perfect children, make delicious meals, work a full-time meaningful job, volunteer, ensure our partner's happiness, and look youthful and attractive throughout this walk through the rose garden. For those of you in this group, accepting that you can't work can be very hard.

Exercise: Exploring the Meaning of Work in Your Life

Take some time now to do some writing in your journal on the following: Who are you if you remove the big piece of the pie assigned to "career woman"? What do you talk about with friends who are still working? What do you say when people ask what you do? What can you do if you're irrationally obsessing that you're being a "bad example" for your daughters? If you loved your career and got prostress and meaning from it, what can you do now? What about real issues of your family's decreased income?

These and many more questions are voiced by my clients. As my client Janet describes "I always immediately hop into bed with anxiety." We catastrophize, personalize, think in black and white . . . we're failures, losers, no good, worthless, unattractive, stupid . . . take your pick. While it's irrational, this self-talk is typical at first. However, you're in danger if you let yourself stay there too long. What can you do? Use your new tools to examine irrational ATs and see how they directly intensify depression, hopelessness, anxiety, and the like.

AT	Feelings	Cognitive Distortions	Revised or New Thoughts
1. I loved that job. I'll never find a good job again.	Depression Anger Helplessness	Forecasting	I'm not ready to work full time now but I'll explore part-time options. I made a lot of good connections throught that job—when I feel better, I can pursue those. I also learned a lot there; I may be able to do some independent consulting now.
2.			
3.			

Do you think it's inevitable that you'll never work again? Is this really true, or what is the likelihood that it's true? When you think of work, are you only thinking of your current job or your previous jobs? What other jobs match your interests and abilities? Write, without censoring, on these questions and on the following: a) your dream job(s); b) skills and abilities you'd like to use or develop; c) elements of past jobs you liked and those you haven't; and d) meaning and values you want in your work. Now, write about new issues and considerations you face associated with your health status. Be honest but not overly critical. Be specific. For example: being a courier involves activities x, y, and z. What might stand in my way, physically and mentally, of doing these? What accommodations could be made by me or the company so I could do the job? If this job seems unlikely, is there any related job in which I might be interested?

Confront your fear head on by spinning out the worst-case scenarios. What happens? Do you get fired? Are you unable to find work? Are you destroyed or might you live through it? What can you do? Get help if you need it, and talk to people who love and respect you and have your best interests at heart.

Legal and Financial issues

Let's use FMS as an ARC example that might interfere with your ability to work. As is typical of ARCs, FMS fluctuates, and some people, despite intermittent or constant but moderate fatigue and pain, can continue working for years, while others are so disabled they can no longer work. FMS is a good example, given its continued controversial nature and the fact that people with FMS may look normal while feeling terrible. If you're working and develop FMS, your employer or insurance company, not wanting to cover this "controversial" condition, might demand to see test results and doctors' reports clearly indicating its presence. Many typical tests show up as normal, so you'll need an FMS expert who knows what tests are best. FMS is also a good example to use because it can result from physical trauma, such as a job-related accident. Here you'll be in for a big battle if you apply for workers' compensation or disability benefits. Don't be surprised if you're sent on rounds of visits to disbelieving doctors. Negative stress may also be a trigger for FMS and other ARCs, and again, you'll need to prepare for a battle if you believe your job or work environment is the distressor. In most of these cases, your best bet is to add to your SHOC team an attorney well-versed in FMS (or your ARC) and experienced in battling with the forces that be. A good reference for these issues for all people with ARC is Devin Starlanyl's *The Fibromyalgia Advocate*.

CHAPTER 17

Tools for the Journey

The real voyage of discovery consists not in seeking new landscapes but in having new eyes.

—Marcel Proust

The first part of this chapter discusses aspects of the pain experience plus general recommendations for reducing pain. Specific tools for pain management are covered in each individual ARC chapter and in appendix II. There are a number of points along the pain pathways at which things can go awry and where you can apply mind-body techniques to reduce pain. One of the reasons for the difficulty in finding effective pain reduction, management, or elimination techniques is that "pain" itself is incredibly complex and refers to multiple aspects of an objective and subjective experience.

The Pain Experience

When an illness or injury causes harm to the body, there are several aspects of the body's natural response that may backfire and worsen the experience of pain. For example, when you have an injury, the nerves in that area and in surrounding areas send signals to the brain advising caution in that area. Thus, nerves around the area may become overly sensitized and begin reacting to stimuli as if they were painful when in fact the level of the stimulus wouldn't typically be experienced as painful. In addition, the neurotransmitter called substance P, in charge of sending signals of pain through your spinal cord's "pain gate," is generally well-balanced by normal, healthy levels of the body's painkillers (endorphins) and serotonin. As you recall, serotonin deficiencies are apparent in various ARCs and endorphins may be low due to lack of exercise. Adding to the imbalance are higher than normal levels of substance P in some ARCs, such as FMS. Dr. Dharma Khalsa explains that pain signals can "'jam open' the pain gates . . . as pain signals become engraved on the nervous system." Pain after physical trauma can also increase when the muscles surrounding the injured area become tense, and over time, may go through structural changes, which themselves can cause pain. Besides injuries, initial pain can also arise as part of the disease process. For example, the growth hormone deficits and sleep disturbances of FMS cause problems in removing waste from muscles and repairing muscle tears. The inflammatory response is another natural body response that's typically part of the body's self-healing. However, it can backfire and increase pain, and it's central in ARCs. The pain response has interesting components as well:

- One central aspect of the pain experience that is generally insufficiently discussed by health professionals and their clients involves the effects of the client's subjective feelings of fear, anxiety, depression, hopelessness, frustration, and the like on her pain level. The mind-body unity is clearly illustrated here, as negative emotional states worsen the physical states, such as through increasing the intensity, frequency, and duration of pain. The process just emphasizes that mind and body are two sides of the same coin.

- Another element of the mind-body equation with respect to pain involves certain beliefs an individual can hold. For example, having information and the belief that one has even some degree of control over their situation and illness (although this may not even be the case) can decrease the perception of the intensity and duration of pain. Telling people that they must continue to exercise at a strenuous pace without giving them any sense of the duration of the painful experience leads to reports of a much higher level of pain than when the people are given some information (and thus also some sense of control) about the remaining duration of the distressing experience.

- There is an aspect of chronic illness that seems to cause a catch-22 situation vis-à-vis the experience of pain: The existing intensity of pain and/or the physical damages resulting from the illness understandably reduce the amount of physical activity and exercise a woman pursues, and as a result, her muscles weaken and her body loses its conditioning. Consequently, when she does participate in even relatively mild activities, she may find her body screaming out in pain. This situation also opens the door for further pain, because reduced muscle strength and body conditioning increase the likelihood of reinjuries or even new injuries.

- Each day it seems we are getting closer and closer to discovering methods to control chronic pain. For example, a recent article, "Scientists Make Pain Relief Strides" by Paul Recer in *AP Science Writer*, November 18,

1999, described a biological "smart bomb" that combines a natural protein with a toxin to permanently block chronic pain without the typical side effects of narcotics. Specific nerve cells that cause chronic pain have been isolated and a drug that interferes specifically with these nerve cells while leaving others untouched has been identified. It's now known that chronic pain stems from less than 2 percent of spinal cord neurons! As mentioned, chronic pain is transmitted through substance P, and when this was combined with a particular neurotoxin, the rats that were studied were totally relieved of chronic pain but still responded to other stimuli. Tests musts still be performed on animals such as monkeys prior to testing with humans, but intial results seem promising!

EMDR (Eye Movement Desensitization Reprocessing)

The last several years have seen a rapid growth in exploration of the therapeutic technique known as eye movement desensitization reprocessing (EMDR). Initially, this technique was used primarily to treat individuals with post-traumatic stress disorder, who had experienced severe trauma or crises. More recently, interest has broadened to include the use of EMDR to treat individuals with chronic pain. EMDR has a strong base in neurological processes, and certain similarities have been found in this arena between PTSD and chronic pain. For example, similar neurological changes and processes have been observed in the brains of individuals experiencing PTSD and those experiencing chronic pain. Brain areas involved include the amygdala, the thalamus, the anterior cingulate cortex, and the right cerebral hemisphere. EMDR seems to work based on the fact that bilateral eye movements or other sensory stimulation, when combined with controlled orienting processes, allows incorrectly processed information to be reprocessed correctly (i.e., involving activation of the whole brain rather than just part of it). I myself have used EMDR to help clients work through moderate to severe traumas, as well as to effectively reduce chronic pain, migraines, and muscle tension. This technique is in its early days, but from my personal experience and reviewing the literature, I highly recommend this procedure for some cases. Remember that you must seek treatment from certified trained professionals. You can search for professionals by contacting EMDRIA (see appendix I).

Pain Clinics

Some of you may want to explore or attend a pain clinic. There are some good, comprehensive pain management treatment centers available these days. Refer to the section in chapter 12 on FMS for a description of some such centers and the range of holistic treatments they offer these days. It's essential that you conduct a thorough prescreening before you spend your time, energy, and financial resources. Firstly, you want to ensure that the center is of high quality and well-staffed with educated, experienced people. Also, given the nature of ARCs, it's essential that you get a comprehensive, holistic treatment regimen with the many components already discussed in this book. In addition, you may want to steer clear of those whose focus is solely on getting clients off their pain medications. While this may be one of a number of admirable goals for you down the road, it's also possible that you require medication at present to get you to a state where you can concentrate and learn so that you can continue functioning in various areas of your life. Very few of us choose to stay on medications for the long term, though many medical professionals don't seem to understand this, particularly when it comes to pain medications. Again, you may need to remind your SHOC doctors that significantly less than 1 percent of patients with chronic pain ever end up abusing their pain medications. You'll also want to ensure that the center is a good one by making sure it's been approved by the Commission on Accreditation for Rehabilitation Facilities (CARF). This provides a minimal guarantee that the center is a good one, not to mention the fact that most insurance companies, if they cover pain management centers at all, don't cover those without such accreditation.

Oh, Sweet Sleep!

Sleep is one of the most effective treatments you'll find, as it's central to mind-body rejuvenation and repair. In some ARCs, like FMS and CFIDS, poor sleep contributes to and maintains symptoms like muscle pain, fatigue, and cognitive distortions. Of course, proper sleep is beneficial to all people with ARCs. While there are several phases of sleep, marked by different brain wave lengths, problems seem to arise primarily from deficiencies of two of these. Insufficient REM (dream) sleep can lead to various psychological problems. Delta sleep deficiencies lead to insufficient growth hormone, which is central in repairing minute tears of our muscles each day as we do our daily activities. When such repairs don't occur, we experience constant muscle aches and pains.

Many of you who are searching for alternative treatments have probably heard about melatonin, a current favorite of the media and health-related vendors. Apparently it is now the top selling product in health food stores, even outselling our favorite long-term panacea, vitamin C. The claims that motivate most people to purchase this substance are promises of improved sleep and help with jet lag. Many people believe melatonin is harmless because it is a natural hormone. But as you know, the body functions best and most healthfully when systems and substances are balanced. It's best to check with your SHOC doctor before including melatonin in your regimen. While melatonin may help you sleep, it has various other effects on the body. For instance, melatonin interacts in certain ways with our immune system as it works through hormones and neurotransmitters, such as serotonin. You have read by now of the importance of having normal amounts of serotonin in the body; when serotonin and other neurotransmitters are out of balance, disorders like FMS and SLE are affected. In fact, decreases in serotonin lead to decreased efficacy of the body's natural pain killers, the endorphins, and lesser amounts of the serotonin-derived neurotransmitters that reduce pain, such as epinephrine and dopamine. In addition, low amounts of serotonin are associated with increased "pain neurotransmitter," substance P.

Some experts don't recommend melatonin for those with ARCs like SLE or RA (Rosenfeld 1996). You must check with your SHOC experts first, because there are too many unknowns about ARCs and melatonin to assume it's a good mix. There are natural ways to maximize your body's melatonin without taking supplements. Follow three simple rules: Don't consume caffeine (coffee, some teas, colas, chocolate, medications) or other stimulants, which interfere with natural melatonin production and disrupt healthy sleep; set a regular schedule for your meals, because your body's melatonin production is linked with its natural cycles and circadian rhythms; and avoid strenuous activites prior to bedtime. If you have sleep problems, avoid medicines like aspirin and ibuprofen, certain muscle relaxants, antidepressants, and seizure medicines. Discuss these with your SHOC docs, as you may need a different prescription or changes in the times you take the medication. Timing your meals is important, because eating large, heavy meals a few hours before bedtime can interfere with good, continuous sleep. Alcohol also greatly disrupts healthy sleep in part by triggering two mechanisms: snoring and obstructive sleep apnea. Both conditions are more likely if you are overweight.

Another great way to ensure a good night's sleep (besides a good pair of earplugs) is exercise. Studies show that even moderate exercise can improve the quality and quantity of sleep. Morning exercise is best, but if that's not possible, make sure you don't exercise later than four to five hours before bedtime. As with all mind-body techniques discussed here, this is based on balance. Obviously, if your body gets the exercise it needs, it's much more likely to balance this by getting the rest and recovery it needs. Several other factors interfere with our ability to sleep well: hormonal and neurotransmitter imbalances; pain intruding into sleep and awakening us or making it difficult for us to fall asleep at all; and our minds' merry-go-round of worries, fears, disappointments, and sadness about our illnesses and life changes. For the latter two reasons for poor sleep, PR, DB, visualization, thought stopping, and cognitive techniques presented in earlier sections are invaluable.

Several nutritional remedies can improve sleep. Many of you may have heard of L-tryptophan, an essential amino acid that used to be available in the U.S. as an over-the-counter remedy for sleep difficulties. It is no longer available as a supplement, but you can derive some from natural food sources: milk, cottage cheese, bananas, peanuts, meat, fish, turkey, and other protein-rich foods. In addition, given the importance of serotonin in REM sleep, you can take vitamin B6 (100 mg) and niacinamide (100 mg), which together produce serotonin. Another option is to take one chelated magnesium and calcium supplement three times per day plus three tabs one-half hour before going to sleep (Mindell 1985). Two herbs with sleep-enhancing qualities are valerian root and skullcap.

Ergonomics and Body-Saving Techniques

Only fairly recently has attention been paid to the impact of poorly designed work spaces on individuals who must operate for hours at a time in these areas. With the onslaught of people developing carpal tunnel syndrome and other injuries from repetitive motions, ergonomics is finally being taken seriously. The design of your work and home spaces is incredibly important in terms of increasing or decreasing your pain experience and fatigue. One of the first questions you need to ask yourself is where you spend the majority of your hours during the day. List average times and activities/locations to get a clear picture for yourself. Then examine the area in which you perform these activities. What are you doing in these areas . . . stretching, lifting, sitting, hunching over, standing on your feet? If you're doing your journaling and noting activities and elements that increase pain, you'll be able to note any associations between activities you do and increased pain and tension. Then examine your living or work space to see if modifications may make your activities physically easier and less strenuous or repetitive.

Some examples to ask yourself include:

- When I am writing or reading correspondence, where do I sit? Does this chair or sofa give me enough back support? What happens to my neck as I read? Am I bending over and straining my neck and back?

- Am I in charge of putting groceries away? If so, do I have to reach to the upper cabinets? You may want to be in charge of items stored lower and have someone else do the upper items. If you live alone, think about relocating where you store items or have a safe stepstool and use it every time you are lifting and reaching up.

- One of the biggest offenders for women with FMS is the vacuum cleaner. Newer models are significantly lighter and more effective than older types. If you can afford it, this purchase would be well worth it. If you can't, find someone—a friend, a loved one, a child who wants his allowance, or a neighbor's child who wants to earn some coins—to help out.

- If you have to pick up even moderately heavy items from the floor or low areas, lower your center of gravity, balance your weight on both legs and lift from your leg and thigh muscles, which are stronger than your back and neck muscles. When possible, get help from others.

- Avoid the tendency to overdo it when you're feeling physically better. Don't do what Cara, one of my FMS clients, used to do when she felt better—washing, drying, and folding four loads of laundry (including blankets and towels)! One day at a time, one load at a time.

- How long do you spend on a computer? This is one of the greatest offenders in increasing ARC pain and fatigue. If you spend more than a few minutes a day on a computer, it's essential that your work space be correctly designed. With respect to the keyboard, your forearms should be parallel to the floor and you should not be reaching down or up. A sign that your chair is too low and that you're reaching up is pain spreading between the shoulders and in the neck. Raise your chair or lower your table. If your feet aren't resting flat on the floor and your thighs aren't parallel to the floor, your chair is too high and you will be straining your back and throwing off your alignment. Through the years, I've used a series of footstools, empty boxes, trashcans on their sides, or a stack of books to keep my feet at the right level. Purchase a wrist rest for your keyboard. Although they're ostensibly for the wrists, I find that using this helps ease the pain from my wrists, up my arms, to my shoulders and neck! Dr. Marilyn Ekdahl Ravicz designed a board with two armrests that lie on either side of your rib cage. The board is held in place by the keyboard and you can rest each entire arm on the "armrests." This tool has made one of the biggest differences to me in terms of the time I can spend on the computer without intensifying my pain. If you use one of these armrest boards, you do not need a chair with armrests. If you don't have such a tool, get a chair with good armrests. Another central factor in either increasing or decreasing your pain and productivity relates to the back support of the chair and where you sit on the chair. Push yourself all the way to the back of the chair so that the backrest supports you. Often, unless you have an ergonomically designed chair that fits you well, there will be insufficient support for your lower back. I have used a roll pillow purchased in an Asian goods store to place right behind my lower back to provide lumbar support. However, I've also used rolled up sweatshirts (generally my husband's as they are larger), as well as towels and bedsheets. As you can tell, there are a variety of tools you can purchase that can be of immense benefit. However, while many of us do not have the financial ability to purchase all of these innovative products, most of us do own things like pillows, books, empty boxes, towels, and the like. Be creative and be careful.

- Whenever you're seated for over fifteen minutes or even briefer periods if necessary, get up, move, walk around, and do stretches, such as gentle neck rolls to the left and right sides. Make sure to hold your chin in as you tilt your head to the right, hold for 20 seconds, and release. Don't go so far that it is painful, just go far enough that you feel a stretch and you don't experience great discomfort. Perform this again for the other side.

- One of the most difficult things for me to accept about my ARCs was how difficult it became to travel. This had been my number-one joy and I had traveled extensively around the world from childhood to my late twenties. After my ARCs worsened, car rides longer than twenty to thirty minutes became painful, and plane rides (let alone trying to drag luggage around the airport) were a nightmare. I've heard similar tales from others with chronic illnesses and pain. There are a number of things you can do to make traveling less of a travail. If it is a car trip, minimize the time you're the driver. Arrange the luggage and children in the car so that you can recline the front seat quite far back, and bring some pillows or towels to place behind your lower back or arrange around your neck and head as discomfort dictates. You may be on a tight schedule, but make sure to take stops to get out of the car and do some stretches. It's really not worth it to arrive a bit earlier feeling fatigued and in pain. You aren't going to get much out of your visit that way! With respect to air travel, the most important thing you can do is pack lightly. After you do this several times and experience the difference in discomfort, you won't need any further convincing. In addition, purchase luggage with rollers . . . what an invention! When you board the plane, don't try to store your luggage in the overhead bins. There are usually friendly passengers who will volunteer or gladly help when asked. If nobody is available, ask the flight attendant to help you. If you are feeling extremely fatigued or in great pain, you may want to speak to the boarding attendant. Tell them what is going on and they will generally let you be among the first to board. This will give you some calm time to locate your seat, place your bag below, locate help for the overhead bin, and find pillows and blankets. Always request an aisle seat so you have room to stretch and can get up often.

- Finally, this may be more difficult than learning to pack lightly, but here goes . . . get rid of your heavy purses. The larger your purse, the more heavy stuff you will cram into it, and the more pain you'll cause yourself. Buy a small purse and carry only *essentials*. Backpacks, lightly loaded, can be helpful in dispersing the weight over both shoulders rather than on one. If men can manage to get around without a purse, we certainly can too.

- There are a number of tools and instruments available that are labor and energy-saving, and that allow you to reassert some of your previous independence without throwing you into a state of extreme pain. See appendix I for referrals and resources.

Assertiveness and Communication Training

A pattern I've often seen in those with long-term or chronic illnesses, particularly women, is difficulties with setting personal boundaries and being assertive. As I saw written on a refrigerator magnet, of all places, "Stress is what happens when your gut says 'no' and your mouth says, 'Of course, I'd love to.'" Does this strike a chord with any of you? Why do a lack of assertiveness and this mile-long valley between our guts and our mouths characterize women so frequently? Recall the discussions about the societal and familial messages ingrained into our impressionable minds as little girls. We are meant to be caretakers, socializers, and above all, nice. These overt and covert messages—beginning in infancy—continue throughout our lives, and combating them can be tremendously difficult. In therapy, I often help women see their involvement in this unhealthy behavioral pattern. Others realize they do it, but have difficulty stopping it. They feel shame and guilt if they "speak from their guts"; subconscious or conscious voices tell them it's wrong and they don't deserve to do it.

You must use your cognitive tools to examine these thoughts and behaviors in a rational manner. Ask yourself why you feel you don't deserve to voice your opinion or your needs, while all around you there are other people who don't feel this way. Are they truly superior to or more worthy than you? Many of my female clients' automatic thoughts would suggest so. One of my clients, Janet, was diagnosed with rheumatoid arthritis. She had already been experiencing severe fatigue and emptiness from a lifelong pattern of feeling unworthy and always helping others. She had never been able to set limits with others, as her automatic thoughts told her she was unworthy and would be unlovable if she didn't keep doing everything for others. When she developed RA and the even greater fatigue and pain "interfered" with her endless giving, she began to feel truly worthless. She became very ill; an inner conflict raged between her efforts to maintain her unhealthy giving and her mind-body needs to set limits and rest. What was important and eventually releasing in Janet's self-sabotaging behavior was her realization of her automatic thoughts: "I can't say no because I'd be a selfish person." As we explored her past as a child, she recalled that her mother viewed selfishness as an evil and damning trait. However, this wasn't the entire story. It turned out that Janet was getting a payback for behaving in this self-demeaning, self-denying way. It allowed her to feel like a martyr, which in her mind was associated with superiority over others. In this case, her mind-body couldn't continue functioning in the way she'd been demanding. When she became very ill, she finally had to listen to her mind-body. Though she had to learn to live with RA, she told me that she felt far freer and more worthy than ever before.

You can shed this unhealthy behavior by examining it cognitively and rationally. Search for the truth of the matter. Look to see if you are getting any benefits or paybacks from continuing to put others first and denying your own needs. Perhaps you're afraid that standing up for yourself will push others away and that you'll be left alone. This fear is particularly evident in people with illnesses who believe they must depend on others to take care of them. Examine the reality of this belief too. The fact is that when you're assertive, others often respect you more. Unless you confuse aggressiveness with assertiveness, it's unlikely that you're going to push your valuable friends and loved ones away unless you really work hard at it. Communicating openly and directly is the key.

What If I'm Not Getting Better?
Facts and Fallacies

You may think you're doing everything possible to improve your health and feel frustrated as you aren't improving as fast as you think you should or really aren't improving at all. If so, you need to ask yourself some difficult but necessary questions. What I'm going to discuss doesn't inevitably apply to you if you aren't improving, for after all, we're talking about real illnesses, illnesses about which, for all of our efforts, we really know very little. We're also talking about the human immune system, a very powerful system that has evolved over hundreds of thousands of years to serve as our primary defense. When this mighty complex turns its destructive power inwards, damage is inevitable. But self-healing is also part of the immune system and you have tools to use for this goal. It's often possible to reduce your symptoms and pain. If this isn't happening even when you've tried the mind-body exercises, dietary modifications, and treatments presented in this book, it's time for some inner exploration.

Illness plays a complex role in our society. The negatives of illness are many and obvious, but there can be potential gains as well. I know what a hot button this is, and you may feel anger at the mere suggestion that you'd ever want to be sick. I know I have felt this way. As I said, this issue may or may not apply to you, but it warrants looking into if you're seriously intent on healing. Nobody is watching . . . just ask yourself if there is anything you have to gain by being "sick." Perhaps there is nothing, and this is as valid a response as any. Quite distinct from this issue is one brought up earlier. Though there may be no psychological "cause" to your illness or to healing, there can still be psychological dynamics to consider when you're healing. These don't necessarily inhibit your healing, but it's best if you can think about them in as objective a way as possible. This brings us again to questions such as: "Who am I without this condition? What am I to do? What if I regress to the unhealthy stressful way of living before I had this ARC? What am I to do without excuses about being ill? With no restrictions, what if I don't become the success I expect of myself?" These are all questions that may or may not pertain to you, as they have pertained to some of my clients but not others. If one or more resonate with you, I hope you've learned the importance of writing these in your journal, holding meaningful internal dialogues, and being confrontational or supportive with yourself as the situations require. As you may have thought many times, "Life isn't fair. Why me?" How about turning such questions inside out and seeing what illness has afforded you? Of course, there is just as strong a possibility that you are striving your utmost to heal and doing everything you've been told to do and aren't improving as much as you'd like. This may be the most frustrating, painful situation of all. With our limited understanding of ARCs and with the nature of ARCs being so complex and multicausal, we just may not have the solution yet for your particular condition. However, if you follow the guidelines prescribed in this book, you will experience some relief and growth. Keep plugging away, keeping up on the most recent research available, making sure you have the best SHOC team possible, and being kind and in tune with your true self, and you'll maximize your chances of self-healing. Remember that many of us with ARCs need to redefine our goals for the here-and-now. Of course, we would all like to be cured and rid of illness, but for now this may not be possible. Until that time arrives and even then, we will gain much by focusing on what we can learn from our illnesses and how we can grow in the most joyful, healthy way possible. When the time comes that total cures are available, those of you who have followed your SHOC paths will be ready to benefit from these but will also have learned invaluable lessons from the daily reality of living with ARCs. You may feel as many of my clients have that though living with an ARC is challenging and difficult, you experience some gratitude for having learned and grown in ways you never would have had you not had such an illness.

APPENDIX I

Resources and Referrals

Certain helpful organizations and referrals transcend any one particular ARC, so it's a good idea to skim through all of the following categories.

General and Miscellaneous Information on Women's Health and ARCs

About.com
Enter this website at http://about.com/ and then go into the "health/fitness" section for extensive information on alternative/complementary medicine, disabilities, ARCs, womens health, and wellness.

Access: The Foundation for Accessibility by the Disabled
Box 356, Malverne, NY 11565 (516) 887-5798
Information on traveling for people with disabilities.

American Academy of Physical Medicine and Rehabilitation
One IBM Plaza, #2500, Chicago, IL 60611-3604 (312) 464-9700

American Association of Naturopathic Physicians
(206) 298-0125 http://www.naturopathic.org

American Autoimmune Related Diseases Association, Inc. (AARDA)
Michigan National Bank Bldg., 15475 Gratiot, Detroit, MI 48205 (313) 371-8600

American Chronic Pain Association, Inc.
Box 850, Rocklin, CA 95677 (916) 632-0922. e-mail: ACPA@pacbell.net

American College of Obstetricians & Gynecologists
409 12th St., SW, Washington, DC 20024-2188 (202) 638-5577
Information useful in making decisions re pregnancy and other issues.

American Dietetic Association
216 W. Jackson, #800, Chicago, IL 60606 (312) 899-0040
Information on nutritional requirements.

American Foundation for Pain Research
505 So. Beverly Drive, #1233, Beverly Hills, CA 90212 (800) 554-3335

American Heart Association
7272 Greenville Avenue, Dallas, TX 75231-4596 (214) 373-6300

American Holistic Medical Association
4101 Lake Boone Trail, Ste. 201, Raleigh, NC 27607 (919) 787-5181
Information, lobbying, referrals for patients.

American Silicone Implant Survivors, Inc.
1288 Cork Elm Drive, Kirkwood, MO 63122   (314) 821-0115
Information and newsletters.

Centers for Disease Control and Prevention Hot Line
(404) 332-4559. Web site with extensive information, including research, definitions, treatment, and prevention techniques, on many illnesses: www.cdc.gov

Columbia Hospital for Women Foundation
2440 M Street NW, Ste. 325, Washington, DC 20037 (202) 293-6045, fax (202) 293-7256. Works to educate and empower women. Serves health needs of all women. Conducts research, designs programs and services for use by other health organizations. Supports the exchange of ideas among health care personnel and the public.

Environmental Dental Association
9974 Scripps Ranch Blvd., Ste. 36, San Diego, CA 92131 (800) 388-8124

Equal Employment Opportunity Commission
1801 L. Street NW, Washington, DC 29507 (202) 663-4900 or (800) 772-1213
You may call this number to obtain social security disability benefits information or you may contact your local social security office and request the following pamphlets: SSA Publication #05-10029, "Disability"; Publication #05-10153, "When You Get Social Security Disability Benefits: What You Need To Know"; SSA Publication #05-11000, "SSI Supplemental Security Income."

Food Allergy Network
10400 Eaton Place #107, Fairfax, VA 22030-2208   (800) 929-4040, fax (703) 691-2713
e-mail: fan@worldweb.net Web site: http://www.foodallergy.org

Foundation for Toxic-Free Dentistry
P.O. Box 608010, Orlando, FL 32860-9010 (407) 299-4149

Healthtouch
Web site: http://www.healthtouch.com

Immune System Information
Web site: http://www.immunesupport.com/bulletins/

Institute for Research on Women's Health
1616 18 St. NW, #109, Washington DC 20009 (202) 483-8643, fax (301) 216-2157
Dedicated to research, education, and policy work related to the health and mental health of women. Gender-sensitive pharmacology and workplace abuse are among the specialties.

Institute of Women's Health, Indiana University School of Medicine
Dept of Obstetrics and Gynecology, 926 W. Michigan St., Indianapolis, IN 46202 (317) 274-2014, fax (317) 274-2014

Advocates self-care and studies women's health practices. Conducts community education research projects and sponsors educational demonstration projects.

Interactive Web site for people with ARCs

http://www.members.tripod.com/lvngwell

Jacobs Institute of Women's Health

409 12th St. SW, Washington DC 20024-2188 (202) 863-4990, fax (202) 484-5107

Works with all issues of women's health, especially with the interaction between physicians and their patients. Workshops for medical professionals and others involved with women's health. Publishes a peer-reviewed journal.

LifeCycles for Women PMS Self-Help Center

101 First St., #441, Los Altos, CA 94022 (800) 862-9876, fax (415) 965-4311

Provides education, programs, and products for women's health. Priority is given to common female health concerns including chronic fatigue syndrome, PMS, fibroids, anemia, estrogen therapy. Publishes a quarterly newsletter.

Medic Alert Foundation

Box 1009, Turlock, CA 95380 (209) 634-4917. Info on Medic Alert products, such as emergency badges for those with diabetes, allergies, etc.

Medical Matrix Guide to Internet Resources

Web site: http://www.medmatrix.org. Register and you can *hear* lectures, read the latest research, ask questions, and more!

MedicineNet

Web site: http://www.medicinenet.com

Melpomene Institute for Women's Health Research

1010 University Ave., St. Paul, MN 55104 (612) 642-1951, fax (612) 642-1871

A nonprofit, membership-based organization that studies and helps women understand links between physical activity and health. Sponsors active research center focusing on women's eating/sleeping habits, menstrual patterns, medical history, psychological well-being, attitudes toward body image, activity, and exercise. Free information to members. Research center open to nonmembers for a small fee.

National Alopecia Areata Foundation

Box 150760, San Rafael, CA 94915-0760

National Chronic Pain Outreach Association

Box 274 Millboro, VA 24460 (540) 997-5004 e-mail: ncpoal@aol.com

National Council on Women's Health

1300 York Ave., Box 52, New York, NY 10021 (212) 535-0031

Works to improve all areas of women's health through public and professional education. Sponsors conferences and publishes educational material.

National Institute of Arthritis and Musculoskeletal and Skin

Disease Information Clearinghouse (NAMISIC)

Box AMS, 9000 Rockville Pike, Bethesda, MD 20892. (301) 495-4484 or (301) 496-8188. Comprehensive information on experimental treatments, research, and more. www.nih.gov/niams/healthinfo

National Kidney Foundation

30 East 33rd St., New York, NY 10016 (800) 228-4483

National Organization of Social Security Claimants Representatives

19 East Central Ave., Pearl River, NY 10965 (800) 431-2804

National Women's Health Network

1325 G St. NW, Lower Level, Washington, DC 20005. (202) 347-1140, fax (202) 347-

1168. Devoted exclusively to women's health issues. Advocates women's involvement in the system and their right to receive informed, unbiased health care. Also seeks to educate policymakers and the public about issues involving older women and women of color.

Road Back Foundation
Important information for patients with RA, SLE, FMS, and other autoimmune diseases and related conditions: www.roadback.org

Social Security Insurance/Social Security Disability (SSD)
National Rehabilitation Information Center, 8455 Colesville Road, Ste. 935, Silver Springs, MD 20910-3319 (800) 346-2742

Traditional Healing
Web site offering information on upcoming free talks, weekend workshops, alternative healing methods and more: www.traditionalhealing.com. You can also hear important information on WBAI 99.5 FM Mondays 8-9 P.M. in New York

U.S. Equal Employment Opportunity Commission
Publication and Info. Center Box 12549, Cincinnati, OH 45212-0549. (800) 669-3362

Wholistic Health for Women
8235 Santa Monica Blvd. #308, West Hollywood, CA 90046 (213) 650-1508. A women's clinic offering a full range of wholistic alternative women's health care.

WebMD
Drug and Herbs: for information on prescriptions and nonprescription medications and herbs, medical encyclopedia, clinical trials information, and much more essential data. my.webmd.com/drug_and_herb

Wise Woman Center, Healing Intensives
P. O. Box 64, Woodstock, NY 12498 (914) 246-8081, fax (914) 246-8081.

Women.com
Women.com provides info on alternative and natural medicine, vitamins, herbs, nutrition. Also explores women's diseases and offers medical advice. www. women. com/health

Women's Health Resources
1003 W. Wellington, Chicago, IL 60657 (312) 525-1177
Offers articles, resource guides, brochures, magazines, and other materials on women's health and mental health. Topics include battered women, disabled women, stress, occupational health, and breast cancer.

Women's International Public Health Network
7100 Oak Forest Lane, Bethesda, MD 20817 (301) 469-9210. An international group of women's groups supporting the exchange of ideas on women's health. Newsletter.

MULTIPLE SCLEROSIS

Huggins Diagnostic Center
5080 List Dr., Colorado Springs, CO 80919 (719) 548-1600, fax (719) 522-0563

Multiple Sclerosis Resource Center
Offers information on MS, medical news, directories, articles, related links, etc. www. healingwell.com/ms

National Multiple Sclerosis Society
733 Third Avenue, New York, NY 10017 (212) 986-3240, (800) 344-4867
For free copies of *Inside Magazine,* for MS clients and their families.

Swank Multiple Sclerosis Clinic School of Medicine
Oregon Health Sciences University, 3181 Sam Jackson Park Road, Portland OR 97201 (503) 494-8370

RHEUMATOID ARTHRITIS

American College of Rheumatology
60 Executive Park South, Ste. 150, Atlanta, GA 30329 (404) 633-3777
Arthritis Foundation
1314 Spring Street NW, Atlanta, GA 30309 (404) 872-7100 or (800) 283-7800
You may call this number to find out about chapters closest to you in addition to a wealth of other information. The Arthritis Self-Help Course is given through this group. Call for cost and availability.
National Institute of Arthritis and Musculoskeletal and Skin Diseases Information Clearinghouse (NAMISIC)
Box AMS, 9000 Rockville Pike, Bethesda, MD 20892 (301) 495-4484 or (301) 496- 8188
Information on experimental treatments and research.
Rheumatoid Arthritis
Comprehensive information on lifestyle, nutrition, medical treatments and products, latest research studies, and more. www.healingwithnutrition.com/disease/arthritis
Rheumatoid Disease Foundation
5106 Old Harding Road, Franklin, TN 37064. Information on hundreds of doctors who work with rheumatoid arthritis and gout patients. They apply various alternative and allopathic remedies and therapies.

SYSTEMIC LUPUS ERYTHEMATOSUS

American Lupus Society
3914 Del Amo Blvd., Ste. 922, Torrance, CA 90503 (310) 542-8891
American Apitherapy Society
Hartland Four Corners, Vermont (802) 436-2708
For information regarding honeybee venom treatment.
Covermark Cosmetics
1 Anderson Ave., Monachie, NJ 07074 (800) 524-1120. Help and information on makeup for those with various skin conditions, rashes, etc.
Lupus Foundation of America, Inc.
4 Research Place, Ste. 180, Rockville, MD 20850-3226
(800) 558-0121 or call (301) 670-9292 for the chapter nearest you.
Lupusline
(212) 606-1952. A phone support/information source run by people with SLE.
Lupus Living Support Group
A supportive place to express pain, fears, and other emotions and to learn about SLE (and FMS). www.medakate.org/lupus.html
National Alopecia Areata Foundation
Box 150760, San Rafael, CA 94915-0760
National Institute of Arthritis and Musculoskeletal and Skin Diseases Information Clearinghouse (NAMISIC)
Box AMS, 9000 Rockville Pike, Bethesda, MD 20892 (301) 495-4484 or (301) 496- 8188.
Information on experimental treatments and research.

Sun Precautions
(800) 882-7860. Information on clothing to protect sun-sensitive individuals. Given the possible associated or coexisting conditions with SLE, the following may also prove helpful:
American College of Rheumatology
60 Executive Park South, #150, Atlanta, GA 30329 (404) 633-3777
The American Heart Association
7272 Greenville Avenue, Dallas, TX 75231-4596 (214) 373-6300
The National Kidney Foundation
30 East 33rd St., New York, NY 10016 (800) 228-4483

SJOGREN'S SYNDROME

Because women with Sjogren's syndrome may also have fibromyalgia syndrome, systemic lupus erythematosus, and/or rheumatoid arthritis, you may wish to refer to the sections covering each of these conditions for further useful information.
Dry.org
Internet resources for Sjogren's Syndrome. Web site: www.dry.org. See also *Sjogren's Syndrome: A Guide for the Patient,* presented by the Scripps Clinic Foundation, La Jolla, California at www.dry.org/ss95gui.html
Sjogren's Syndrome Foundation
382 Main Street, Port Washington, NY 11050 (516) 767-2866
Web site: http://www.sjogrens.com
Sjogren's Syndrome Guide for Patients: Scripps Clinic
Website: http://www.dry.org
Sjogren's Syndrome Home Page
Web site: http://www.tp.net/tonym

GRAVE'S DISEASE/HASHIMOTO'S THYROIDITIS

The Thyroid Society
7515 South Main St., #545, Houston, TX 77030 (800) 849-7643 Web site: http://www.the-thyroid-society.org e-mail: help@the-thyroid-society.org

TYPE I DIABETES

American Diabetes Association National Service Center
1600 Duke Street, Alexandria, VA 22314 (800) 232-3472
Web site: http://www.diabetes.org Call for the most recent version of the Association's dietary guidelines, which contain important information about: what types and how much of various nutrients you should include in your diet, weight loss diets, frequency of meals, consequences of exercise, and the like.
American Dietetic Association
430 North Michigan Avenue, Chicago, IL 60611 (800) 877-1600
Web site: http://www.eatright.org
Diabetes Center
Web site: http://www.allhealth.com/diabetes/types
General info; support groups and chat rooms.

Diabetic Forum

To subscribe to this mailing list, e-mail listserv@lehigh.edu. You will receive regular updates and important information automatically.

Diabetes Interview Newsletter

e-mail: listserv@netcom.com

International Diabetes Center

3800 Park Nicollet Boulevard, St. Louis Park, MN 55416 (612) 983-3393

International Research Project on Diabetes

e-mail: listserv@kamikaze.com

Joslin Diabetes Center

1 Joslin Place, Boston, MA 02215 (617) 732-2440

Web site: http://www.joslin.harvard.edu

Medic Alert Foundation

Box 1009, Turlock, CA 95381 (800) 432-5378

National Diabetes Information Clearinghouse

Box NDIC, Bethesda, MD 20892   (301) 468-2162

National Institute of Diabetes and Digestive and Kidney Diseases (NIDDK)

Web site: http://www.niddk.nih.gov/health/diabetes/diabetes.htm. Extensive services, studies, federal programs, medications, education, etc.

FIBROMYALGIA SYNDROME (also see CFIDS)

American College of Rheumatology

60 Executive Park South, #150, Atlanta, GA 30329 (404) 633-3777

American Fibromyalgia Syndrome Association

6380 E. Tanque Verde Rd., #D, Tucson, AZ 85715 (520) 733-1570

Arthritis & Fibromyalgia Care Program

800 East 28th St., Minneapolis, MN 55407-3799 (612) 863-4774

Arthritis Foundation

1314 Spring St., NW, Atlanta, GA 30309 (404) 872-7100 or (800) 283-7800. A pamphlet on FMS is available.

Fibromyalgia Alliance of America

Mary Anne Saathoff, RN, BSN, Box 21988, Columbus, OH 43221-0988 (614) 457-4222 e-mail: MaSAAThoff@aol.com

Fibromyalgia Association of British Columbia

Box 15455, Vancouver, BC, Canada V6B5B2

Fibromyalgia Network

Kristin Thorson, Box 31750, Tucson, AZ 85751-1750 (800) 853-2929, fax (520) 290- 5550 Web site: http://www.fmnetnews.com

Publishes a quarterly newsletter on FMS/CFS ($19 for 4 issues). Other educational materials: *Getting the Most Out of Your Meds; The Fibromyalgia Help Book; Understanding Post-Traumatic FMS; Arthritis Information Pack*. They also provide listings of referrals to support groups and treatment professionals.

Fibromyalgia Nutrition Resource Center

(800) 229-3376

Goldstein, Jay, M.D.

701 No. Glassel St., Orange, CA 92867 (714) 516-2830 Web site: http://www.DrJGoldstein.com. Dr. Goldstein is a brilliant, knowledgeable, and compassionate doctor with

respect to comprehending and treating conditions such as FMS and CFIDS. His success rate in dealing with people with either or both conditions is amongst the highest there is.

Guaifenesin treatment
Dr. Paul St. Amand, (310) 577-7510

Healthlink USA
Wide range of information regarding FMS treatments, diagnoses, e-mail groups, personal stories, support groups, etc. www.healthlinkusa.com/Fibromyalgia.html

International Foundation for Bowel Dysfunction
Box 17864, Milwaukee, WI 53217 (414) 241-9479

ImmuneSupport.com
Immune support and chronic pain specialist—latest news of CFIDS & FMS.
www.immunesupport.com/bulletins

Lupus Living Support Group
A supportive place to express pain, fears, and other emotions and to learn about SLE (and FMS). www.medakate.org/lupus.html

National Institute of Arthritis and Musculoskeletal and Skin Diseases Information Clearinghouse (NAMISIC)
Box AMS, 9000 Rockville Pike, Bethesda, MD 20892. (301) 495-4484 or (301) 496-8188. Information on experimental treatments and research.

National CFIDS Foundation, Inc.
103 Aletha Road, Needham, MA 02492-3931 (781) 449-3535
A nonprofit organization that produces one of the most informative, well-researched newsletters available. *National Forum* is a newsletter covering FMS, CFIDS/ME, multiple chemical sensitivity, and related illnessses. Dr. Jay Goldstein is the medical advisor ($25.00/year).

National Chronic Fatigue Syndrome & Fibromyalgia Association of America
352 Broadway, Ste. 222, Kansas City, MO 64111 (816) 931-4777

National Fibromyalgia Research Association
Box 500, Salem, OR 97308 (503) 588-1410, (800) 853-2929, or (520) 290-5508
Free information packet.

National Foundation for Fibromyalgia
Box 3429, San Diego, CA 92163-1429 (619) 291-8949

National Headache Foundation
5252 No.Western Ave., Chicago, IL 60625 (800) 843-2256 or (312) 878-7715

National Sleep Foundation
1367 Connecticut NW, #200, Washington DC 20036 (202) 785-2300

USA Fibromyalgia-Fibrositis Association
Robert Ryan, CEO, D.B. Miskimen, Chair
2671 Sawbury Blvd., Columbus, OH 43235 *or* Box 20408 Columbus, OH 43220
(614) 764-8010, (614) 442-8344, fax (614) 558-9370

CHRONIC FATIGUE IMMUNE DEFICIENCY SYNDROME (See also FMS above)

American College of Rheumatology
60 Executive Park South, #150, Atlanta, GA 30329 (404) 633-3777

Arthritis & Fibromyalgia Care Program
800 East 28ᵗʰ St., Minneapolis, MN 55407-3799 (612) 863-4774
Arthritis Foundation
1314 Spring St., NW, Atlanta, GA 30309 (404) 872-7100 or (800) 283-7800
Chronic Fatigue Immune Deficiency Syndrome Association
Box 220398, Charlotte, NC 28222 (800) 442-3437
CFIDS Buyer's Club
1187 Coast Village Road, #1-280, Santa Barbara, CA 93108 (800) 366-6056
Connecticut Chronic Fatigue Immune Deficiency Syndrome Association
Box 9582, Forestville, CT 06011 (203) 582-3437
Gulf Coast Chronic Fatigue Syndrome/CFIDS
752 J Ave. Estancias, Venice, FL 34292-2316 (813) 484-0706
Haworth Press, Inc.
10 Alice St., Binghamton, NY 13904-9981 (800) 895-0582. Produces the only peer-reviewed medical journal on CFIDS for doctors ($32.40/year).
Healthlink USA
Enter "healthlinkusa.com/71feat.htm" for CFIDS links to websites, information on treatments, diagnoses, prevention, support groups, e-mail lists, message boards, personal stories, and research.
National Chronic Fatigue Syndrome & Fibromyalgia Association of America
352 Broadway, Ste. 222, Kansas City, MO 64111 (816) 931-4777
National CFIDS Foundation, Inc.
103 Aletha Road, Needham, MA 02492-3931 (781) 449-3535
A nonprofit organization that produces one of the most informative, well-researched newsletters available. National Forum is a newsletter covering FMS, CFIDS/ME, multiple chemical sensitivity, and related illnesses. Dr. Jay Goldstein is the medical advisor ($25.00/year). www.ncf-net.org
National Chronic Pain Outreach Association
Box 274 Millboro, VA 24460 (540) 997-5004 e-mail: ncpoal@aol.com
National Headache Foundation
5252 No. Western Ave., Chicago, IL 60625 (800) 843-2256 or (312) 878-7715
National Sleep Foundation
1367 Connecticut NW, #200, Washington, DC 20036 (202) 785-2300

MIND-BODY TECHNIQUES
General

For a search engine covering publications on acupuncture, traditional Chinese medicine, holistic medicine, and other topics, go to: http://homepage.tinet.ie/~progers/rogfindco.htm

Acupuncture and Acupressure

Acupressure Institute
1533 Shattuck Avenue, Berkeley, CA 94709 (510) 845-1059
American Academy of Medical Acupuncture
5820 Wilshire Blvd., #500, Los Angeles, CA 90036
(800) 521-2262, fax (213) 937-0959 e-mail: KCKD71@prodigy.com

National Acupuncture & Oriental Medicine Alliance
14637 Starr Rd., SE, Olalla, WA 98359   (206) 851-6896
American Association of Oriental Medicine
433 Front Street, Catasauqua, PA 18032 (610) 433-2448

Chiropractic

American Chiropractic Association
1701 Clarendon Blvd., Arlington, VA 22209 (703) 276-8800
International Chiropractors Association
1110 No. Glebe Rd., #1000, Arlington, VA 22201 (703) 528-5000

EMDR

Eye Movement Desensitization Reprocessing Institute, Inc.
Box 51010, Pacific Grove, CA 93950-6010   (831) 372-3900, fax (831) 647-9881
For information on receiving training and becoming certified.
Eye Movement Desensitization Reprocessing International Association (EMDRIA)
Box 141925, Austin, TX 78714-1925   (512) 451-5200, fax (512) 451-5256. e-mail:
emdria@aol.com EMDRIA maintains a register of qualified EMDR clinicians, supports
research, informs the public, and develops guidelines.

Ergonomics

Abbey Medical
17390 Brookhurst St., Ste. 200, Fountain Valley, CA 92708
Arthritis Self-Help Products
3 Little Knoll Court, Medford, NJ 08055
Enrichments
145 Tower Dr., Box 579, Hinsdale, IL 60521
HAS Health Suppliers
Box 288, Farmville, NC 27828

Herbs

American Herbalist Guild
Box 746555, Arvada, CO 80006 (303) 423-8800
Herb Research Foundation
1007 Pearl St., #200, Boulder, CO 80302 (303) 449-2265
Women's Herbal Conference
P.O. Box 6, Shelburne Falls, MA 01370(413) 625-6875
Offers workshops and retreats that teach women how to use herbs for medicinal use.
Holds an annual herbal conference.

Hypnosis

American Society of Clinical Hypnosis
2200 East Devon Ave., #291, Des Plaines, IL 60018
Society for Clinical and Experimental Hypnosis
128-A Kingspark Dr., Liverpool, NY 13090 (315) 652-7299
Both organizations are cautious in terms of member qualifications. You can call or
write to them (send a self-addressed, stamped envelope) for referrals to a quality professional in your area. There are many self-instructional tools available in the market,
such as audiotapes, videotapes, and books. Check on their quality.

Milton H. Erickson Foundation
3606 No. 24th St., Phoenix, AZ 85016 (602) 956-6196, fax (602) 956-0519

Meditation

Esalen Institute
Big Sur, CA 93920 (408) 667-3000
Insight Meditation Society
1230 Pleasant St., Barre, MA 01005 (508) 355-4378, fax (508) 355-6398
Insight Meditation West
Box 909, Woodacre, CA 94973 (415) 488-0164
Institute for Noetic Sciences
475 Gate Five Road, Ste. 300, Sausalito, CA 94965
(415) 331-5650, fax (415) 331-5673

Massage and Other Types of Bodywork

American Massage Therapy Association
820 Davis St., Ste. 100, Evanston, IL 60201 (847) 864-0123
Bonnie Prudden Pain Erasure
7800 East Speedway Blvd., Tucson, AZ 85710 (520) 529-3979 or (800) 221-4634
Feldenkrais Guild
524 SW Ellsworth St., Box 489, Albany, OR 97321 (800) 775-2118
National Certification Board for Therapeutic Massage and Bodywork
8201 Greensboro Dr., Ste. 300, McLean, VA 22102 (703) 610-9015
Reiki Alliance
Box 41, Cataldo, ID 83810-1041 (208) 682-3535
Reiki Outreach International
Box 609, Fair Oaks, CA 95628 (916) 863-1500, fax (916) 863-6464
The Rolf Institute
205 Canyon Blvd., Boulder, CO 80306 (800) 530-8875 e-mail: RolfInst@aol.com
The Trager Institute
21 Locust Ave., Mill Valley, CA 94941-2806 (415) 388-2688
e-mail: TragerD@aol.com

Qi Gong

Qigong Institute
East West Academy of Healing Arts, 450 Sutter Place, #2104, San Francisco, CA 94108
(415) 788-2227, fax (415) 788-2242
World Natural Medicine Foundation
College of Medical Qi Gong, 9904 106th St. Edmonton, AB T5K 1C4, Canada (403) 424-2231, fax (403) 424-8520

CAREGIVER RESOURCES

When You're Ill or Incapacitated/When You're the Caregiver (1995) by James Miller Willowgreen Publishing, Box 25180, Fort Wayne, IN 46825 (219) 424-7916

Helping Yourself Help Others (1994) by Rosalyn Carter & Susan Golant. Times Books, Random House, 201 East 50th St., New York, NY 10022. (800) 733-3000
When I contacted this company, I was told that they now have the book available only in paperback. The book code is #812-925-91-2 and the quoted cost was $14.00

plus tax; shipping is $3.00. This sounds like a thorough, helpful book which discusses burnout, isolation, finding meaning, and perhaps most difficult of all, dealing with doctors.

Overextended and Undernourished: A Self-Care Guide for People in Helping Roles (1996) by Dennis Portnoy
Johnson Institute, 7205 Ohms Lane, MN 55439-2159 (800) 231-5165
At the time of writing, the following item number was given: 3279. The quoted cost was $5.95 and the address to submit requests was: Hazelden, Box 176, Center City, MN 55012-0176. Phone number as above.

The Caregiver Survival Series (1995–96) by James R. Sherman
Mosby Lifeline, 11830 Westline Industrial Drive, St. Louis, MO 63146 (800) 667-2968. Includes four large-print books discussing how to achieve balance between caretaking and one's own self-care. The titles include: *Positive Caregiver Attitudes; Preventing Caregiver Burnout; Creative Caregiving;* and *The Magic of Humor in Caregiving.*

There are also a number of particularly helpful organizations for caretakers:

Children of Aging Parents (CAPS)
1609 Woodbourne Rd., #302A, Levittown, PA 19057
(800) 227-7294 or (215) 945-6900, fax (215) 945-8720

National Family Caregivers Association
9621 E. Bexhill Dr., Kensington, MD 20895-3014
(800) 896-3650 or (301) 942-6430, fax (301) 942-2302
Web site: http://www.nfcacares.org e-mail: info@caregiver.org

Family Caregiver Alliance
425 Bush St., #500, San Francisco, CA 94108 (800) 445-8106 (in CA) or (415) 434-3388 Web site: http://www.caregiver.org e-mail: info@caregiver.org

A P P E N D I X   I I

More Tools to Help You Thrive

Acupuncture and Acupressure

These methods were recommended in the ARC chapter. They have far-reaching benefits and implications, and the more we know about them, the more we see how they may be beneficial.

Acupuncture

Acupuncture is one of several alternative techniques making significant progress toward acceptance by Western doctors and our scientifically based, empirically driven health field. This results from several forces: the public's increasing use of acupuncture and decreased dependence on Western physicians; much evidence supporting acupuncture's efficacy; and the realization by many doctors that all of their scientific progress and technological innovation can't help some patients.

In addition to pain management, acupuncture help ARC patients in several ways. For example, many people with ARC also experience irritable bowel syndrome (IBS). Evidence suggests that acupuncture can reduce IBS symptoms. It also helps MS patients who have developed paralysis. For cigarette smokers with TID, one of the most important changes they must make is to stop smoking, and acupuncture has been found to assist people in this area.

So, what is acupuncture all about? According to the view of the traditionalists, qi, the essence of energy, flows along interrelated meridians (sort of like pathways) that weave in and out throughout the entire body. In general, practitioners are concerned with twelve so-called regular meridians and two out of eight extra meridians. Each meridian serves particular organs, including the heart, liver, kidneys, and so on, and they surface at the body at hundreds of locations called acupuncture points. These locations are where practitioners try to intervene and reestablish a harmonious balance between yin and yang. A diseased state arises from either a meridian disruption causing an imbalance, or because a disturbance in the organ connected to a meridian has destroyed the harmonious nature of that meridian. What causes disruptions? These days it is thought that injuries to the body, infection, debilitating illnesses, diet, and omnipresent stress are responsible. In addition, forces described in metaphorical language, such as cold, heat, fire, wetness, and dryness, can also disrupt the meridians.

The central tenet in Chinese medicine is that illness and distress arise from an imbalance of yin and yang, so treatment strives to reestablish the balance that is necessary for good health. Inserting needles along acupuncture points can reestablish that harmony because they affect qi and blood to boost deficits, reduce excesses, and change stagnation into movement, all of which reestablish balance between yin and yang. A more contemporary view is that the imbalance between yin and yang, together with other presences, leads to the pooling of substances like carbon monoxide and excess lactic acid in the body's muscular system. Inserting needles at select acupuncture points stimulates these areas and thus disperses these substances. Accordingly, balance between yin and yang is again established. While we lack objective evidence about meridians, there are interesting findings about these locations. Examination of acupuncture points under a microscope shows a more dense concentration of nerve endings compared to other parts of the body. Also, acupuncture points emit detectably greater electromagnetic energy than other body areas (Rosenfeld 1996).

Not surprisingly, Western physicians and researchers have a different view of how acupuncture works. In fact, there are several theories about its ability to reduce pain and improve healing. One of these theories is called the gate theory, and it stems from the work of Ronald Melzack and Patrick Wall. Their theory is complex and I'm presenting only the general idea here. The model suggests that pain sensations don't come from a single nerve system but from the entire nervous system. One of the main principles stems from their gate-control theory of pain. Basically, this states that there is something like a gating system that controls the amount of information that will be accepted from parts of the body, often at the surface or close to the surface where an injury or problem has occurred. The information regarding pain that is allowed to pass through the gate is then sent to certain structures in the brain, which transform the information into the experience of pain with which we are all familiar! One additional point is all that is needed to understand the explanation of how acupuncture works according to this theory: There are two different types of fibers, thick fibers and thin fibers, that "fire" and thus send information to the gate. It is thought that the gate allows more pain information to pass through *as the amount of information conveyed by the small fibers becomes greater than that conveyed by the large fibers.* Thus, acupuncture is effective in reducing the pain experience because the insertion of the needles triggers more information to be conveyed by the large fibers. Accordingly, it is much more difficult for the thin fibers to exceed the thick fibers, which means that the gate will no longer let more pain information pass through to be processed and then experienced as pain.

One of the leading theories today maintains that there is a relationship between acupuncture and endorphins, our body's natural, self-generated painkillers. Acupuncture may reduce pain because the needle insertion into the acupuncture points causes the body to release endorphins, which act in similar ways to various painkillers, most typically morphine. If when acupuncture is performed a chemical known to block the effects of morphine is ingested, the increased pain tolerance usually caused by endorphins is also blocked and is not effective (Pomeranz and Chiu 1976). There does seem to be one significant difference between endorphins and morphine: Endorphins are thought to be anywhere from 3,000 to 10,000 times more powerful than morphine! Pomeranz also found that when mice who had been born without sufficient opiate receptors were given acupuncture, they did not experience a pain reduction as did the normal mice from the same treatment. There has been a great amount of research into this theory over the brief span of its history and while additional research is certainly required, there is a significant body of evidence supporting this theory. There has also been significant research into this on the Chinese side. Unfortunately, many of these studies have not been conducted in the rigorous scientific method demanded by Western researchers and physicians. However, this is not to say that important information regarding the efficacy of acupuncture with relation to humans has not been gained. Kaptchuk's 1983 book, which explores Chinese medicine, offers a description of some of these findings:

- Inserting a needle into acupuncture point Stomach 36 strengthens intestinal peristalsis (as seen in the transport time for barium in humans). Other related acupuncture points establish the opposite reaction, namely, they relax the intestinal functioning.

- Of particular interest to the readers of this book is that it seems that acupuncture can stimulate the immune system. Evidence used to support this involved monitoring patients with bacillary dysentery before and after they received acupuncture. After three hours, there was an evident increase in phagocytosis, the engulfing and digestion of bacteria or other foreign invaders by white cells, and this effect actually continued to increase until peaking twelve hours after treatment. In this case, while regular acupuncture was effective, electric acupuncture was more effective.

- Inserting needles into Large Intestine 4 and Triple Burner 5 leads to vasodilation and lowers elevated blood pressure. On the other hand, inserting needles into Pericardium 6 leads to vasoconstriction, which helps increase excessively low blood pressure.

You can refer back to chapter 5 for a discussion of the typical assessment performed by acupuncturists and other alternative health professionals. These days most acupuncturists use very thin, disposable needles to prevent the transmission of any diseases or infections from one person to the next. However, it is definitely worth your while to ensure that disposable needles are being used. Because the needles are so thin and your professional is experienced, acupuncture is generally not painful, although you may experience some discomfort when the acupuncturist twists particular needles to increase their effectiveness. If you have this feeling, tell the acupuncturist so they can unscrew the needles somewhat.

There are several different types of acupuncture available, including "electric" acupuncture, in which a weak electrical current is run through the needles to activate their effect. I myself have not had this type of acupuncture, although I have spoken with a number of women with fibromyalgia who vouch for its efficacy. Some acupuncturists may use sound waves and light rays at the acupuncture points to enhance the effects of the needles. The length of treatment is variable, and depends on your particular symptoms, disorder, relative physical health, constitution, negative stress level, and other factors. Your primary goal should be to locate an acupuncturist who is licensed, well qualified, and very experienced with your ARC (see appendix I). A growing number of health care professionals in the pain-management field are using acupuncture as an adjunct treatment with physical therapy, pain medication, and other methods. Of course, acupuncture does not work for everyone, nor does it work for every type of disorder or pain. However, it has helped many people with various auto-immune-related conditions in myriad ways. It's worth your while to consult with an expert, as well as your primary caretaker if she knows anything about acupuncture, to determine if this may be a good treatment into incorporate in your SHOC.

Acupressure

Acupressure is also important in treating ARCs and associated symptoms or disorders. Acupressure actually predates acupuncture, and thus the same beliefs and concepts discussed above apply to this method. As with acupuncture, this treatment is intended to heal by reestablishing the proper flow of qi throughout the body's meridians. Rather than needles, pressure applied through the fingers and hands is intended to release and restore the appropriate balance of energy. Relief is obtained as the pressure leads to the release of specific neurotransmitters interfering with the onset of pain.

One of the most important things about acupressure is that you can do some of it to yourself. This is the kind of technique that goes along perfectly with this book's theme regarding the importance of self-care and self-reliance to whatever degree is appropriate to your condition, and the assumption of an active, growth-oriented role in dealing with your whole health and well-being. You may obtain the services of an experienced professional at times, particularly in the beginning stages of learning the method, but you can also apply it by yourself to obtain immediate relief. There are various self-acupressure techniques, such as Acu-Yoga, Do-In, and Tui Na, from which you can choose (Balch and Balch 1997). See appendix I for resources and referrals. Fnd a certified practitioner for your SHOC.

Biofeedback

This mind-body technique is useful for pain and stress reduction and is an interesting synthesis of eastern treatments and mechanized, measurable techniques characteristic of conventional medicine. For centuries it was believed that many of our body's reactions, particularly those linked with the autonomic nervous system, were "automatic" or beyond our conscious control. Technology has shown that giving people data about their heart rate, skin temperature, muscle tension, or brain waves helps them consciously change these variables. Biofeedback equipment offers data on one or more of the following: skin temperature, brain waves, muscle tension, and heartbeat. The information is in auditory or visual form, and the recipient uses her mind to change presented signals. Biofeeedback is effective for people with ARC because it can improve insomnia, anxiety, menstrual pain, muscular tension and pain, cardiac arrhythmia, migraines, Raynaud's phenomenon, high blood pressure, incontinence, nerve damage, and GI problems. Let's look at Raynaud's phenomenon, a disorder in which blood vessels in the fingers and toes are excessively constricted and cause extremely cold skin. In thermal biofeedback, temperature monitors are placed on fingers and toes and temperature data is made accessible to the client. She learns with the benefit of continuous feedback to raise the temperature of her fingers and toes. Studies show a 66 percent decrease in symptoms, and when this method is combined with a cold stressor challenge (in which the temperature around the client is lowered as she simultaneously learns to raise her skin temperature), an amazing 92 percent symptom decrease can occur (Schwartz and Schwartz 1993). Biofeedback is also effective in treating the migraines and chronic headaches that accompany many ARCs. It also helps you learn how to relax your muscles thoroughly, as compared to just sitting or lying down and telling yourself to relax. As tense muscles are part of the vicious cycle of pain, biofeedback teaches you to truly relax the muscles in the neck, shoulders, and back and reduce chronic pain and stiffness. The type of biofeedback used to reduce headaches and muscle tension is electromyographic (EMG) biofeedback, which measures muscle tension. You can find biofeedback organizations in large cities or through local colleges and universities.

Bodywork

Self-Bodywork

The first type of bodywork we'll discuss here is a yoga stretch that reduces back tension and back and upper leg pain. Lie face down with your hands at your sides. If possible, turn your head to one side. If not, roll a towel and form it into a circle, placing it under your face so it supports your chin, face, and forehead while allowing easy breathing. Take some DBs and focus on relaxing your back and legs. You may visualize the muscles in your legs and back as if they were taut bands that lengthen and relax. Rest this way for one to two minutes then place your hands beneath your shoulders, making sure back and legs stay relaxed, and slightly raise your head and upper back so that you are resting on your forearms. Stay in this position for several minutes and continue focusing on relaxing your leg and back muscles. Now you will perform what looks like a cat stretch. From the position on your forearms, slowly raise your upper body by working to extend your arms as straight as possible. You will probably be able to straighten your arms a bit more with each of the several repetitions of this movement. It's essential that you maintain that relaxation in your back and legs, and keep your hips aligned, resting on the floor. Stop if you feel any pain and return immediately to your forearms. If you feel fine, arch your back for five seconds and then return to the forearm resting position. Repeat the cat back stretch three to four times until your arms are extended as straight as possible. *Don't go to the point of pain!*

You can use your body's self-healing abilities to reduce pain, based on physiological principles like "reciprocal inhibition." When you contract and hold a muscle, the opposing or antagonist muscle relaxes and is easier to stretch. This is a backwards-in approach to getting relief in a region. A second principle is "post-isometric relaxation," meaning that the muscle you just contracted and held becomes easier to stretch. Hold the contraction for at least ten seconds. If you can barely turn your head over your shoulder from tightness and pain, you can start to work here. For your left shoulder, place your left hand against your left cheek and *gently* push your cheek toward your left shoulder for fifteen to twenty seconds. This uses reciprocal inhibition; as you're contracting but not allowing the muscles on the left to move, the tense right-side antagonist muscles that cause pain when you turn left become flexible and relaxed. The post-isometric principle also reduces pressure and tension in left-side neck muscles. Do the same with the right hand and cheek, pushing toward the right shoulder. Then turn your head to the left as you first tried to do and it will turn further and less painfully.

Massage

Massage is a form of bodywork and represents a form of natural treatment that relies on the physical connection and interaction between provider and client. It involves the systematic manipulation of the body's soft tissues. As with other forms of treatment, it is essential that you find somebody who is properly trained, as well as knowledgeable about and experienced in treating your autoimmune-related condition. Ask about the masseuse's training and education. They may provide you with names of past clients so that you can contact them and ask directly about the masseuse's abilities and any relevant strengths and weaknesses they may have. It is very important that you do find a good masseuse who is well-informed about your particular autoimmune-related condition because, as with chiropractic work, great damage can be done by someone who is not sufficiently educated and experienced. There are some individuals who should not choose massage at all, and for those who can, the type of massage should be matched to their health concerns and conditions. It's important that you talk to your physician or other qualified health professionals before you obtain this treatment. They can tell you whether massage is safe for you, and if so, what type(s) of massage are most effective for your condition. I will discuss the types of massage available below. Keep in mind that many of those who remain skeptical of these methods of treatment base their arguments on the fact that evidence of their efficacy comes generally from anecdotal evidence rather than from controlled scientific studies. However, anecdotal support has often been an important step in triggering further scientific exploration and as such research continues, these skeptics may well find that their arguments no longer hold water.

There are a number of ways through which massage is believed to reduce pain. For example, massage increases blood flow through muscles and circulation through the lymphatic system. It also helps relax tense, painful muscles and increases the range of motion. All of these effects are important in the treatment of autoimmune-related conditions. Difficulties with tight, tense muscles cause a great amount of pain in various autoimmune disorders, and individuals with pain in certain areas of the body tend to compensate by using other areas more or by restricting their movements (and consequently their range of motion). The pain and restricted range of motion can be greatly improved through the increased blood flow and relaxation of the muscles provided by massage. In addition, improved lymphatic circulation helps reduce the inflammation that is a real source of difficulties in autoimmune disorders. Massage is also helpful in aiding in the healing of soft-tissue injuries and in improving one's general feelings of well-being.

Here are some other popular types of massage:

1. A Swedish massage is probably what most laypeople think of when they hear the word massage. This therapy has been used in the United States since the mid-nineteenth century. Swedish massage involves the use of a range of motions in order to assist in muscle relaxation, as well as in the reduction of inflammation and pain. In addition, Swedish massage is often used in cases of accident and injury, as it is an effective method to include in an overall rehabilitation plan.

2. A deep tissue massage is often a component of different types of massage. Basically, the approach has some similarities to the Swedish massage; however, deep tissue massage involves targeting deeper muscles and using more pressure. This difference arises in part because the goal of deep tissue massage is to reduce the level of long-term tension, which causes great damage and pain in the muscle groups involved. Such long-term stress and tension are frequently associated, and perhaps causally at times, with autoimmune-related conditions.

3. A similar form of deep tissue massage is known as neuromuscular massage. It shares with deep tissue massage the element of focusing the manipulations and pressures on specific areas of the muscle. As in shiatsu massage, the use of finger pressure is a central component. In particular, neuromuscular massage generally focuses on working specific trigger points in order to increase blood flow and reduce tightness and pain. Trigger points are particular areas in the muscles that are sensitive to pressure; when pressed, they send out pain signals to distant locales from the region pressed. While trigger points can appear in a variety of

disorders, you frequently hear about them in association with FMS and sometimes CFIDS. For more on pain reduction treatments and trigger points, you can refer to the What You Can Do section in chapter 12.

4. Rolfing is cyclical in its acceptance. At present, Rolfing has regained its place of popularity, perhaps due to the general surge of interest in all alternative/complementary techniques. The underlying principle will sound familiar if you read the section on Chinese medical treatments and/or the brief introduction to chiropractic services above. It states that in essence, health is obtained when the body parts are in alignment. Ida Rolf, the woman who developed this therapy in the late 1940s–early 1950s, believed that physical and mental problems arose when the body was out of alignment with gravity. She believed that by deeply massaging the fascia, or connective tissues covering the body's muscles, alignment would be reestablished. This massage is thought to improve both physical and emotional problems. It can reduce chronic pain and stiffness as well as distress and anxiety, all of which are important elements in ARCs. In addition, Rolfing has been used to treat carpal tunnel syndrome, a disorder often found in people with FMS. The technique is usually time-limited, with approximately ten sessions offered. The use of fingers is important, as in the other forms of massage discussed. However, the elbows and knuckles are also used to free fascia tightness and produce body alignment. If the words "elbows and knuckles" give you pause, then you must think carefully prior to selecting Rolfing, because it can be painful at times. Additionally, clients are also taught how to move their bodies to retain alignment and improve efficiency of movements.

5. Finally, two types of massage will be discussed together here, as they share similarities and differ somewhat from those discussed above. These include the Feldenkrais method and Esalen massage.

   The Feldenkrais method is a form of massage falling within the category of bodywork. For readers of this book, the Feldenkrais techniques are known to provide a number of benefits of great interest to those with ARCs. Practitioners typically focus on relieving chronic musculoskeletal pain, a symptom that is an unfortunate marker in many ARCs. Furthermore, it offers improvements in sleep, greater energy and mental acuity, and improved responses to stress. This type of bodywork can provide some rehab benefits in individuals with chronic illnesses, such as MS and other ARCs. The system focuses on modifying bad postural habits, breathing, and movement. The procedure may be learned in two ways. One may attend group sessions in which participants follow slow, guided movements in order to replace their habitual, unhealthy movements with new, healthier ones. There's also an individual portion called functional integration in which the practitioner uses similar movements and exercises, although she or he also physically guides the client, who then realizes just where she is holding her tension, how often, and what unhealthy movements she need to change. This method truly employs a holistic model, as the central point is to reduce negative movement styles and muscular patterns, thereby reducing negative feelings and thoughts. Recall that the model I use in this book conveys that thoughts generate associated emotions and physical/emotional behavior, but that there is feedback because emotions and physical behavior also affect thoughts. The Feldenkrais method fits in well as it correctly maintains that physical behavior affects thoughts and emotions. Unlike the types of massage discussed above, this method includes goals of working on one's self–image through touch rather than through any attempts to manipulate the body back to some normal, healthy arrangement. This approach is effective in treating MS, one of the ARCs discussed in this book, as well as targeting ARC symptoms like chronic pain, stress, and sleep problems.

Esalen massage is similar to the Feldenkrais in its perception of a holistic mind-body unity. The self and physical/emotional well-being is again a central issue, and the goal is to allow the individual to access deep states of consciousness through the intense relaxation attained through this technique. Also as with Feldenkrais, the treatment consists of slow, gentle touch and rhythmic movements.

6. Myotherapy can be of great benefit for ARC patients. You will read in the What You Can Do section of chapter 12 on FMS about a treatment developed in the 1940s that is called trigger point injection. This treatment involved injecting saline and procaine directly into the trigger points and painful muscles to get them to relax. Since these earlier times, trigger point injection treatment has changed. Some thirty years later, Bonnie Prudden showed that injections were not effective in and of themselves. In fact, she found that using deep pressure massage to target tender trigger points resulted in comparable results to those found with trigger point injection. Thus, Bonnie Prudden Myotherapy (now known simply as myotherapy) was born. It consists of using deep-pressure massage targeting specific painful (tender) and pain-referring (trigger) points in muscles to decrease pain and excessive body tension. It's clear why this treatment can be useful for a range of ARCs. The treatment of muscular conditions in myotherapy is very useful in treating neck, shoulder, and back pain (typical in SLE, FMS, CFIDS, RA, and MS, to name a few). In addition, myotherapy has successfully been used with TMJ syndrome (frequently manifest in FMS). Furthermore, headaches and carpal tunnel syndrome (both of which may occur in conjunction with various ARCs) can be handled successfully with myotherapy. Myotherapy is specifically labeled as a successful way to reduce the pain of RA, MS, and SLE (Editors of Time-Life Books 1997).

The treatment begins after a thorough assessment of your lifestyle, work, illnesses, and so on. After your muscles are tested for flexibility and strength, the trio of elbows, fingers, and wrists are employed in applying pressure to the offending trigger points. After passive stretching of your muscles, the therapist will give you a series of exercises to do at home. It's essential that you do these. I'm always a bit skeptical of therapists working with the body who do not give exercises to do at home, in the office, or elsewhere. This is because work-outs and bodywork that are limited to time spent in sessions are simply not able to provide the client with sufficient practice and knowledge regarding her body and how to apply newly learned techniques in novel situations outside the four walls of the treatment room.

Qi Gong

Qi gong, a Chinese medical technique with a 4,000-year-old oral history (and a 2,000-year-old recorded history) develops integration of body, mind, emotions, and spirit. It also includes some very practical daily tips that those who experience chronic pain, muscular weakness, and the like can easily include in their daily routines. Qi gong relies on a synthesis of techniques about which you've read, such as meditation, DB, and particular movements. The more research into alternative techniques I do, the more I see the growing popularity of this type of healing. While numerous studies have been carried out in China to substantiate the efficacy of this technique, researchers in the U.S. don't always accept these studies as valid and may discount the potential of qi gong. For those familiar with and accepting of the discipline's effectiveness, there are widespread claims for its ability to solve many ills. Qi gong can help with asthma, allergies, back pain, carpal tunnel syndrome, circulatory system problems, depression, insomnia, menopause, neuralgia, chronic pain, and TMJ syndrome. The basic purpose of qi gong is to increase the strength and balance of one's qi or, in rough translation, one's essential life energy. As noted throughout this book and particularly exemplified in the aforementioned discussion of Chinese healing theory, the concept of balance is central to health. In fact, qi gong is associated with balance and healing in two ways; namely, through internal qi and external qi. Internal qi is worked with as an attempt to increase internal energy and balance. This involves performing consistent meditation and qi gong's specific exercises intended to create balance in energy and increase internal health. The use of external qi is harnessed only by masters who learn to create this healing energy, which can be transferred to individuals with physical and emotional illness in order to improve their health and well-being.

The practice of qi gong is based on a variety of different philosophies, including Taoist, Buddhist, and Confucian. Together they contribute their respective beliefs and perspectives and form this discipline, which attempts to improve well-being through attaining a strengthening and balance of the body's energies. If you plan to use this technique as part of your SHOC, it's important to do two things: first, consult with your SHOC doc and other experts regarding this decision, and second, make sure you find a teacher with extensive training and experience in this technique. In addition, remember that serious illnesses should not necessarily be treated only by either conventional or alternative approaches. Most ARCs are serious, and you would want to combine Western methods with alternative approaches. If you decide to learn more about qi gong, you must find a legitimate, knowledgeable teacher. This person will teach you the correct exercises to perform, watch you do them, and offer suggestions and corrections. You will be expected to perform exercises at home between classes. It requires a commitment of your time and energy if you truly desire to obtain results from this technique. There are countless exercises in qi gong, most of which fall under four categories: sitting, lying down, standing, and walking. It's important that your teacher understand your particular ARC, as there are specific exercises you should practice more frequently to focus on your special needs. Besides internal qi, there are many who also seek the experience of external qi. This involves visiting a qualified master who may touch specific points on your body or allow their hands to hover above your body. It is believed that the hands of a master generate energy that enters the client's body and causes her own qi to balance and her body to heal. Overall, though, qi gong is viewed as a practice that an individual should learn to maximize her qi and her body's ability to heal. In the same manner as mindfulness meditation, qi gong is not just a temporary approach to cover up the appearance of a particular symptom or pain. It is thought to work best if incorporated into one's life and practiced daily, although it may be used to assist with the onset of particular problems or pains.

Shiatsu and Reiki

The philosophy or beliefs upon which these types of bodywork are based are highly similar to those of acupuncture and acupressure. What follows is a brief explanation of these techniques and their benfits for ARC patients: Shiatsu, meaning "finger pressure" in Japanese, is based on the view that blockages are interfering with the ability of one's energy (or as described above, qi) to flow freely throughout the body. Therefore, pressure is applied to the various acupressure points in order to unblock any areas in which energy can be stuck and thus not flowing freely through the meridians. The hands and fingers are used to produce a strong repetitive pattern of pressure maintained over specific points for up to ten seconds. The goal of shiatsu is to help the individual reclaim her health and then to stay in this state over time. One is healthy when she is in balance and her energy is able to flow in an easy, unimpeded way throughout the meridians of her body.

It is thought that reiki was initially used in Tibet thousands of years ago but then died out until 1850 or so, when it was rediscovered by an educator in Japan. Reiki is thought of as a way to use a physical method (application of one's hands on the body of the health seeker) to use universal energy to produce healing (Editors of Time-Life Books 1997). Reiki's conceptualization of healing is similar to those above that are based on ancient philosophical and spiritual beliefs held by Eastern cultures for centuries. As with acupuncture, acupressure, and other related treatments, Reiki practitioners maintain that illness comes from two sources: disharmony and the imbalance of universal energy. In order to restore health, both of these abnormal characteristics must be restored to balance and harmony. Reiki involves a certified master or practitioner placing her hands over the chakras (centers of energy) of your body. Under these conditions, healing energy is expected to more easily flow into your unhealthy body. The scheduling of sessions varies depending on your condition and the healer's assessment. You also are directly involved in the healing process, as you are advised to consume great amounts of tea and water to help eliminate the toxins from your body. Reiki can be an important treatment for ARCs and related symptoms. For example, two ARCs thought to be directly improved through the use of reiki are CFIDS and RA. In addition, reiki alleviates a number of symptoms related to a variety of ARCs: insomnia, heartburn, indigestion, irritable bowel syndrome, and, of course, the old chronic pain and negative stress. Again, you must find practitioners of this technique who are properly trained, experienced, and certified. Often there are a prescribed number of hours of training that individuals must have completed before they can be certified. You can refer to the resource list in Appendix I to obtain further information and referrals to appropriate practitioners.

Chiropractic Treatment

This treatment focuses on manipulations of the spine, most often in order to reduce pain. It is interesting to note the similarities between how chiropractors and acupuncturists perceive treatment. Chiropractors view health as arising when impulses generated in the brain can flow freely through the spinal cord to serve their various organs. For this to occur, the vertebrae along the spinal cord need to be in alignment. If they are not, the impulses cannot flow freely and various symptoms, including pain, result. In order to restore health, chiropractors use various methods of manipulation to assist in realigning the spinal vertebrae. They will move various parts of the body and will ask the client to move, stretch, and gently push through particular motions. While chiropractors may discuss nutrition and exercise with you, they do not prescribe medication and thus represent a more natural approach preferred by some people. The majority of scientific studies conducted on chiropractors have examined the efficacy of this form of treatment with various types of low back pain. In fact, chiropractic services are gaining the air of legitimacy in part because these studies have shown that this method is at least as effective for low back pain as conventional treatment provided by medical doctors. Besides relief from back pain, a frequent unwanted companion of many ARCs, chiropractic techniques can also reduce other ARC symptoms like neck pain, shoulder pain, and carpal tunnel syndrome, among others.

Collagen Formation and Connective Tissue Repair

Some health experts believe foods from the nightshade family contain alkaloids that interfere with collagen formation. Removing foods like eggplants, peppers, tomatoes, and potatoes one by one from your diet will let you know if and how they affect your ARC. Much press is being accorded to glucosamine sulfate, which is thought to help in collagen generation and cartilage repair. L-cysteine is a detoxifying amino acid that is central to immune functioning and also an element of collagenous tissue. Take 500 mg twice per day on an empty stomach with water or juice (not milk); it's most effective when taken with 50 mg vitamin B6 and 100 mg vitamin C. Other substances involved in collagen formation, connective tissue repair, strengthening, and rebuilding include: silica (supplies silicon); copper (best when taken with 2,000 mg calcium, and 1,000 mg magnesium daily); coenzyme Q10, 60 mg daily; free-form amino acid complex; multivitamin complex with 10,000 IU vitamin A and 15,000 IU natural beta-carotene daily; and pycnogenol or grape seed extract (Balch and Balch 1997). You can try the supplement MSM or foods like onions, eggs, and garlic that contain sulfur, which is central to connective tissue repair. Vitamin C, when taken with B6, E, and zinc, is believed to improve the repair of connective tissue and boost collagen generation. These are essential processes in ARCs and connective tissue disease because collagen is the material of which cartilage is composed. Also, having low levels of vitamin C and lower than normal levels of pantothenic acid are associated with symptoms such as pain and stiffness.

References

Abraham, G. and J. Flechas. 1992. Malic acid, energy and fibromyalgia. *Journal of Nutritional Medicine* 3:49–59.

Ali, M. 1994. *The Canary and Chronic Fatigue.* Denville, NJ: Life Span Press.

American Autoimmune Related Diseases Association. 1998. ARCs, though common, are understudied, reports new study. *INFOCUS* 6(3):1–3 September.

American Autoimmune Related Diseases Assn, Inc. 1998. Autoimmunity: A Major Women's Health Issue. National Conference, Detroit, Michigan. Cosponsored by AARDA, Detroit Newspaper Agency, Every Woman, Michigan's Year of Women's Health, Wayne State University School of Medicine, and the U.S. Public Health Services Office on Women's Health.

Andersen, M. L. 1993. *Thinking About Women: Sociological Perspectives on Sex and Gender.* Macmillan Publishing Company: New York.

Andrews, L. 1989. Mirroring the Life Force. In *Healers on Healing*, edited by Richard Carlson and Benjamin Shield. Los Angeles: Jeremy P. Tarcher, Inc.

Appiah R., S. Hiller, L. Caspary, K. Alexander, and A. Creutzig. 1997. Treatment of primary Raynaud's syndrome with traditional Chinese acupuncture. *Journal of Internal Medicine* 241(2):119–124.

Arthritis Foundation. 1983. *Rheumatoid Arthritis.* Atlanta, Ga.: AF.

Balch, J. F., and P. A. Balch. 1997. *Prescription for Nutritional Healing.* Second Edition. Garden City Park, NY: Avery Publishing Group.

Baldry, P. E. 1993. *Acupuncture, Trigger Points and Musculoskeletal Pain.* London: Churchill Livingstone.

Banks, P. A., D. H. Present, and Penny Steiner, editors. *The Crohn's Disease and Ulcerative Colitis Fact Book*. National Foundation for Ileitis & Colitis. New York: Charles Scribner's Sons.

Barnett, R. C., and G. K. Baruch. 1985. Women's Involvement in multiple roles and psychological distress. *Journal of Personality and Social Psychology* 49:135–145.

———. 1987. Social Roles, Gender, and Psychological Distress. In *Gender & Stress*, edited by R. Barnett, L. Biener, and G. Baruch. New York: The Free Press.

Baruch, G.K., and R. C. Barnett. 1986. Role quality, multiple role involvement, and psychological well-being in midlife women. *Journal of Personality and Social Psychology* 51:578–585.

Bennett, K. M., S. R. Clark, S. M. Campbell, and C. S. Burkhardt. 1992. Low levels of somatomedin C in patients with the fibromyalgia syndrome: A possible link between sleep and muscle pain. *Journal of Arthritis and Rheumatism* 35(10):1113–1116.

Berman, B. 1998. Exploring the alternatives. *INFOCUS*: Newsletter of the American Autoimmune Related Diseases Association, Inc. 6(3).

Blau, S. P., and D. Schultz. 1984. *Lupus: The Body Against Itself*. Garden City, NY: Doubleday.

Burton Goldberg Group. 1997. *Alternative Medicine*. Tiburon, Calif.: Future Medicine Publishing, Inc.

Campbell, K. R. 1998. Diabetes. *Medizine*. MediZine, Inc.: 10–11. April/May.

Chaitow, L. 1995. *Fibromyalgia & Muscle Pain: What Causes It, How It Feels, and What to do About It*. San Francisco, Calif.: Thorsons.

Cheney, P. 1991. "Is CFS caused by a virus?" Conference on Chronic Fatigue Syndrome: Current Theory and Treatment presentation. Bel-Air, Calif. May 18.

Chopra, D. 1993. *Ageless Body, Timeless Mind: The Quantum Alternative to Growing Old*. New York: Harmony Books.

Cleary, P. 1987. Gender Differences in Stress-Related Disorders. In *Gender & Stress*, edited by R. Barnett, L. Biener, and G. Baruch. New York: The Free Press.

Cohen, C., W. J. Doyle, D. P. Skoner, B. S. Rabin, and M. Gwaltney. 1997. Social ties and susceptibility to the common cold. *Journal of the American Medical Association* 277:1940–1944.

Collinge, W. 1993. *Recovering from Chronic Fatigue Syndrome: A Guide to Self-Empowerment*. The Body Press/Perigee: New York.

Conkling, W. 1996. "Are Women the Weaker Sex?" *American Health* July/August, 54–58.

Courmel, K. 1996. *A Companion Volume to Dr. Jay A. Goldstein's 'Betrayal by the Brain': A Guide for Patients and Their Physicians*. New York: The Haworth Medical Press.

Cousins, N. 1989a. *Head First: The Biology of Hope*. New York: E. P. Dutton.

Cousins, N. 1989b. The Healing Equation. In *Healers on Healing*, edited by Richard Carlson and Benjamin Shield. Los Angeles: Jeremy P. Tarcher, Inc.

Csikszentmihalyi, M. 1990. *Flow: The Psychology of Optimal Experience*. New York: HarperCollins.

Culverwell, M. 1995. Putting diabetes on the map. *JDF International Countdown.* Winter: 28–37.

Cunha, B.A. 1992. *Infectious Disease News* 5(11):8–9.

Dauphin, S. 1995. *Understanding Sjogren's Syndrome.* Tequesta, Fla.: Pixel Press.

Dauphin, S. 1987. *Sjogren's Syndrome: The Sneaky Arthritis.* Tequesta, Fla.: Pixel Press.

DeFreitas, E., B. Hillard, P. Cheney, D. Bell, E. Kiggundu, D. Sankey, Z. Wroblewski, M. Palladino, J. Woodward, and H. Koprowski. 1991. Retroviral sequences related to human T-lymphotropic virus type II in patients with chronic fatigue immune dysfunction syndrome. *Proceedings of the National Academy of Sciences U.S.A.* 88:2922–2926.

Dibner, R., and C. Colman. 1994. *The Lupus Handbook for Women.* New York: Simon & Schuster.

Editors of Prevention Magazine Health Books and Sharon Faelten editor. 1998. *The Doctors Book of Home Remedies for Women.* New York: Bantam Books.

Editors of Time-Life Books. 1997. *The Alternative Advisor.* Alexandria Va.: Time-Life Inc.

Edwards, J. R., and C. L. Cooper. 1988. The impacts of positive psychological states on physical health: a review and theoretical framework. *Social Science Medicine* 27(12):1447–1459.

Fibromyalgia Network. *Fibromyalgia Syndrome (FMS): A Patient's Guide,* Tucson: Fibromalgia Network.

Fransen, J., and Jon J. Russell. 1996. *The Fibromyalgia Help Book: Practical Guide to Living Better with Fibromyalgia.* St. Paul, Minn.: Smith House Press.

Friedberg, F. 1995. *Coping with Chronic Fatigue Syndrome.* Oakland, Calif.: New Harbinger Publications, Inc.

Fromer, M. J. 1993. *Healthy Living with Diabetes.* Oakland, Calif.: New Harbinger Publications, Inc.

Gardner, Pierce. 1998. Lyme disease vaccines. *Annals of Internal Medicine* 129(7): 583–585.

Glass, D. C. 1982. Psychological and physiological responses of individuals displaying type A behavior. *Acta Med Scand (Supplement),* 660:193–202.

Glynn, L. 1999. *Psychosomatic Medicine* 61:234–242.

Goleman, Daniel, Ph.D., and Joel Gurin, editors. 1993. *Mind-Body Medicine.* Yonkers, NY: Consumer Reports Books, A Division of Consumers Union.

Goldenberg, D. 1993. Fibromyalgia, chronic fatigue syndrome and myofascial pain syndrome. *Current Opinion in Rheumatology* 5:199–208.

Goldstein, J. 1996. *Betrayal by the Brain: The Neurologic Basis of Chronic Fatigue Syndrome, Fibromyalgia Syndrome and Related Neural Network Disorders.* New York: The Haworth Medical Press.

———. 1993, 1994. Fibromyalgia Network Newsletters. *Journal for Action for ME.*

Granges, G., and G. Littlejohn. 1993. Prevalence of myofasical pain syndrome in fibromyalgia syndrome and regional pain syndrome: A comparative study. *Journal of Musculoskeletal Pain* 1(2):19–35.

Grisso, Jeane, Michelle Battistini, and Lesley Ryan. 1988. Women's health textbooks: codifying science and calling for change. *Annals of Internal Medicine* 129(11):916–918. December.

Hernandez, Yvonne L., and Troy Daniels. 1989. Oral candidiasis in Sjogren's syndrome: Prevalence, clinical correlations, and treatment. *Oral Surgery, Oral Medicine, Oral Pathology* 68(3):324–329.

Hirshberg, C., and M. Barasch. 1995. *Remarkable Recovery: What Extraordinary Healings Tell Us About Getting Well and Staying Well.* New York: Riverhead Books.

Hoffman, Ronald. 1993. *Tired All the Time: How to Regain Your Lost Energy.* New York: Poseidon Press.

Isenberg, D. and J. Morrow. 1995. *Friendly Fire: Explaining Autoimmune Disease.* Oxford: Oxford University Press.

Jacobson, D., S. Gange, N. Rose, and N. Graham. 1997. Epidemiology and estimated population burden of selected autoimmune diseases in the united states. *Clinical Immunology and Immunopathology* 84(3):223–243.

Jason, L., J. Richman, A. Rademaker, K. Jordan, A. Plioplys, R. Taylor, W. McCready, C. Huang, and S. Plioplys. 1999. A Community-based study of chronic fatigue syndrome. *Archives of Internal Medicine* 159(18):2129–2137.

Kabat-Zinn, J. 1993. Mindfulness Meditation: Health Benefits of an Ancient Buddhist Practice. In *Mind/Body Medicine: How to Use Your Mind for Better Health*, edited by Daniel Goldman and Joel Gurin. Yonkers, NY: Consumer Reports Books.

Kanner, A. D., J. C. Coyne, C. Schaefer, and R. S. Lazarus. 1981. Comparison of two modes of stress measurement: Daily hassles and uplifts versus major life events. *Journal of Behavioral Medicine* 4(1):1–39.

Kansky, G. 1999. Pondering Evidence and Reality. *The National Forum* 2(4):19–20. The National CFIDS Foundation, Inc., 103 Aletha Road, Needham, MA 02492–3931.

Kaptchuk, T. 1983. *The Web That Has No Weaver: Understanding Chinese Medicine.* Chicago, Ill.: Congdon & Weed.

Karasek, R. 1979. Job demands, job decision latitude and mental strain: implications for job redesign. *Administrative Science Quarterly* 24:285–308.

Kasper, A. 1997. *Textbook of Women's Health.* Philadelphia: Lippincott-Raven.

Kemeny, M. 1998. Lecture on the Immune System. Los Angeles: Cortext.

Khalsa, D. S., and C. Stauth. 1999. *The Pain Cure.* New York: Warner Books.

Kiecolt-Glaser, J. K, R. Glaser, et al. 1987. Marital quality, marital disruption, and immune function. *Psychosomatic Medicine* (49):13–34.

Konstantinov, K., A. von Mikeca, D. Buchwald, J. Jones, L. Gerace, and E. M. Tan. 1996. Autoantibodies to Nuclear Envelope Antigens in Chronic Fatigue Syndrome. *Journal of Clinical Investigation.* 98(8):1888–1896.

Kroll-Smith, S., and H. Floyd. 1997. *Bodies in Protest: Environmental Illness and the Struggle over Medical Knowledge.* New York: New York University Press.

Kubler-Ross, E. 1969. *On Death and Dying.* New York: Macmillan.

LaCroix, A. Z., and S. G. Haynes. 1987. "Gender Differences in the Health Effects of Workplace Roles" in *Gender and Stress.* R. Barnett, L. Biener, and G. Baruch (Eds.). New York: The Free Press.

Lahita, R. G., and R. H. Phillips. 1998. *Lupus: Everything You Need to Know*. Garden City Park, NY: Avery Publishing Group.

Lang, D. 1997. *Coping with Lyme Disease: A Practical Guide to Dealing with Diagnosis and Treatment*. New York: Henry Holt.

Larsen, R. J., E. Diener, and R. S. Cropanzano. 1987. Cognitive operations associated with individual differences in affect intensity. *Journal of Personality and Social Psychology* 53(4):767–774.

Levine, S. 1987. *Healing into Life and Death*. New York: Anchor Books.

Lorig, K., H. Holman, D. Sobel, D. Laurent, V. Gonzalez, and M. Minor. 1994. *Living a Healthy Life with Chronic Conditions*. Palo Alto, Calif.: Bull Publishing Co.

Manthorpe, R., et al. 1981. Sjogren's syndrome: A review with emphasis on immunological features. *Allergy* 36:139–153

Manthorpe, R., et al. 1986. Sjogren's syndrome. *Scandinavian Journal of Rheumatology* Suppl. 61:237

Marcus, N. and J. Arbeiter. 1994. *Freedom from Chronic Pain*. New York: Simon & Schuster.

McKay, M., M. Davis, and P. Fanning. 1981. *Thoughts and Feelings: The Art of Cognitive Stress Intervention*. Oakland, Calif.: New Harbinger Publications, Inc.

Maclay, P. 1999. Ask the experts. *Fibromyalgia Wellness Letter* 2(2):8.

Mairs, N. 1996. *Waist-High in the World: A Life Among the Nondisabled*. Boston: Beacon Press.

Meichenbaum, D. 1985. Stress Inoculation Training. New York: Pergamom Press.

Melzack, R., and S. G. Dennis. 1978. *Neurophysiological Foundation of Pain in the Psychology of Pain*. New York: Raven Press.

Metagenics. 1993. Nutritional breakthroughs against fibromyalgia. *Nutritional Pearls* 17. Aug/Sept.

Milton, J. 1667. *Paradise Lost* 1.254

Mindell, Earl. 1985. *Earl Mindell's Vitamin Bible*. New York: Warner Books, Inc.

Mountz, J., and L. Bradley. 1993, 1994. Fibromyalgia Network Newsletters. *Journal for Action for ME*.

Myss, C. 1997. *Why People Don't Heal and How They Can*. New York: Harmony Books.

Nass, T. *Lupus Erythematosus: A Handbook for Nurses*. Lupus Society of Wisconsin, Inc.

National Institute of Mental Health. The Office of Scientific Information and the Depression Awareness, Recognition, and Treatment (D/ART) Program. National Institute of Mental Health, Rm. 10–85, 5600 Fishers Lane, Rockville, MD 20857.

Nechas, E., and D. Foley. 1994. *Unequal Treatment*. New York: Simon & Schuster.

Nelson, P. 1988. *Autobiography in Five Short Chapters* in *The Courage to Heal*, edited by Ellen Bass and Laura Davis. New York: Harper & Row Publishers.

Olness, K. 1993. Hypnosis: The Power of Attention. *Mind/Body Medicine*, edited by Daniel Goleman and Joel Gurin, New York: Consumers Union.

Osler, W. 1980. From an article in *Lancet*, 1910, in Joan Arehart-Treichel, *Biotypes: The Critical Link between Your Personality and Your Health*. New York: Times Books.

Pacini, F., T. Vorontsova, E. Molinaro, E. Kuchinskaya, L. Agate, E. Shavrova, L. Astachova, L. Chiovato, and A. Pinchera. 1998. Prevalence of thyroid auto-antibodies in children and adolescents from Belarus exposed to Chernobyl radioactive fallout. *The Lancet,* 352(9130):763–766.

Padus, E., and the Editors of *Prevention* Magazine. 1986. *The Complete Guide to Your Emotions & Your Health.* Emmaus, Pa.: Rodale Press.

Pavlidis, N., et al. 1982. The clinical picture of primary sjogren's syndrome: a retrospective study. *Journal of Rheumatology* 9:685–689.

Peck, S. 1997. The effectiveness of therapeutic touch for decreasing pain in elders with degenerative arthritis. *Journal of Holistic Nursing* 14(2):176–198.

Phillips, R. H. 1984. *Coping with Lupus.* Wayne, N.J.: Avery Publishing Group, Inc.

Pincus, T. 1993. Arthritis and Rheumatic Diseases: What Doctors Can Learn From Their Patients. *Mind/Body Medicine: How to Use Your Mind for Better Health,* edited by Daniel Goleman and Joel Gurin. Yonkers, New York: Consumer Reports Books.

Pollin, I., and S. Golant. 1994. *Taking Charge: Overcoming the Challenges of Long-Term Illness.* New York: Times Books.

Pomeranz, B, and D. Chiu. 1979. Naloxone blockade of acupuncture analgesia: Endorphin implicated. *Life Sciences* 19(11):1757–1762.

Ravicz, S. 1998. *High on Stress: A Woman's Guide to Optimizing Stress in Her Life.* Oakland, Calif.: New Harbinger Publications.

Ravicz, S. 1996. *Distress and Eustress Among Healthy and Unhealthy Type A Personalities.* Ann Arbor, Mich.: UMI.

Reich, J. W., and A. Zautra. 1981. Life events and personal causation: Some relationships with satisfaction and distress. *Journal of Personality and Social Psychology* 41(5):1002–1012.

Riskin, Peter. *On the Brain.* Harvard Mahoney Neuroscience Institute.

Rose, J., et al. 1993. Genetic susceptibility in familial multiple sclerosis not linked to the myelin basic protein gene. *Lancet* 341(8854):1179–1181.

Rosenfeld, I. 1996. *Dr. Rosenfeld's Guide to Alternative Medicine.* New York: Random House.

Rosner, L., and S. Ross. 1992. *Multiple Sclerosis: New Hope and Practical Advice for People with MS and their Families.* New York: Simon & Schuster.

Royal, P. 1982. *Herbally Yours.* Hurricane, Utah: Sound Nutrition.

Ruble, T. 1983. Sex Stereotypes: Issues of Change. *Sex Roles* 9:397–401.

Schemmer, K. E. 1988. *Between Life and Death.* Wheaton, Ill.: Victor Books.

Schwartz, R. S. 1989. Fatigue and the lupus patient. *Lupus News* 9(2):1–2.

Schwartz, M., and N. Schwartz. 1993. *Mind Body Medicine.* Edited by Daniel Goleman and Joel Gurin. Yonkers, NY: Consumer Reports Books.

Shlotzhauer, T. L., and J. L. McGuire. 1993. *Living with Rheumatoid Arthritis.* Baltimore, Md.: The Johns Hopkins University Press.

Shuman, R., and J. Schwartz. 1994. *Living with Multiple Sclerosis: A Handbook for Families.* New York: Collier Books, Macmillan Publishing Company.

Shuman, R., and J. Schwartz. 1988. *Understanding Multiple Sclerosis: A Guidebook for Families.* New York: Charles Scribner's Sons.

Siegel, B. 1993. *How to Live Between Office Visits: A Guide to Life, Love and Health.* New York: HarperCollins Publishers.

Siegel, B. 1989. *Peace, Love & Healing.* New York: HarperPerennial.

Siegel, B. 1986. *Love, Medicine & Miracles.* New York: Harper & Row.

Simonton, O. C., S. Matthews-Simonton, and J. L. Creighton. 1978. *Getting Well Again.* New York: Bantam Books.

Smith, J. M. 1992. *Women and Doctors: A Physician's Explosive Account of Women's Medical Treatment, and Mistreatment, in America Today and What You Can do About It.* The Atlantic Monthly Press.

Snyder, S., J. Steiner, M. Connolly, G. Hamilton, H. Valentine, T. Dawson, and L. Hester. April 3, 1997. *Hopkins: New Variations on Old Drugs Promote Nerve Regeneration.* InteliHealth (web site): Home to John Hopkins Health Information.

Sobel, D., and R. Ornstein, editors. 1998. *Mind/Body Health Newsletter* VII:3.

Starlanyl, D. 1998. *The Fibromyalgia Advocate.* Oakland, Calif.: New Harbinger Publications, Inc.

Sumner, D. 1999. FMS gene found! *The National Forum* 2(4):1, 19. The National CFIDS Foundation, Inc. 103 Aletha Road, Needham, MA 02492–3931.

Surks, M. 1993. *The Thyroid Book.* Yonkers, NY: Consumer Reports Books.

Susser, M. 1997. Chronic Fatigue Syndrome in *Alternative Medicine: The Definitive Guide,* edited by The Burton Goldberg Group. Tiburon, Calif.: Future Medicine Publishing, Inc.

Swank, R. L. 1950. Multiple sclerosis: Chronicle of its incidence with dietary fat. *American Journal of Science.* 220(2):421–430.

Swank, R. L., and B. B. Dugan. 1990. Effect of low saturated fat diet in early and late cases of multiple sclerosis. *Lancet* 336(8706):37–39

Swedo, S., and H. Leonard. 1996. *It's Not All in Your Head.* San Francisco: HarperSanFrancisco.

Szasz, S. 1995. *Lupus: Living with it.* New York: Prometheus Books.

Teitelbaum, J. 1996. *From Fatigued to Fantastic!* New York: Avery Publishing Group.

Thomas, C. and K. R. Duszynski. 1974. Closeness to parents and the family constellation in a prospective study of five disease states: Suicide, mental illness, malignant tumor, hypertension and coronary heart disease. *John Hopkins Medical Journal* 134(5):251–270.

Vanfossen, B. E. 1986. Sex Differences in Depression: The Role of Spouse Support. In *Stress, Social Support, and Women,* edited by S. E. Hobfoll. New York: Hemisphere.

Van't Land, M. 1994. *Living Well with Chronic Illness.* Wheaton, Ill.: Harold Shaw Publishers.

Vliet, E. L. 1995. *Screaming to Be Heard: Hormonal Connections Women Suspect and Doctors Ignore.* New York: M. Evans and Company, Inc.

Walker, W. R., and D. M. Keats. 1976. An investigation of the therapeutic value of the "copper bracelet." *Agents Actions* 6:454.

Wall, P., and R. Melzack, editors. 1989. *Textbook of Pain.* New York: Churchill Livingstone.

Wallis, L. A., editor. 1997. *Textbook of Women's Health*. Philadelphia: Lippincott-Raven.

Werbach, M. 1993. *Healing Through Nutrition*. New York: HarperCollins Publishers.

Whitacre, C., S. Reingold, P. O'Looney, and the Task Force on Gender, Multiple Sclerosis, and Autoimmunity. 1999. *Science* 283:1277–1278.

Williamson, M. E. 1996. *Fibromyalgia: A Comprehensive Approach*. New York: Walker and Company.

Wolfe, F., et al. 1990. The american college of rheumatology 1990 criteria for the classification of fibromyalgia: Report of the multicenter criteria committee. *Arthritis and Rheumatism* 33:160.

Zautra, A., and J. Reich. 1980. Positive Life Events and Reports of Well-being: Some Useful Distinctions. *American Journal of Community Psychology* 86:657–670

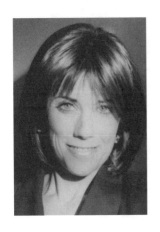

Simone Ravicz, Ph.D., M.B.A. is a licensed clinical psychologist. She earned her B.A. in Psychology at Brown University in Rhode Island, her M.B.A. at U.C.L.A., and her Ph.D. at the renowned school for Psychology, United States International University in San Diego, California. In addition, she is certified in Mind-Body Medicine through the National Institute for the Clinical Application of Behavioral Medicine and in the new Eye Movement Desensitization Reprocessing technique (EMDR). She also has diplomate status in medical psychology and trauma/PTSD.

At present, Dr. Ravicz is an adjunct professor at Saybrook Graduate School in Northern California, and has private practices in Santa Monica and Pacific Palisades, California. She also writes for various journals, and instructs corporate and private groups through a variety of workshops, including stress management, assertiveness, and communications training, mind-body health, balancing work and family, and developing positive stress (prostress) lifestyles. Much of her research and clinical work focuses on female psychological and physical health issues, ranging from children through adults.

Her previous book is *High on Stress: A Woman's Guide to Optimizing the Stress in Her Life*, New Harbinger Publications, 1998.

More New Harbinger Titles

HIGH ON STRESS
A Woman's Guide to Optimizing the Stress in Her Life
Helps you rethink the role of stress in your life, rework your physical and mental responses to it, and find ways to boost the positive impact that it can have on your well-being. *Item HOS $13.95*

LIVING WELL WITH A HIDDEN DISABILITY
Provides a wealth of resources for healthy living, including advice on navigating the health care system and suggestions for strengthening the body, mind, and soul. *Item HID $15.95*

PERIMENOPAUSE
Changes in Women's Health After 35
Perimenopause begins with subtle physiological changes in the mid-thirties and forties, and it can encompass a bewildering array of symptoms. This self-care guide helps you cope and assure your health and vitality in the years ahead. *Item PERI $16.95*

BREAKING THE BONDS OF IRRITABLE BOWEL SYNDROME
Shows how to identify troublesome foods, monitor symptoms and develop strategies for managing flare-ups, and challenge thoughts and emotional reactions that prevent recovery. *Item IBS $14.95*

OVERCOMING REPETITIVE MOTION INJURIES THE ROSSITER WAY
This system of easy-to-learn stretches has brought pain relief to thousands who suffer from carpal tunnel syndrome and other repetitive motion injuries and everyday aches and pain. *Item ROSS $15.95*

THE FIBROMYALGIA ADVOCATE
Shows you how to assemble a functional health care team, deal with the legal aspects of the health care system, and fight for your right to receive effective care for fibromyalgia and the related condition of myofascial pain syndrome. *Item FMA $18.95*

Call **toll-free 1-800-748-6273** to order. Have your Visa or Mastercard number ready. Or send a check for the titles you want to New Harbinger Publications, 5674 Shattuck Avenue, Oakland, CA 94609. Include $3.80 for the first book and 75¢ for each additional book to cover shipping and handling. (California residents please include appropriate sales tax.) Allow four to six weeks for delivery.

Prices subject to change without notice.

Some Other New Harbinger Self-Help Titles

Multiple Chemical Sensitivity: A Survival Guide, $16.95
Dancing Naked, $14.95
Why Are We Still Fighting, $15.95
From Sabotage to Success, $14.95
Parkinson's Disease and the Art of Moving, $15.95
A Survivor's Guide to Breast Cancer, $13.95
Men, Women, and Prostate Cancer, $15.95
Make Every Session Count: Getting the Most Out of Your Brief Therapy, $10.95
Virtual Addiction, $12.95
After the Breakup, $13.95
Why Can't I Be the Parent I Want to Be?, $12.95
The Secret Message of Shame, $13.95
The OCD Workbook, $18.95
Tapping Your Inner Strength, $13.95
Binge No More, $14.95
When to Forgive, $12.95
Practical Dreaming, $12.95
Healthy Baby, Toxic World, $15.95
Making Hope Happen, $14.95
I'll Take Care of You, $12.95
Survivor Guilt, $14.95
Children Changed by Trauma, $13.95
Understanding Your Child's Sexual Behavior, $12.95
The Self-Esteem Companion, $10.95
The Gay and Lesbian Self-Esteem Book, $13.95
Making the Big Move, $13.95
How to Survive and Thrive in an Empty Nest, $13.95
Living Well with a Hidden Disability, $15.95
Overcoming Repetitive Motion Injuries the Rossiter Way, $15.95
What to Tell the Kids About Your Divorce, $13.95
The Divorce Book, Second Edition, $15.95
Claiming Your Creative Self: True Stories from the Everyday Lives of Women, $15.95
Six Keys to Creating the Life You Desire, $19.95
Taking Control of TMJ, $13.95
What You Need to Know About Alzheimer's, $15.95
Winning Against Relapse: A Workbook of Action Plans for Recurring Health and Emotional Problems, $14.95
Facing 30: Women Talk About Constructing a Real Life and Other Scary Rites of Passage, $12.95
The Worry Control Workbook, $15.95
Wanting What You Have: A Self-Discovery Workbook, $18.95
When Perfect Isn't Good Enough: Strategies for Coping with Perfectionism, $13.95
Earning Your Own Respect: A Handbook of Personal Responsibility, $12.95
High on Stress: A Woman's Guide to Optimizing the Stress in Her Life, $13.95
Infidelity: A Survival Guide, $13.95
Stop Walking on Eggshells, $14.95
Consumer's Guide to Psychiatric Drugs, $16.95
The Fibromyalgia Advocate: Getting the Support You Need to Cope with Fibromyalgia and Myofascial Pain, $18.95
Healing Fear: New Approaches to Overcoming Anxiety, $16.95
Working Anger: Preventing and Resolving Conflict on the Job, $12.95
Sex Smart: How Your Childhood Shaped Your Sexual Life and What to Do About It, $14.95
You Can Free Yourself From Alcohol & Drugs, $13.95
Amongst Ourselves: A Self-Help Guide to Living with Dissociative Identity Disorder, $14.95
Healthy Living with Diabetes, $13.95
Dr. Carl Robinson's Basic Baby Care, $10.95
Better Boundries: Owning and Treasuring Your Life, $13.95
Goodbye Good Girl, $12.95
Fibromyalgia & Chronic Myofascial Pain Syndrome, $19.95
The Depression Workbook: Living With Depression and Manic Depression, $17.95
Self-Esteem, Second Edition, $13.95
Angry All the Time: An Emergency Guide to Anger Control, $12.95
When Anger Hurts, $13.95
Perimenopause, $16.95
The Relaxation & Stress Reduction Workbook, Fourth Edition, $17.95
The Anxiety & Phobia Workbook, Second Edition, $18.95
I Can't Get Over It, A Handbook for Trauma Survivors, Second Edition, $16.95
Messages: The Communication Skills Workbook, Second Edition, $15.95
Thoughts & Feelings, Second Edition, $18.95
Depression: How It Happens, How It's Healed, $14.95
The Deadly Diet, Second Edition, $14.95
The Power of Two, $15.95
Living Without Depression & Manic Depression: A Workbook for Maintaining Mood Stability, $18.95
Couple Skills: Making Your Relationship Work, $14.95

Call **toll free, 1-800-748-6273,** or log on to our online bookstore at **www.newharbinger.com** to order. Have your Visa or Mastercard number ready. Or send a check for the titles you want to New Harbinger Publications, Inc., 5674 Shattuck Ave., Oakland, CA 94609. Include $3.80 for the first book and 75¢ for each additional book, to cover shipping and handling. (California residents please include appropriate sales tax.) Allow two to five weeks for delivery.

Prices subject to change without notice.